Dying to be Heard

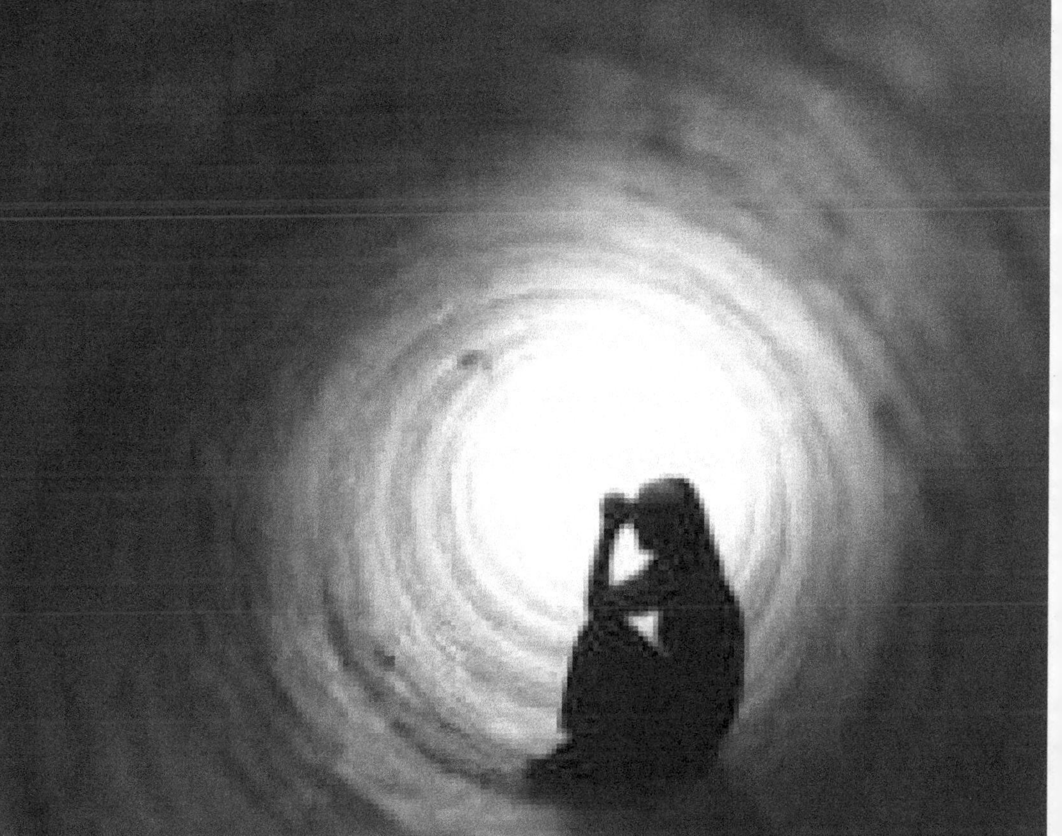

By Paula

Published by
Chipmunkapublishing
United Kingdom

http://www.chipmunkapublishing.com

ISBN 978-1-78382-5271

About Chipmunkapublishing

Mental health books give a voice to writers with mental illness around the world. At Chipmunkapublishing we raise awareness of mental health and the stigma surrounding mental health problems by encouraging society to listen. We are documenting mental health literature as a genre so history does not forget the survivors and carers of people with mental illness and disabilities.

Dedicated to Martyn Geary
If I hadn't met you Martyn, I wouldn't be where I am today. I probably wouldn't be here at all.

And to Jayne Yeates
Thank you for wearing my cloak every week, you make sure that I am never alone even in the darkest of times.

And also to you Kelsang Norpel
It turns out that you were and still are a constant thread weaving through the fabric of my mind, although I couldn't see it at the time.

Thank you all – I will never forget.

I'm writing this to YOU - the therapist, the counsellor, the psychiatrist.

I'm writing this to YOU - the survivor, the inquisitive one, the interested.

AND

I'm writing this to YOU - the perpetrator, the paedophile, the abuser

AND FINALLY

I'm writing this to ALL OF YOU who neglected me, ignored me and rejected me.

How many beans make 5? That's what my Dad used to say to me and then my children after I'd grown up. They would look at him puzzled, not wanting to state the obvious and wait patiently until he enlightened them and it was the same answer every time.

A bean, 2 beans, a bean and a half, and half a bean.

Or is it?

It could be, 2 beans, a bean, a bean and a half, and half a bean.

It could be any variation on the above. What matters is the answer is always 5.

We don't know what colour the beans are, what environment they grew in, how old they are, what type of bean they are, or if we can eat them.

What's important is that we get the answer 5, no matter how we get there. I just wanted to put that in as a little tribute to my Dad.

When my world fell apart and my mind quite simply collapsed in on itself, people were constantly telling me I would get there. "You're getting there" they would say, or "You'll get there". This scared and frustrated the hell out of me. What could they see that I couldn't? Where is there? What did there look like? How will I know when I get there?

When I separated and later divorced my first husband I was 26 years old and I had lost everything. My home, the life I knew, my direction, my everything and I ended up sleeping on a mattress on the floor at a friend's house. Having lost all direction and feeling frighteningly overwhelmed a friend took hold of my hands, looked me in the eyes and told me I would find my level. I liked that. I knew what that meant. Finding my level meant finding the life I wanted to live, the home I wanted, the people I wanted to be around, the life that just fit. But in order to find all of that I needed to clear out all the rubbish, renovate the soul, just like you would renovate an old run down house. It was many, many years later before I did this.

It gets messy, so very messy before it can be restored and sometimes in the process of clearing out, more pieces fall apart and have to be restored, or dealt with and thrown away as they are no longer useful, or serve any helpful purpose.

So wherever you are in 'getting there', whether that's moving home, changing career, job, relationships, or dealing with something that's stopping you from living the life you want to live, I hope you find your 'there'. Because for some people tragically, getting there means quite simply not being here anymore.

If you feel like that, or work with somebody who does, then please read this, because believe me you will find your there.

The purpose of this book is to take you with me through my experiences leading up to and including sexual abuse, the devastating impact that had on my life and the consequences when people completely let me down.
I begin this book giving the reader a broad understanding of my life and how I came to write in my journal for almost four years. It's not an autobiography, it's not intended to be. My purpose is to make you see as explicitly as possible what lead to the events that destroyed my life and then what happened to begin to turn it around. Almost like a text book, but with real emotional insight.
The main body of this book looks specifically at a period of almost 4 years where I documented my inner most thoughts and feelings, when eventually the impact of everything that had happened took its toll on me and I was ready to end my life. It's not an easy read and at times it will challenge its reader. But stick with it because you couldn't fail to learn from reading this book, from whichever perspective you are approaching it.
The final part of this book will simply reflect on my understanding of my life which lead up to my decision to end it by suicide and how that understanding was gradually and gently re-moulded to my understanding of my life now.

In the beginning there was an Angel.

I was born on the 18th December 1969 in an ambulance on the way to the Royal Gwent Hospital in Newport. My birth was rather undignified as I made my appearance when the ambulance pulled up at traffic lights and I decided I wasn't going to wait any longer. This being the week before Christmas the street lights were decorated with stars and Angels and the street light I arrived under was lit with an Angel. A beautiful Christmas Angel looking down on my arrival. And there the image ends!

My rather rapid arrival took everybody by surprise, not least the ambulance technician who took one look at me covered in blood and decided against wrapping me up in his coat. My Mother articulated her disgust also and repulsed at having me anywhere near her, the ambulance guy decided to wrap me in paper towels. As the story goes, by the time we arrived at the Maternity Unit, I was in a poor condition, I had turned blue, I was hypothermic and not expected to survive. The neonatal staff asked my Mother what she wanted to call me and she replied 'Barry Jon' after the Welsh rugby union player. It was pointed out to her that I was in fact a girl and not expected to survive, but my Mother's only response was that she wanted a boy. It was suggested that I was christened as soon as possible and perhaps Angela would be a suitable name given the circumstances around my arrival. My Mother was disgusted by this suggestion as she stated that she hates the name Angela and instead chose the name Anne after establishing the name of the nurse who was looking after me. Following my recovery we returned home to my Father and my older sister Stephanie, who grew to be my world.

My Sister was 13 months older than me and had Spina Bifida. She couldn't walk but other than that she was absolutely perfect. We played, we fought and I looked after her. She was my best friend, she was my world. We didn't go to the same school, but other than that we did everything together. I have never forgotten that people would often come to the house to talk to her and ask her questions. I was sad that nobody wanted to talk to me or ask me questions, I didn't understand why she hated it and I wished people wanted to talk to me. Every week we would visit my Nana and Grandad. My Auntie and Cousin Jason lived with them and Jason was 4 years older than me. It would usually end up that one of us would fall out with Jason and the other would take his side. It only lasted for the few hours we were visiting and when we got home me and my Sister would be friends again.

We would often play Nurses for hours and my Sister always had to be the patient because she couldn't stick her tongue out. Every time she tried, she would retch and that was great fun because it made her the perfect patient. She could be sneaky too. She would hit me and if I hit her back she would start crying and I would get the blame. It was my fault because she was disabled. I didn't get it, I didn't see it. She was just Stevie, my big Sister. At night I would help her onto her potty, because my Mother wasn't awake to take her to the toilet. She would wake me up and she would edge herself to the edge of the bed and I would grab her before she fell on the floor. When she had finished, I would empty her potty into the toilet and then help her get back to bed. At that time she loved Gary Glitter and I loved the Bay City Rollers and we would sing their songs in bed. Sometimes my Mother and Father would go out drinking. They couldn't always get a baby sitter, so my Mother would tell me they were going out, but not to tell Stevie because she would be frightened. I said I was scared, but she reminded me that it was okay for me because I wasn't disabled. I had a lot to be grateful for. Life went on pretty normally as far as I was concerned, but I was getting tired of every time we went to my Nanas, Jason my cousin, would start picking on one of us and then we would fall out. The last time we went to my Nanas we made a pact. If Jason fell out with one of us, we would stay together and we would try to be friends all week with no arguments. As predicted Jason starting picking on Stevie this time, he wasn't her friend and he asked me who I wanted to be friends with and I chose her. We had a great afternoon together and went home really happy and we did stay friends all week. I wish I had never suggested that pact between us. The following Sunday morning I was watching TV with Stevie. Church on Sunday, or Sunday Worship or Cricket. That was kids TV then. Anyway, Stevie was quiet and really moody with me. She was holding her head over to one side and I asked her if she had a headache. She shouted at me and told me not to tell my Mother and Father. I was scared, she was behaving differently and I was sad because we had been friends all week and now she was angry with me and I didn't know why. I woke my Mother and Father then told them that Stevie had a headache and was behaving strange. They got up and lay her on the settee with the sick bowl and called a Doctor. The Doctor told my Father she needed to go to hospital and said he was calling an ambulance, but my Father said he would take her himself. Stevie was lying on the settee with her eyes closed and she wouldn't talk to me. We all went in the car to Alder Hey Hospital and I waited on my own in a corridor for hours. Nurses kept running in and out of the room and nobody would talk to me. I was terrified. I just wanted to talk to Stevie, to let her know I was still her friend. I never had a chance to say goodbye.

On 12th June 1977 Stevie died. I had been taken back to my Nanas earlier in the day and my Mother and Father went back to the hospital. Nobody was talking to me. It had just gone five 0'clock in the morning when there was knocking at the door. Knocking, knocking, knocking. I didn't want anybody to answer it. I didn't want anybody to let the news in. Nobody did answer the door. My Nan and Grandad, Auntie and cousin all stayed in bed then I answered the door. My Mother told me that Stevie had died. She told me nothing would be special anymore.

After her death I was taken to stay with relatives who I didn't really know. Nobody talked to me and my Mother and Father went away and I didn't know if they were ever going to come back. I don't know to this day where they went, but at some point there would have been my Sisters funeral, they later told me they had gone on holiday for two weeks. When they took me home my Sister's stuff had gone. Everything. There were no clothes, no toys, expect tiny tears. Her bed had gone, even the potty. There was nothing of her, nothing. I had nothing to hold on to, I couldn't even smell her. The bedroom had been re-decorated and I was expected to be happy. If I didn't respond as my Mother wanted she would get angry with me then I would become frightened of her and my Father. It was the first time in my life I had experienced loss. I was achingly lonely, the bedroom was missing my Sister. Everything was different. Nobody came to the house anymore, I had nobody to play with and I was told now that Stevie had gone nothing was special anymore. I was 7 years old and I understood that because Stevie was now gone, nothing was special anymore.

I continued to feel sad and very lonely. My Mother and Father would go out 3 nights a week at the weekend, but they no longer attempted to get a baby sitter, they said they didn't need to now because I was strong, independent and I could look after myself. I was terrified. They would go out and I would sit and watch television too afraid even to go to the toilet. When they came home they would be very, very drunk. My Mother would drool all over me, by Father would be looking for an argument with my Mother and often they would scream and shout at each other. My Mother would tell me all of her problems the next day , how horrible my Father was to her and how he would hit her. I grew to feel very frightened of my Father and I also began to hate him.

I was very lonely at home. My Mother had taken a job and I was given a key to let myself in at home. I would clean the house and get pocket money for it. I would plead with my Mother not to leave me in the house on my own whilst they went out drinking, but she told me she had to otherwise my Father would be very angry with her. I was scared of him and I didn't want him to hurt her.

My Mother and Father were very materialistic and they bought me jewellery and expensive presents. If I complained that I was bored, or that I was lonely I was reminded by my Mother about just how much money they had spent on me to make me happy. All I wanted was them to play with me, or take me to the park, or on days out like my friends parents did. I asked my friends if their parents went out drinking and left them at home on their own and they told me they didn't. I felt very lonely.

I loved babies, I have always loved babies. All I ever wanted to do when I was young was get married and have babies. My Mother was disgusted with me for saying that. I just wanted somebody to love. One day whilst out playing with my friend Sharon we saw a couple having a picnic on the grass with their daughter. She looked to be less than a year old, but she was crawling around and playing with toys on the blanket. We went over and asked if it was okay to play with her. They told us her name was Sarah-Jayne. She was the cutest baby I have ever seen. We played for a while and asked if it would be okay to take her for a walk some time. They told us we could and a lovely new relationship was about to be born.

Accepted at last.

Jack and Emily Kilbourne were the parents of Sarah-Jayne. What happened after that first meeting was both myself and Sharon walked back to their flat so we knew where they lived so we made an arrangement to call again the next day to take Sarah-Jayne for a walk. It was the school holidays so we had plenty of time. It was 1980 and I was 10 years old, just about to go into my last year at primary school. Sharon came with me the first couple of times. We knocked at Emily's and she would bring the Buggy outside, she lifted Sarah-Jayne into the buggy and we would take her for a walk around the block. We soon realised that not long into the walk Sarah-Jayne would fall asleep and when we took her back this appeared to really please Emily. I was keen to do this more. Sharon got fed up very quickly though and after a few times she stopped coming, but I enjoyed taking Sarah-Jayne out and I loved that Emily was pleased that I had got her to sleep. She even started letting me carry her upstairs into the flat so I could put her down in her cot. I loved that. Emily would give me a drink and a snack and I would go home. I felt sad to be going back to school, but Emily told me that I could come over and play with Sarah-Jayne which I would do at the weekends and after school whenever I could. I'd told my Mother about Sarah-Jayne, but she had shown no interest, she was glad that I was out of the way. I was always in the way. Of what I didn't know.

Over time my visit to Jack and Emily's became more regular. I would be invited to go for a Sunday Roast and I was allowed to feed Sarah-Jayne which I loved. Jack's Dad would also come for Sunday lunch after he had been to the pub and we all sat down together. I loved it, I was part of a family. I would play with Sarah-Jayne after lunch, until she went for her nap. Sometimes I would knock early on a Saturday or Sunday and we would go swimming. Jack suggested that because we went swimming so early, instead of having to get up early, perhaps I could stay the night. I asked my Mother and she agreed. I was in my element. I no longer had to feel frightened of being on my own at home. Jack and Emmily wanted me to stay and Jack would sometimes kiss me and Sarah-Jayne and I felt complete. I had a family again and they loved me. They wanted to be with me and Jack gave me special kisses. I couldn't be happier.

The Nightmares begin.

The first time Jack sexually abused me I had gone round to their flat and Emily was in bed. It was early December, not long before my 11th Birthday and Jack was in the living room with Sarah-Jayne. Jack had a dressing gown on and the lounge was set up so the sofas were opposite to each other and the television was to the left as I sat opposite Jack. Jack was sat with his legs wide open and his dressing gown was gaping. It was very hard not to look where it was gaping as I was facing him. It tried to focus on the television, but he was moving his legs a little so my attention was drawn to the darkness under the dressing gown in between his legs. Jack left the room for a minute or two, possibly to go to the toilet, possibly to check if Emily was sleeping. Whatever the reason he wasn't gone for long. When he came back he sat next to me and put his arm across the back of me. I felt uncomfortable, I couldn't really tell why. He was close to me, a bit too close and I felt a little bit anxious. He asked me if I could see, I leaned forward a little and told him I couldn't really see the television. He told me he didn't mean the television and he squeezed my shoulder pulling me towards him and told me to look. He wanted me to look at him, so I glanced really quickly in the direction he was pulling me towards. It was the gap in his dressing gown where his legs were open. I told him I couldn't see and again looked away. Jack laughed at me and gave me a friendly tickle in my stomach. Only it wasn't a friendly tickle, he was pressing my stomach with his fingers and I didn't like it. I wriggled but he took that to mean I was ticklish and he told me he hadn't realised I was ticklish. He continued to move his fingers down my stomach and he started to press and wriggle is fingers over my knickers. My heart was thumping so hard I could hear it in my ears. I told Jack I didn't want to play, he laughed at me. I told him again I didn't want to play but he carried on until I moved away from him. I was shaking with fear, but Jack was laughing. I didn't know what to do. Sarah-Jayne was playing on the floor in front of us and I got down to play with her. I made my excuses very soon after that and I went home.

When I arrived home I was shaking so much. I was really frightened and really confused. Jack had just asked me to look at him naked between his legs and he had touched me where nobody had touched me before. I didn't like it, I didn't want to do what he was trying to make me do and I didn't like him touching me over my knickers. But he laughed. He laughed like it was just a game. He laughed at me because I didn't like it and that made me feel bad. Thoughts began racing round in my head. "Jack loves me, so I shouldn't feel bad, I'm bad for not liking what he did. He wanted to carry on playing, it was me that didn't. Maybe it was my fault. Maybe I should have touched him and he would have liked me to do that". These thoughts raced round and round in my head continually. I didn't tell my Mum or Dad. I didn't feel close enough to tell them and I thought it was my fault. I didn't know why I thought it was my fault, but Jack loved me so it must have been my fault because I didn't like it. The more I thought about it the more confused I became. Then I settled on the fact that Jack must have done that to me because maybe he didn't love me anymore. Maybe he didn't like me going to his house all the time. Maybe he did it because he wanted me to stop going. I decided that I would only go to see Sarah-Jayne when I got home from school, before Jack arrived home from work. That way I wouldn't be in the way. I wouldn't annoy him, but I could still see Sarah-Jayne.

The second time Jack sexually abused me I had gone round after school, whilst I was waiting for my Mum to cook my dinner. I was sat on the front step, I was feeling lonely and sad. My Mum told me not to go away as my dinner wouldn't be long, but I forgot that and I wanted to go and see Sarah-Jayne, I would only stay for a few minutes I thought. When I arrived Emily told me that she was pregnant and that she wasn't really feeling very well. She stayed with me for a while whilst I played with Sarah-Jayne, but she a short while later she asked me if I would play with Sarah-Jayne whilst she went for a lie down. I didn't know what to say. I didn't want Emily to be angry with me if I said no and I couldn't tell her that I didn't want to stay until Jack came home, because I was frightened that she would ask me why. So I agreed and Emily went to lie down in her bedroom.

I have always had a sense of 'things'. I can't really describe it. I feel anxious, or scared, or unsafe and my instinct is right more often than not. On this particular day after Emily went to bed I felt really frightened. I was frightened to see Jack when he came home from work. I had a real dread that something was going to happen when he got home. I hadn't seen Jack since he had sexually abused me and I didn't know if he would be angry that I was there when he arrived home. I felt really frightened.

Jack arrived home some time later and he sat on the sofa next to me. He was fiddling with his zip on his trousers. He stood up with his back to me and was fiddling with his zip. He sat down next to me and told me that the zip on his trousers was broken. He had his arm around the back of me and he was talking to me. After a few minutes he told me he wanted to play the tickling game again. Only this time he said that I had to touch him where he touched me. He started off tickling my stomach and he said that I had to tickle him on his stomach. Then he started to move his hand down, but this time he put his fingers inside my knickers and he was fiddling with me. I wasn't tickling him, or fiddling with him I was 'touching' him on his thigh, either side of where I could see his penis poking through his zip. Jack was pressing his fingers on me inside my knickers, he was moving his fingers lower and lower and he kept telling me to touch him where he was touching me. I now understand that his penis was erect. I could see it was hard and whilst I couldn't see the end, the whole shaft of his penis was exposed through his open zip. He was pressing hard and moving his fingers inside my knickers. He kept telling me that I had to touch him where he was touching me. I could see his erect penis, but I didn't touch him. I didn't believe he wanted me to touch his penis. He couldn't mean that and what if I did and he got angry with me and shouted at me. I told Jack that I didn't want to play anymore. He laughed at me and said that if I didn't want to play with him then he would carry on playing with me. Jack was pressing his fingers hard inside my knickers and it was beginning to hurt. He was trying to push his fingers inside me and he was hurting me. I sat forward quickly and told him I didn't want to play anymore and said I had to go home. I stood up and I felt dizzy, I didn't know why. My heart was pounding and I was shaking so badly. Jack just sniggered as I got up. I raced home and I could hear my Mum shouting me.

When I arrived home I wanted to tell her what Jack had done to me, but she was shouting at me, shouting at me for going away when she had told me to stay near because my dinner was nearly ready. I started crying, I couldn't stop shaking and that made her even angrier. She told me that if I didn't stop crying then she would give me something to really cry about. Meatballs, chips and peas I had for dinner that night. I was so frightened. I didn't understand why Jack didn't love me anymore. I didn't sleep at all that night, I didn't sleep again, except when exhaustion got the better of me and I would eventually nod off. Every night I went to bed I would be too scared to close my eyes just in case Jack climbed in my bedroom window and 'got me'. I was so sad and lonely. I didn't understand why Jack didn't love me anymore, My Mum and Dad didn't love me and now Jack and Emily didn't love me anymore. I had ruined everything by going round too much and I was just in everybody's way. I couldn't understand why nobody loved me anymore. I felt so sad, so lonely. I was such a bad person. My Sister left me, my Mum and Dad didn't love me, I seemed to annoy them, now I had annoyed Jack and Emily. Jack had 'touched' me because he didn't want me to go round anymore, because he didn't love me anymore. I was devastated. Every night I would dread going to bed and every morning I would wake up shaking, not only outside, but it felt like I was shaking inside too. I thought I must be a very bad person if nobody loved me. My Mum had told me that nothing was special anymore after my Sister died and she made sure I knew that. Jack had made me feel so special and now I wasn't his special little girl any more. Nobody loved me and I didn't know why. Maybe I was just a really bad person, I didn't know.

Jason was 4 years older than me and I would see him most weekends, more now that I didn't see Jack and Emily anymore. I loved Jason, he was my good looking older cousin and I looked up to him in every way. Jason told me that he was going to marry me and my Mum said she didn't think it would be allowed, but Jason said he would get special permission so we could.

One evening Jason, my Nana, Grandad and my Auntie came over and stayed with us for the weekend. I was 11 years old at the time, making him 15. It could have been Easter time, I'm not entirely sure but they only ever stayed when something was going on. Either Christmas, Easter, or if there was an event on at the Royal British Legion. Anyway, they all went out with my Mum and Dad and Jason stayed with me. I was so relieved to have somebody with me, so I wouldn't be on my own. Jason told me that he loved me and asked me if I knew what it meant to have sex. I told him I did, but I didn't tell him about Jack. Jason was excited and asked me if we should 'do it'. I was excited and told him I wanted to 'do it' with him. He told me he was frightened that he might hurt me, but not knowing what that meant I told him he wouldn't. We got undressed in the living room and Jason lay on top of me. I could feel his hard penis pressing against me and it felt like it had when Jack had been pressing his fingers against me inside my knickers. Before I had chance to say anything we heard footsteps and Jason jumped up. We both quickly dressed just before my Mum came through the living room door. She looked at us both. We must have looked really shocked and she asked us what we had been up to, but we denied anything and she was too drunk to pursue anything further and she let it go.

It wasn't long after that that we were at my Nans again. Me and Jason were playing in the back yard which wasn't very big and housed an air-raid shelter. There was a ladder against the wall of the house and Jason dared me to climb up the ladder and step across to the roof of the air raid shelter. He showed me how easy it was by completing this task first. I then climbed up the ladder and went to step across to the roof, but I lost my nerve. I had my leg out half way across the gap to the roof. I told Jason I couldn't do it. He laughed at me and told me I had to as he stuck his fingers up my skirt and started fiddling with me where Jack had. I screamed at him to stop it, he just laughed and told me he would stop if I stepped across and onto the roof. I told him I couldn't do it and said I wanted to get down. I was trying to kick his hand away, but he was pressing his fingers against my knickers. I was shouting at him and telling him I wanted to get down. He just laughed at me and told me that he would just carry on 'doing this to me' until I got down. I was shouting at him and he was just laughing. I was trapped again and there was nothing I could do to make him stop. There was nothing I could do stop him pressing his fingers against me, trying to force his fingers hard against me over my knickers. He was hurting me just like Jack had done. That same feeling again. The same feeling when he had pressed his penis against me. Hard pressure that was beginning to hurt.

I was so angry, I was shaking and Jason was laughing at me. He had forced his fingers hard against me and I couldn't stop him. Exactly the same as Jack had done and I was trapped. I felt like I couldn't breathe. I was trapped and I felt like I was being crushed, I was struggling to get my breath, I thought I was going to suffocate. Why did Jack do that to me and why did Jason do that to me? I thought it was all my fault, Jack didn't like me and I'd agreed a few weeks earlier to have sex with Jason. It was all my fault. I shouldn't have agreed to have sex with Jason, but he said he loved me and now he didn't love me anymore because he wanted to hurt me. I couldn't understand why nobody loved me and why everybody just wanted to hurt me. I thought I must be a really, really bad person. I hated myself. I hated myself because people didn't like me. I always appeared to be in the way and all I wanted was to be loved, but I just ended up annoying people and then they didn't love me anymore. Jason didn't love me anymore because I wanted him to have sex with me, but now I didn't want him to hurt me. Why wouldn't anybody listen to me telling them to stop. Jack and Jason just laughed, so I believed it was my fault. Nobody ever listened to me and nobody loved me. They could do what they liked to me and my feelings didn't count and I didn't know why. I really believed I must be a very bad person. I hated myself so much.

Secondary school.
I went to a Secondary Comprehensive School from September 1981 until July 1986 and that was about it. I learned very little, I took in even less of what the teachers were trying to teach me and I made a decision that by the age of 14 I would have had enough of life and I was going to kill myself. *"Nobody loves me, nobody listens to me when I tell them to stop. I am a useless, worthless person and I hate myself so much. My existence makes people want to hurt me."* My best friend at the time was Karen Berry. Karen would knock for me on our way to school and one day she brought a medicine bottle over and it had Martini in it. Karen thought it was funny that she had sneaked it out and we drank it between us. I liked the affect it had on me. It made me feel warm inside and calm. I told Karen I wanted her to bring it again and so it began. Every morning Karen would bring a medicine bottle full with Martini and I would drink it to myself before we went to school and if she ever forgot it, I would send her home to fetch some. I liked the way this was making me feel. I didn't really care what people thought about me when I had a drink and I found it got me through the day. The only time I struggled a little was if we had PE first thing and that became a bit of a challenge, but other than that I felt fine. I went to school every day and I learned nothing. Every day and every night I was replaying what Jack had done to me. I was reinforcing my belief that he did it because he didn't like me and I was constantly terrified that he would come and 'get me'. I was constantly reinforcing my belief that I was worthless, useless. Nobody would listen to me. My Mum and Dad didn't care about me and I was just here to be used. I knew I didn't matter. Nothing about me mattered. I hated myself so much. I made people not like me and I didn't know why. I believed it would be better off if I was no longer here. Roll on 14.
A couple of years later my Mum bumped into Emily, she had moved address and had just given birth to her third child a couple of weeks earlier. Emily had invited us both round to meet the baby and to have a catch up. I told my Mum that I wasn't interested any more in going back, I told her I wasn't bothered about baby's any more, but she ignored me and she contacted Emily and arranged for us to visit. I was petrified to go back, but my Mum ignored me. Why wouldn't she, I was worthless anyway. Emily made me feel really welcome and told me that she'd missed me. She told me I could go round and stay over if I wanted to get the bus to hers. I felt under pressure. I felt I couldn't say no. Why would I say no and what excuse would I give when sat with Emily and my Mum staring at me. So it began again. I started staying over on a Friday or Saturday night. Jack was pleasant and I was never alone with him. Then there was one night. I slept in Sarah-Jaynes bed, Emily told me that Sarah-Jayne and her younger brother Jack always started off in their own bed, but would end up getting into hers and Jack's bed. On one particular occasion when I was staying at Jack and Emily's, I woke up sometime in the early hours. As I turned round Jack was just getting out of bed. He whispered he had to get back before anybody woke up. I never went again. Emily had asked me at one point during the time I was visiting why I had stopped going suddenly and I told her that my Mum and Dad didn't like me going around to her house all the time. Emily didn't believe me, I saw it in the way she looked at me, but she didn't pursue it.

Friendship groups changed and I became friends with a girl called Kim. I confided in Kim what had happened with Jack. Kim told a teacher. Her name is Brenda Smith, she was my Maths teacher and helped run the netball team I played in. Kim went across to tell Brenda Smith one afternoon practice at netball. Kim came back to me and told me she had told Brenda what I had told her. I asked Kim what her response had been and Kim told me she had said *"these things happen"*. I was absolutely destroyed. Everything that I had believed about myself was true. This is what men did and I was expected to put up with it. What the hell was wrong with me. Everybody else seemed to be fine with it, everybody else appeared to be fine, so what was wrong with me. Why didn't I like it. That's why nobody listened to me when I told them to stop. That's why they just laughed at me, because these things happen. *"Not only am I a worthless piece of rubbish, but there is something really, really wrong with me because I don't like what men do to me, I can't cope with it. I am rubbish. I hate myself so much."*
I used to call for Kim regularly at the weekends. I lived quite a distance from Kim and the walk involved crossing Town Park a huge expanse of fields between one estate and another. On one occasion I was walking across Town Park and a man approached me. I was 13 years old and he started talking to me and he held my hand. I held his hand and I walked with him whilst he took me across the fields away from the view of the housing estate. We sat on the grass and talked for a little while and then he put his hand down my trousers. *"these things happen"* okay I was frightened and he was kissing my neck. I didn't like it and I didn't like the smell of him. He was kissing my mouth and he forced his tongue in my mouth. I remember looking at my trainers at one point thinking what is it he likes about me, my trainers are horrible. He was hurting me, he was forcing his fingers hard against me. I had that pressure feeling I had with Jack and Jason and it was really hurting, but then there was a sharp pain and he entered me with his finger. He was hurting me so much, but I have to remember *"these things happen"*. I tried not to make a sound as he raped me. I only managed to get away by promising to meet him again the next day. I promised him I would go back the next day if he let me go because my friend would be worried about me because I was late. I never told Kim, why would I? *"These things happen"*.
I couldn't help it though I really hated what was happening to me. What was wrong with me why didn't I like it. I wished I was dead, I couldn't bare to live like this. I hated myself for not being able to cope with what was happening to me. I hated being forced to do things I didn't want to do. I didn't tell him to stop, Jack didn't stop, Jason didn't stop, now I understood even though I hated it. *"These things happen"*. Why would I tell him to stop, he wouldn't have stopped anyway and that would have made me feel worse. That would have meant I was going to be ignored again. I would have said out loud that he was hurting me and I would have been ignored. I would know that my feelings meant nothing and that would make me feel even worse about myself. *"I hate myself so much, I'm a worthless piece of rubbish and I just want to die."*
I hated school, I couldn't take anything in. I didn't have boyfriends, if I did I would make an excuse to finish with them because I didn't want to be touched by them, hurt and be made to feel even more worthless than I already did. I left school with

no qualifications and I went on a YTS course, a Youth Training Scheme it was known as. I loved that. I worked in a library and I felt safe. I was 16 years old surrounded by adults who looked after me. Who asked me if I was okay and they were kind to me. I didn't want to leave, but sadly placements only lasted for 6 months and then I was expected to take a new placement. At the end of placement we had a disco put on by the College. I went with my friend Karen and we had a good night. At the end of the night Karen told me that a lad called Carl Collins wanted to walk us home. I told her I didn't want him to and she laughed at me. She asked me what was wrong with me. Stating I didn't like boys and I didn't like girls, so what was wrong with me. I felt crushed, everybody knew there was something wrong with me. I didn't like my body being used by men and that meant I was abnormal, I felt so ashamed so I agreed to let him walk with us. Carl Collins walked Karen home first and then said he was going to walk me home. I had a very, very bad feeling about this. Carl walked me to a place near my home. He started kissing me and I didn't like it. He pushed hard against me and he placed his feet between mine and forced my legs apart. He then pushed me into the bushes and forced his fingers hard inside me. I couldn't help but scream he hurt me so much and then he raped me. I couldn't help crying and he had blood on him and afterwards he ran away. I was left crying and in pain, I was bleeding and I could hardly stand up. I managed to get myself home and I crept into the house. My Mum and Dad were in bed, I couldn't have a shower, that would draw attention to myself and wake my Mum and Dad. I could hardly wipe myself in the toilet I was in so much pain. So, I got rid of the blood off my legs and climbed into bed crying. I hid my bloodstained knickers until I could get them in the washing machine myself. I could feel him inside me for days afterwards. When Karen asked me how I was the next day, I couldn't hide how I felt and I told her everything. She told me I needed to go to the Police, but how could I? He had done something to me that I was supposed to like and I didn't and it hurt and I was bleeding. Why would I want anybody to know how abnormal I was? Why was I so abnormal? I wished I was dead, my shame and humiliation was too much to live with. I hated myself so much. I clearly wasn't mapped out for this world. My drinking became heavier, I was spiralling out of control. I was going to any pub I could get in and be served at. My friends would go to the bar, because I was often turned back. I would drink as much alcohol as I could to escape the same feeling every single day. That feeling was continuous flashbacks of being sexually abused, continuous feelings of self-hatred and self-loathing. I hated myself more than I can articulate. What was it about me that made men want to hurt me. I just wanted to die. I just wanted to get so drunk and spaced out that I never came back again. But I did, I woke up every single day and the flashbacks and self-hatred and self-loathing were with me every single minute of every single day. Unless I was passed out drunk, I couldn't sleep.

Despite all of these feelings, I was beginning to panic that I wouldn't be able to lead a 'normal' life, get married and have children. I was panicking that I would have to meet somebody and get married before I was too old. I'd had 'dates' with lads before, but I always ended it before it got any further than the kissing stage. I hated it as soon as they put their tongue in my mouth, I felt repulsed and sick, so I made up excuses, I didn't care what they were, or what they thought, I was panicking too much to carry on.

I met Stewart Watts as I remember at a wedding, I worked with his sister-in-law and she arranged for us to get together. He told me not long after we had started going out that he was going to marry me. I couldn't believe it, he wanted me. There was only one thing for me to do and that was to be brave and tell him what had happened to me when I was a child. I told him everything and he was very, very quiet. Our relationship developed quite quickly and it very quickly got to the stage where he started to 'maul' me. But of course it wasn't, it was 'normal', it was me that wasn't normal. He would kiss me and touch my breasts in the car before dropping me off, I hated it, he made my skin crawl. He whispered to me to tell him what that man did to me when I was a child. He would stop what he was doing and listen whilst I 'reminded' him what Jack had done to me and then he would start 'mauling' me again, with more energy. It wasn't long before we attempted to have sex. Stewart couldn't get his penis inside me and I felt so awful, I felt guilty. He was trying to push his penis inside me and it just wouldn't go. He told me he didn't know how anybody could have raped me. I felt there was something really, really wrong with me. I told him if he wanted to do it he would have to 'make it go' and he did. The pain was like nothing I had experienced before. With Carl it was a ripping pain, a sharp ripping pain and then it was all over, but this. This was like having sand burn, like when as a child your parents would wipe the sand off your feet and it would burn. Well this was sand burn that went on and on and on. Time and time again. Afterwards, it felt so hot inside and then I would start bleeding. Every single time he would force his penis inside me and every single time it was like sand burn, then bleeding. Sometimes he would take his penis out and then force it back in again and I would cry out in pain and he would tear the skin as he entered me. I had sand burn and paper cuts in my vagina. It would hurt to pass urine, it would hurt to sit down and then 2 or 3 days later he would do it again and often the tear hadn't healed enough and as well as sand burn and bleeding it would sting, it would sting so much and he would do it again. He would take his penis out whilst he was 'doing it' and then force it back in and I don't have the words to articulate that pain. I started to tell him that he was hurting me and he told me that he couldn't stop until he 'came'. So I knew every time we had sex I had to endure it too the end. I was starting to panic and realise that I wasn't going to be able to cope with this every couple of days for the rest of my life, so I started asking him to stop. I started telling him that he was hurting me and said I wanted him to stop and then he stopped responding. He started ignoring my pleas for him to stop. I started crying because he was hurting me and completely ignored me, like I wasn't even there. All the time I was bleeding, It was stinging and burning, I couldn't cope. I went to see my Doctor, I told him that I was very sore down below. He took a look and after he had examined me he told me it was very red inside. He said I was torn and bleeding. He asked me if there was something I wanted to tell him. I was horrified, how could I tell a Doctor that I couldn't have sex normally, how could I tell a Doctor that there was something wrong with me. I was mortified, I told him there was nothing and I left. Stewart was already humiliating me, he whispered to me during sex to tell him what that man did to me when I was a kid. He told me I didn't like it because there was something wrong with me and he told me that what he was doing was normal and everybody did it. I felt so embarrassed, so inadequate, so worthless. I couldn't behave normally and I was devastated, so I let it go on. Stewart progressed to having sex with me in all positions, all of which were incredibly painful and some of which made me feel physically sick. He would force me to perform oral sex on him and if I turned away he would lower himself onto my face so I couldn't breathe. The only way I could breathe would be to grab his penis and put it in my mouth.

Hello Control – Welcome Anorexia.

I knew I couldn't live like this, I had to do something to take back some control. Something of me that he wasn't physically or emotionally able to violate. I decided the only thing I could control that he wouldn't know about was food. It began so subtly and it made me feel great. I had this brilliant secret and it was just between me and me. I began by cutting out snacks, just the regular stuff you might eat between meals, like biscuits, or crisps, even fruit. I found it remarkably easy, so I decided to progress it a bit further. I would be up and downstairs first in a morning, so I would give myself less cereal and pretend I had just finished when he came down, after a couple of weeks of doing this I realised that he didn't notice anyway so I would come downstairs and put his cereal in a bowl and put an empty clean bowl and spoon in the sink. He didn't notice a thing. This was easy and I was feeling pretty good about my little secret. He had no consideration for me at all now in relation to sex, he had grown tired of explaining why I wasn't normal and he would just fuck me whenever the mood took him. If I pretended to be asleep he would fuck me, if I cried he would fuck me, if I asked him to stop he would fuck me. I had to do something about the pain. Alcohol was my very best friend. I would drink so heavily that when it came to my regular fucking I was so drunk, the pain was dulled. I was still torn and bleeding and sore, that all came back the next day, but whilst it was going on, I would laugh at him, mock him, tell him he was crap and he would fuck me all the more and all the time I had my secret.

Going without breakfast and snacks had become too easy, I wasn't getting that rush I'd got at the start. I took sandwiches to work, cut into four and I would eat three and leave one in the back of my draw at work. Easy peasy. So, I developed it further. I would eat two and leave two in the back of my draw at work. I started to lose weight and people would comment on my slim figure, they would say I was doll like and Stewart said I looked like a child. I felt like a child, I felt like a child being raped by all those men who had raped me before. If I felt like a child and I looked like a child, then I wanted to do everything I could to get back to that child. I started to exercise. If I exercised and didn't eat, then I could get so tiny, I would be me again. Stewart didn't notice anything, nothing at all. He liked the petite figure before him, I was so easy to manipulate, fuck, do pretty much what he liked with. I would run every day and exercise at home, the weight was dropping off and I loved it. Something started to happen though after a while. I could starve and exercise all week, but around once a week, I would get this really, really sweet taste in my mouth. My blood sugars would drop, I would be shaking and I would crave anything and everything. I used to go food shopping on a Wednesday morning and that tended to be when it happened. I would buy bread, so much bread and stuff it in my mouth until I felt so full and so sick and my heart would be beating, no thumping so hard in my chest, I thought it was going to explode. I didn't like it when this happened and it made me feel like I had to exercise even harder, because I felt like I'd just eaten a week's worth of food in the space of probably half an hour. This went on for a few weeks, but I started to loathe myself for doing it, so I had the wonderful idea. Denying myself food was no longer giving me that rush of adrenaline, that rush of elation, Stewart was still fucking me, but I no longer had that good feeling that the secret gave me, only the escape of alcohol. I decided I need something else and I knew exactly what to do. When I got the craving I would wait until Stewart was beginning to maul me and I would tell him that if he went to the shop and bought me some chocolate, or ice-cream or whatever it was I fancied, then I would let him do whatever he liked to me. This couldn't have been a bigger turn on for him and he would be out of the door before I knew it. Whilst he was out, I would start eating. I would eat anything I could get my hands on whilst he was out. Bread, cake, biscuits. I would eat and eat and eat until I felt so sick, my heart was pounding in my chest. Then Stewart would come back from the shop with treats and I would eat it on top of everything else I had just stuffed down my neck and then he would start. The pain I felt being at Steweart's mercy did not quite match the pain I felt in my chest, stomach and the nausea from everything I had just eaten. I could laugh at him again, I felt so much worse than he could make me feel. I was back in control. Now I had alcohol and food to make me feel much worse than he could. Alcohol to distance me from the pain and food to cause me more physical pain than he was doing. I continued to exercise, binge and drink and my weight was dropping off. Stewart loved it, my Mum and Dad loved it because people would tell them how petite, doll like I looked. It motivated me more and more and more, but I was beginning to get tired. I was running out of energy. Stewart was becoming more and more adventurous with his sexual demands and I had stopped reaching those highs again. I couldn't cope, I hated what Stewart was doing to me and I hated what I was doing to me because it wasn't working any more. It wasn't giving me any respite, any high. It wasn't taking me away from the physical pain he was inflicting on me. I started to come down. I started to realise again, that this was the life I would have to live with for the rest of my life and I knew I couldn't do it. I knew I wanted to die. If only I could exercise hard enough and lose enough weight then maybe I would go to sleep and not wake up in the morning. My heart really thumped hard in my chest, maybe I would have a heart attack and die in my sleep. I continued to exercise hard, I starved myself of almost everything, only eating an evening meal because nobody could see me skip breakfast and lunch and I decided to hurry the process of my death up, instead of binging on biscuits and bread, which would put all that weight back on, I would binge on lettuce and I did. Whenever I got the craving I would binge on lettuce, or tomato. I was desperate to die, I couldn't cope with the pain Stewart was inflicting on me. I couldn't bare to live being so worthless, I hated myself so much, I was so tired, so weak. Tired of getting drunk all the time, it made me feel weak, tired of having no energy, tired of being cold, tired of living in hell, being forced to have sex, the pain, the bleeding. I just couldn't cope with living any longer. Every single night I would look at the side of my wrists and whisper, "*please let me be thin enough to die tonight*". All in all this took place over about a period of 5 years, but then something happened. When I was running, I started to notice a funny pain in my ankles, I was also getting pain in my wrists. It was a bit like a pinching pain. It was affecting my speed when I was running and I didn't like the feeling, so I went to see my GP. I told her my symptoms and she stood me on the scales. She told me I weighed 40kg. I had a BMI of just over 14.5. She told me that if I lost any more weight then she would be carting me off to hospital. I told her that I had probably just overdone the exercise. She advised me to tell family so they could support me and like an innocent fool, I did.

The Humiliation begins.

I told Stewart that I had been to the Doctor and that she had told me I was underweight. I told him that she said she thought I had anorexia. I told my Mum and Dad the same. Stewart looked at me with absolute disgust. He humiliated me, told me that I looked like a freak and told me I was the ugliest thing he had ever seen. My Mum and Dad went pretty much along the same line. My Dad told me I looked disgusting and said I just looked like a skeleton with skin stretched over. I have never regretted being alive so much in my life. From that day on I was force fed, I was humiliated, I was rejected and I was repeatedly told how disgusting I looked. One night after we had all been to the pub, I was obviously very drunk as was my Mum and Dad, My Mum asked me why I had lost so much weight and I told her. I told her I had been sexually abused when I was a child and I couldn't cope with it. I couldn't cope with living anymore and I told her that I wanted to die. She told me that she was really disappointed in me. She told me that she thought I was made of stronger stuff and that I should have told her when I was a child. I was crying and I told her that I wanted to die and she told me we could do it together. She told me that if I wanted to commit suicide, then she would do it with me. She told me if I ever wanted to talk about it then I could. And she never mentioned it again! Instead both her, Stewart and my Dad used this new found knowledge to continue to humiliate me, tell me how disgusting I looked and how disappointed they were in me. Stewart, who had wanted us to try for a baby, didn't come near me after that. He would look at me with revulsion and not many months later we separated. My relationship with food has never fully recovered, I continued to starve myself on and off for many years afterwards and I avoid certain foods that remind me of binge eating and I feel very uncomfortable when I feel full as it reminds me of binge eating. I prefer to eat enough not to feel hungry, but I try to eat enough and I dislike buffets immensely because I never know how much is going to be enough and then I end up not eating enough. It's become less of an issue as years have gone by, but I will only ever eat to live, rather than live to eat. It's a necessity, that if I don't monitor will only become a stressor, particularly after being force fed.

Falling Apart.

After Stewart and I split I went to live with a friend. She had separated from her husband so drinking heavily was perfectly acceptable. The flashbacks continued and my friend and I would talk for hours and the conversation came round to Stewart. I explained the more physical aspects of sex, most definitely not the emotion, or my abnormality. One evening during a conversation about Stewart, my friend suddenly interrupted me and stated that what Stewart had been doing all these years was rape! I did not believe her for one minute. We were both drunk. But no, apparently forcing a penis inside you when you are telling them to stop is rape. Causing you physical harm whilst trying to force their penis inside you when you are telling them to stop is rape. Asking somebody to stop and they don't is rape. Telling somebody you don't want to have sex and then them forcing their penis inside you is rape. Well fuck me if you'll pardon the pun!

As if I didn't have enough already to fall apart about, then this really took the lid off. I went to counselling and sure enough, somebody forcing you to have sex without your consent is rape! Now that put a whole new perspective on things for me. Now I was loaded with guilt. I allowed him to do it for all those years because Brenda Smith said "*these things happen*". If I didn't have enough to be ashamed of then this really took the biscuit. It dawned on me that since the age of 10 I had been gradually violated more and more until not only did I have no body left, I had no mind. I had been physically, sexually and emotionally violated and I had nothing left. I had confided in those I trusted and they had used that to absolutely destroy me. I was drinking more than ever and the flashbacks when I was drunk. Well, they weren't flashbacks, they were real time over and over again. I was being raped over and over again. I didn't want to live, I was broken and I'd started having panic attacks. I didn't die though, but I was constantly giving myself deadlines. If I don't feel better by the end of the month then I would kill myself. I was going to get incredibly drunk, then I was going to take a load of pills and just before I passed out, I was going to drink a bottle of bleach. And that thought and that pressure grew stronger and stronger as the end of every month neared, it was torture. Should I, shouldn't I? I started counselling at Rape Crisis. Chris Wroe. She was great and she listened and she listened and she listened and I don't remember a single thing that she said, but I could talk and cry and cry and talk and then I would go back and do the same. But then she told me she was leaving. The lid had come off and she left. I had started my midwifery training and I was struggling with panic attacks, flash back, just living in general. I confided in my personal tutor her name was Annie Cropston. I told her about Stewart and Rape Crisis and we met regularly, she said she was concerned about my weight and she introduced me to Judith Ross a mental health nurse who was teaching at De Montfort University. I spoke with her a couple of times, but not really about anything in great depth. It was Annie that I met with regularly, she listened whilst I talked about my struggles, but in spite of this I did well during my training, worked throughout my course and secured my own living accommodation, without any support at all from my Mum and Dad who told me I had caused them enough stress, they made it clear they wouldn't help me move house and said they couldn't understand why I wanted to do a shit shovelling job anyway. I was completely alone.

I focused on my training, with training and work I didn't have to worry about the possibility of meeting anybody else, because I was having sex with Melvyn, who would come and see me and listen to my problems and I appreciated that. Even if it meant having to have sex. It was a small price to pay. I didn't need anybody. I had passed my training and secured the job that I loved, I didn't have to worry about meeting anybody. Melvyn was a mental health social worker who I had confided in one day at work and he visited me regularly to listen to my nightmares.

New Beginnings.

My Son was born in 2002. As already stated at the beginning of this text book. I have deliberately left life details out of this because it isn't an autobiography, it's a text book to illustrate my life experiences and the impact that they have had on my life. However, it is relevant to mention this about my Son. Firstly, because he was conceived through donor insemination. I wanted a baby, but I had decided I didn't want a man, ever again. I spoke with close friends and Annie Cropston and asked for their opinion. Annie was clear that she didn't think this was a good idea. But I did and I knew I could love and support a child on my own. The happiest time of my life was when me and my Son were together on our own. Having my Son relaxed my anxieties about life in general as I had him and work to focus on and nothing else. So, when I met Alan in 2005, I felt I had grown and healed as a person. Alan was very, very attentive when we met. He showered me with gifts, he considered my every need, he said he was a virgin, which was even better, he didn't drink very much at all and the best thing of all was he didn't want to know about my past. Finally, I had met somebody who wasn't going to abuse me.

In 2005 I had an ectopic pregnancy. I cried after my surgery and Alan hugged me and told me not to cry. We didn't talk about it and I was told I shouldn't tell anybody because it was nobody else's business so I didn't. It was the beginning of being isolated from friends. I later realised that when he was telling me not to cry, it was because he really meant it. He didn't want me to cry, he didn't want to me express any emotion at all. To the point where I was lying in bed the day after I came home and he stuck his dick in my mouth. Oral sex to make him feel better and to shut me up. I had 2 pregnancies after that, but I didn't connect with them at all. I had flash backs of sexual abuse, I felt exposed, I couldn't talk about how I was feeling and I did not bond with my unborn babies at all. I just wanted them out. Every experience throughout pregnancy and after triggered flash backs of sexual abuse and I couldn't talk about any of it. I wasn't allowed to talk about any of it.

2015 The year all that ended.

The longer time went on the harder it was getting to live without flashbacks. I was isolated in my relationship and mocked and ridiculed so my self-esteem was continually being knocked and I felt like I couldn't move on. It was becoming harder and harder to leave the past behind. I was never allowed to express emotion or discuss my past, but I couldn't make it go away.

June 2015 I had been enrolled on a communications course. I wanted to improve my communication skills as I was looking after a vulnerable client group and I was always looking at ways I could be better in caring for these young people. I enjoyed the course, there was only about eight of us on the course and we were asked to do role play. I don't know anybody who likes role play, but we had professional actors who were given scenarios from our speciality, chosen by us and then they would play the part of the client and we would assume our own professional role.

I decided to choose a scenario that was very relevant to my practice and one that I had encountered several times. My scenario was a young person who had been raped and was struggling with flash backs and the effects of being pregnant. I began my response by asking the young person if they had accessed counselling, if they had informed the police and if there was any specific support they felt we could offer as well as advising a referral to our specialist mental health service for ongoing support. I thought I'd done rather well.

Martyn Geary was my tutor and he held his hand up to stop me and then he said. *"somebody has just disclosed something to you, you need to ask them more about it"*. In that very instant my whole world fell apart. *"No I don't"* I was thinking. *"I don't want to hear anything about it"*. In that moment Martyn was looking at me and what I heard was, *"I know you have been sexually abused, I can see it and if you ask them to describe what has happened, they are going to describe exactly what happened to you"*.

I don't remember much about any of what happened next, because all I had going round in my head was all the abuse that I had been subjected to and it was suddenly right at the front of my head, like too many televisions being switched on all at once, really loud, demanding attention. I was shaking, I was terrified, I couldn't make them stop and I couldn't make them go away. I was absolutely terrified. I didn't know what was happening to me. I was shaking every day at work, I was telling people I felt stressed, I was concerned that I had too many cases of sexual abuse on my caseload, but when I went through it, it was about 4 out of 40. I was identifying with my client group. When they were telling me their experiences all I could think was, that's happened to me. That's happening to me right now. I was functioning and I appeared normal, but I had been transported back and was living physically and emotionally the sexual abuse I had been subjected to. I asked for Supervision at work, but I was told it wasn't possible, it was too expensive. I had completely tuned out of the present. I was functioning, I don't know how, but I wasn't present at all in the here and now and I was absolutely terrified, because I was trying to get back and I couldn't. I told Martyn I was struggling with the course, I told him that I was overwhelmed with my client group and he referred me to a Supervisor. I spoke with Mira and I was telling her that my role was very stressful and that I had asked for Supervision and I was told I couldn't have it. I gave an example of another health care professional who had become traumatised by a clients history and the response

I received was if they can't cope with the job, then they shouldn't be doing it. All the time I was screaming inside, that I needed help. I needed the people I was approaching to see what I was seeing. I thought I was telling them. To me it was obvious. I was asking for help and nobody was listening. I wasn't even having flash backs, I was just there, right back there when it was all happening. I knew I was there and I was asking for help to get me back, but nobody was listening. I was physically present, but I had gone inside.

I was about to start a clinic one morning and a colleague came in to talk to me. She asked me if I was okay and I told her I didn't know. I was just staring at her because I didn't know what else to say. I was almost catatonic, my physical being was present, but it was like I'd been invaded. Invaded by all the sexual abuse and it was happening right there, it was all playing out in front of me over and over again, I was totally consumed by it and I couldn't stop it. She then asked me if I was going to do anything silly and again I replied that I didn't know. I was completely unable to articulate anything. All I knew was I'd been invaded and I knew I couldn't handle it. *"I would be better of not being here."* I had tried and tried to get back but I couldn't and I was frightened that I couldn't get back, but I thought it was permanent and I knew I had to go. I had planned the next time I was on my course that I would open the window and jump out, we were on the 6th floor, so absolutely no chance of survival. That didn't frighten me at all. What frightened me was what was happening right then. I'd been invaded and I couldn't get back. I couldn't function, I couldn't do anything but I was being abused over and over again the physical and emotional feelings were happening over and over again.

She asked me if she could talk to Martyn about how I was feeling and I said she could. That same day Martyn called me and arranged a meeting for the next day. He sounded very kind. I don't know what she told him, but when I met with him he began by saying he was concerned that I had thoughts of self-harm. That really jolted me back into the present. We were in a room with high windows, it was quiet and warm and I felt safe. There was nothing in that room that made me feel anxious or made me feel that I might have the opportunity to kill myself. Martyn was very calm and unhurried and I started to tell him that I was finding the course difficult, because it was bringing back some difficult memories. I told him I felt scared and that I had been trying to tell people that I was struggling, but nobody was listening. I told him about my plan to throw myself out of the window. Martyn was really calm and I started to calm down for the first time in weeks. Everything began to slow right down. Martyn listened whilst I talked and I don't know what I talked about, but all I remember was he was very calm and unhurried. At the end he asked me if I would go and talk to my GP about how I was feeling and I agreed. I agreed because he had taken his time with me, he didn't panic me or rush me and asking me to talk to my GP made me feel like it came from a place of genuine care and concern, so I didn't feel frightened to talk to my GP. I did make an appointment and I did tell my GP how I was feeling. He prescribed medication and asked me to see him again. I continued with my course and never sat near the window. Every time I was in that room the temptation was high. I even passed the course with a great grade. I remained at work for a couple of weeks more, but I couldn't cope with the overwhelming emotion and I referred myself to occupational health, I told Alan and a few friends how I had been feeling and then I went off sick from work. My life had finally caught up with me and it had really taken its toll. I decided through all the mire that I would keep a journal and write in it every day, because I knew even then that I wouldn't remember anything that was about to happen. I knew it would become a black abyss and it has. I don't remember much about the next 2 years at all and I am glad I still had a tiny bit of insight glowing inside and despite everything I didn't understand, some how I did understand that I would use it one day.

Part 2

The journal

This part of the book is purely taken from entries I have made in real time. I wasn't sure whether to put reflections in this part, or leave it for you the reader to understand. So, I have decided that some pages will include some of my reflections, how I perceive things now, or the reflections will just help by putting some context around what I am saying. Some entries will be left for you to just absorb. That way you can choose to read or ignore my own reflections as I can't decide whether they will be helpful to the reader, or influence their own thoughts and original reflections and I don't want to do that.

24.07.2015

I lasted less than an hour at work today. I met with my Manager and told her I was totally distracted and not focused at work anymore.

This thing has beaten me, it's time to stop running and to meet this thing head on.

I am shattered, I am shaking and I can't concentrate on anything.

I have Sertraline 50mg, but I don't know what good it is doing. I just want to cry and sleep. This is day one of my focus on healing me.

Reflection: I had no idea what was happening to me. I was terrified. I walked into work that morning and sat talking to a colleague just swinging my legs. She told me I didn't look very well and said she thought I should go home. I opened my diary and showed her everything I had to do, but she persisted and told me I should talk to my manager. She told me a long time later that, that day I had looked like a small child sat there swinging my legs. And I did that day. I felt 10 years old. How on earth did I look like I felt?

After speaking to my Manager, I gave her my diary and I went home. I threw all my work clothes in the bin and I went to bed. I just needed to sleep. I needed to escape the physical feelings as well as the emotional feelings. I didn't understand what was going on. I was completely overwhelmed.

When I woke up later that day, I was asked what time dinner would be and asked when was I going shopping. I had no idea what was to come.

Notes:

25.07.2015
Still shaking and shattered, had supportive texts. Waiting for counselling assessment on Tuesday. I am going to document how my healing goes no matter how hard it becomes to pick up a pen.

Reflection: Everything had shut down. I couldn't think straight, I couldn't process anything. I had no control at all over making my mind function normally. It was the most terrifying experience. I just wanted to sleep. I felt so incredibly tired.

Notes:

26.07.2015
I have been hiding behind my Kindle and sleep all day. I was shaking this morning even turning the page on my kindle made me shake, but as I became engrossed in my book I stopped shaking.
I had to supervise the kids having showers and that made me start to shake, so I picked up my Kindle and became engrossed again.
My friend Carol called me and I started to get hot, I started to feel panicky and just wanted to get off the 'phone. Why? Because I had to think! I had to make conversation and I was struggling.

Reflection: This felt very strange. If I had to think, or look at anything at all I would begin to shake uncontrollably. It was like my head had completely shut down. If I wasn't able to escape into another world, i.e. my book, I literally couldn't cope. I was even trying to physically overcome the feeling inside me, but I couldn't. I had no control at all over what my brain, my mind was doing. Talking on the 'phone was equally as bad, because I couldn't think, it felt too hard. I really did feel broken, like a computer, I just couldn't process, no matter how hard I was trying. At this stage I still didn't know what was happening and I was really frightened.

Notes:

27/07/2015
I went for a jog this morning. I was terrified before I went out, but felt much better when I got home. We took some recycling to the charity shop and bought some lunch. I had a sleep in the afternoon. Felt very shaky at dinner time, had a panic attack.

Reflection: I was absolutely exhausted. I was still trying to fight through it, but my body had other ideas. For the first time in my life I couldn't control it.

Notes:

28/07/2015
I went to Quetzal today for my counselling assessment, I didn't sleep well last night worrying. I cried throughout the whole assessment, but it was actually a relief to tell someone exactly how bad I feel. Talked about feelings, abuse, anorexia, self-harm. When I got home my mind was fuzzy. I was told there would be a 4-6 week wait for counselling. I couldn't think straight, I couldn't concentrate. I went to a friend's house to talk and talk and talk. It really does feel good to tell people exactly how you feel. It relieves the pressure, for a short time at least. Still shaking. I just want the shaking to stop. I don't feel in control, yet friends keep telling me I am because I am doing something about it. I'm not used to not being in control. I want to be strong again for my family so I know I have to do this and do it properly - and I will, because I never want to feel like this again. Maybe shaking is my body telling me I am not okay. I keep being told I will be okay. The woman at Quetzal was confident I will put this matter to rest when I deal with it properly. I think I will be different after this. I will be whole. A strong whole, not a fragile whole. My friends are getting me through and my family too.

Reflection: I was beginning to realise I couldn't make this go away any longer. I had spent 35 years keeping a lid on everything and being very much in control of my emotions. I started to realise I couldn't fight it any longer. I had no idea where this was going. I had no idea how to repair myself, but what I did know was nothing was going to be the same ever again.

Notes:

29.07.2015
Today was a quiet day. I cancelled my tutorial, I concentrated on my assignment this afternoon. I saw a friend tonight, she was very supportive, also telling me to look after myself, put myself first. Still shaking, but went for a jog. When I am jogging I am not shaking.

Reflection: This was the first of many days when I felt numb. It was like my body and mind just couldn't panic, stress, or fight so I just felt numb. Like it was regrouping. I had no idea what it meant to put myself first. I felt like I was completely falling apart, but I had this awful sense of dread. I didn't know how far I was going to fall and worst of all, I couldn't control how far, or how fast it was happening. I was falling down a big tunnel and I just couldn't grip the sides.

Notes:

30.07.2015
I saw my GP this morning. He gave me a sick note for 2 weeks. I rang Occupational Health, they are making me a Consultant appointment in 6 weeks. Quetzal rang, appointments start next week, Tuesdays 5.30 pm. Had an appointment this afternoon. All in all a very shaky, very emotional day. I feel like I am about to start making myself whole again. I am terrified to start , I feel okay until I start talking and then I cry. I am not okay, but I am beginning to believe I will be okay. I am shaking, I am terrified and I am not thinking straight. I don't feel right now that I will ever be able to think about anything again. I am so scared, but I don't feel alone anymore. When I got back from my appointment my head was spinning I didn't know what to do. Sit, stand, walk, talk. I felt agitated, but at the same time physically very weak. I felt dizzy and panicky. It passed when I was persuaded to play with the kids in the garden. What will happen tomorrow?

Reflection: I realised it was time to surrender to it, I thought if I surrendered to it, stopped fighting it, everything would slow down. But it didn't. It was like everything wanted to be heard at once, all at the same time and every single traumatic experience I had had was causing a physical and emotional response. All those experiences screaming to be heard at once and I couldn't make them stop, I couldn't make them slow down. Every single flashback and emotional reaction wanted to be heard all at once and even when I felt I had surrendered to it, it consumed me all the more. My head was so aggressively busy and I couldn't make the thoughts slow down, I couldn't make them queue to be heard. It was like every single experience had had enough of being suppressed and they were all having this massive tantrum in my head, screaming and shouting, forcing themselves to be heard.

Notes:

31.07.2015

Feeling very subdued today. Still shaking. I look forward to the day I write no longer shaking. Only a fleeting suicidal thought today. Wasn't thinking of anything or anyone. Got to the traffic lights by the library and really started shaking. I feel hot now thinking about it. I stepped back from the road because I just felt like I was being pulled out. I crossed the road as quickly as I could, but then suddenly felt exactly the same in the same place walking back. I felt okay afterward, I think it is an association with that place, because it's there that I started to feel really bad a couple of weeks ago. It's always an image of walking into the path of a car. It's good to be able to write it down without feeling guilty. This is my shit and I am determined to get rid of it. I feel very, very flat. Up until today I have felt I could cry at any moment, but today I feel empty. Increased my Sertraline today to 100mg on GP advice.

Reflection: Feeling the pull of suicide is very, very strong. Even if the thought is only fleeting. I felt very impulsive, should I, shouldn't I? A fleeting thought that could cause an action that had permanent consequences. I think fleeting thoughts are sometimes scarier than ongoing thoughts in that the spike in energy and impulse is incredibly strong. A split second decision that could change everything. Thankfully it still scared me and that's what made me pull away. But I knew that the fear was being taken over by willpower and I was being sucked further and further away from reality and I could see it, but I couldn't do anything to stop it. It was absolutely terrifying.

Notes:

01.08.2015

Had a massive panic attack. I don't think I can do this. I just want everything to be okay. I can't work, I feel terrible, the kids want me to play but I have a crashing headache. Still shaking, I want to feel better, I'm not used to being out of control and I'm scared.

Reflection: It was scary because I had surrendered to it, but it, being the flashbacks and emotional reactions were just becoming stronger, more powerful and very, very threatening. These ghosts were so angry now. They wanted out and they weren't going to wait their turn and they were angry because they had been silenced. Very violent and very aggressive.

Notes:

02.08.2015
Today was a very bad day, that ended better. I remembered something. I was 11years old and he was 15. He wanted to have sex with me. I'd already been abused so I was up for it, but then family returned after a drunken night out and we almost got caught. A short while later when I'd started to feel really bad about myself we were playing in the yard. You dared me to climb the ladder onto the air raid shelter, but I bottled out. As I was climbing down you stuck your hand up my skirt and started fingering me. I shouted at you to stop and I climbed back up the ladder. You laughed at me telling me I had to come down eventually. I started crying as you fingered me all the way down the ladder. You bastard, why did you have to do that to me? You helped destroy my childhood. You abused me.
I remembered today age 13 walking across the field to a friend's house, an older male started walking with me and asked me to go with him so I did. He kissed me, felt my budding breasts and put his hand down my knickers. He wanted to take me further away to have sex with me. I told him I would be late for my fried and agreed to meet him the next day. I didn't go back. All the time I remember looking at the trainers I was wearing thinking why does he want to do this to me when I have horrible trainers. You made me hate men and myself even more.
I was walking home one night and a boy came up to me and told me to walk with him. I told him I didn't want to and he said he had a knife and would use it if I didn't go with him. We passed a shop as we were walking and I ran out into the road to get away from him. I waited in the shop for a while and ran home terrified.
Walking across the same park a man exposed himself to me. He ran and hid behind the trees and I ran home terrified.
I was already terrified after being sexually abused and this just reinforced my terror. I do not remember a time in my life when I was not scared.
I saw Carol tonight, I have been shaking badly all day with the sudden memory recall. We talked and talked and she made me feel better for a while until I got home. But it was lovely for a while.

Reflection: I grew up in a new town built in the late 60's, a dreadful place in the North West. It was the most terrifying place to live and being exposed to and threatened by men and boys was something I grew up experiencing, but after I was told 'these things happen'. I never thought to question it, I just hated life.

Notes:

03.08.2015

Bad, bad day, shaking. Just me and the kids, they entertain themselves now. Charlie says he misses me. He wants me to get better. That makes two of us. I almost lost it today, started panicking about tomorrow. I text a colleague from work, that fended off a panic attack, but then I just wanted to cry. I wanted to sob and sob, but I couldn't. I have never been able to, never the right time, never safe! I felt like crying again tonight so I asked Alan to play badminton in the garden. It distracted me whilst we were playing. I am so scared that I will fall apart tomorrow. I see panic attack, paramedics, hospital. To comprehend what has happened makes me want to scream, go mad, vomit. Like a mother losing a child, I lost my child. The pressure is building, I feel hot and I want to hurt myself to relieve the pressure, but I am in bed and I will stay in bed. I am thinking hard about my friends who believe in me and I will stay in bed, but it is so hard!

Reflection: This mounting pressure was becoming unbearable. Nothing was feeling any better, it felt like it was getting worse. Panic attacks make you feel like you are going to die and I really didn't think my body would be able to survive this. It was being battered.

Notes:

04.08.2015

Shit, shit, shit; It's so hard to write tonight. Went with the kids to arrange my tattoo. First counselling tonight and panicking so much. Vicky her name is. We talked about the contract. Then! 35 years of sick gut wrenching emotion started to pour out. My throat started to tighten and I felt like I couldn't breath and then the tears came, my throat relaxed and I cried as I told her about the abuse. Then I told her I still felt guilty. I told her I had ongoing thoughts of self-harm. I'd been anorexic, I'd tried to drink myself to death and in the last two weeks I had twisted my rings so forcibly around my finder it had blistered. She told me self-harm was a coping mechanism I had always used. We talked about medication, I am not going to take it anymore. I was shaking, dizzy and feeling sick before I started taking it and I am the same now. I couldn't stop crying, I was feeling such a rush of emotion in my head I just told her everything. It needed to come out. I was abused when I was 10yrs old, 11yrs old, 13yrs old and 16yrs old. Then from the age of 20 until I was 26. Each time the abuse got worse, from fingering to rape. She summed up by saying I'd been terribly neglected and suffered horrendous abuse. I came out of the session and completely fell apart. How I was feeling has just been validated and hearing those words thumped me in the stomach, almost took my breath away. Thirty five years of pushing something that massive down and then in that one sentence BANG! The enormity has hit me. I couldn't go home, I couldn't stop crying. I text Carol, a mutual friend called Daryl and Melvyn and they all responded supportively. I went to Carols, she called me and invited me over. I cried and told her everything. I told her I still feel guilty about EVERYTHING she knew already. She told me it would be hard. She just knows what to say. I told her about my thoughts of self-harm and explained that the counsellor had told me that it was my way of coping. I told Carol that I wouldn't self-harm because she, Melvyn, Daryl and Vicky were supporting me. I said I needed to say it though, because I was thinking it and I want to say it's how I feel because of the pressure behind the thoughts. I need to talk about the pressure. It builds up in my head and I don't know how to release it. It's so powerful right now. God this is shit. Carol was right it is shit and it hurts like hell! I feel like I have laid myself bare to Vicky and I feel completely exposed, totally vulnerable and blown wide open, but I can't deal with this any longer. Please let it be okay.

Reflection: I went to see Vicky at the Quetzal Project. It is a counselling service supporting adult victims of child sexual abuse. I was sat in a chair in a very large room and Vicky sat facing me and she hardly responded to anything I said. In fact, the more I was talking, the more afraid she looked. I talked and talked and talked and I felt worse when I came out. Not because I was releasing everything for the first time, but because apart from the odd sentence she didn't talk at all. Also those words she said. "You have been terribly neglected and suffered horrendous abuse". Shit! now that was a sickening blow to the gut. I had a terrible reaction inside to that statement. I felt sick, I felt shocked, it took my breath away. How the hell could somebody say that. Imagine you have suffered horrendous burns to your face. You know you are scarred for life, you imagine how you look, you know how you feel. But then somebody unexpectedly shoves a mirror in your face and all the images you had are suddenly thrust in front of you and you can't take it in. You suddenly don't know if that's what you believed you looked like, it's horrific, but now there is no hiding from it, because you have been shown exactly what you look like. Vicky using those words was telling me exactly what I had experienced. Savage, absolutely savage.

The pressure of the flashbacks diminished for a short time, but the pressure for somebody to respond to me at the very least was incredibly strong. I didn't feel comfortable with Vicky, but I had nobody else. I went to Carols because Alan told me not to come home until I had stopped crying and I could behave normally.

Notes:

05.08.15

God this hurts! I slept badly last night, re-living the session. I've been terribly neglected and suffered horrendous abuse. I feel gut wrenchingly sick. I want to scream and fall apart. Fuck, Fuck, Fuck, I have squashed that down for 35 years. All the energy, all the fighting, battling, living on guard and suddenly it all comes crashing down. I am destroyed, I am broken, I am totally exposed. Fucking hell I want to scream. I am completely consumed with memories and true feelings of being trapped, frightened, sexually abused, fingered, raped. Guilt, shame, embarrassment, disgust, scared, isolated, terrified, tormented, completely devastated. Today has been a really bad day. At lunch time I had some really scary thoughts. I'd got it into my head that Alan was punishing me for not coping. Not wanting to hear my nightmare, not wanting to share my pain. He thinks that I'm just off work and can carry on as normal. I thought about the guilt I feel for being a terribly person. I thought about the red handled knife we have in the kitchen. If I scored down my arm and ripped it open, then, there; I have punished myself for being a bad girl, a naughty, useless, in the way burden, who would be better off dead. I was shaking so badly, I couldn't think of one reason why doing it was the wrong thing to do. Then I thought about the kids. They are not punishing me, they love me dearly and I love them. But I'm hurting so much, so very much. I have Carol, Melvyn and Daryl and my memories are trapped in my head, desperate to be heard. All of them at once, so much noise, the television irritates me, the radio is too loud. I just want peace. I want to feel at peace. I want to be held and cuddled and healed, I want my life the way it should have been. I just want to be okay.

Reflection: Although I was consumed, it later turned out that I was right about being punished by Alan for not coping. I didn't realise it then, but there was worse to come from him. It was like he could see I was falling apart and he was going to do everything he could to finish me off. I just didn't realise it at that time. The self-harm thoughts were very powerful. The pressure I keep referring to felt like a physical pressure, a pressure inside my body that I couldn't get out and I felt I needed to release it, make an opening to let it escape. I couldn't deal with the emotional pressure, my head was too full, so I had to physically release it. This is also why the television, radio and noise felt too overwhelming. There was already a lot of loud, aggressive, flashbacks constantly racing through my head and anything else was just too much.

Notes:

06.08.2015

I feel so sad tonight. Today was a busy day and I had my tattoo. I was actually thinking about it all day, although still shaking. Then tonight we all went to see Darly in his new house and normal conversation ensued. But the longer normal conversation went on, the more disconnected I felt, because I don't feel normal. I don't feel normal at all. I feel out of place, nothing fits anymore. I don't know who I am. I am laughing, but feel sick inside. I don't know how I feel, I just feel all wrong. I feel so, so sad, I just want to be okay. I just want to sit and cry with my head in my hands. I feel so lost.

Reflection: Daryl was a mutual friend of mine and my now ex-husband. We met him and his wife when they moved in 2 doors away from us. They had since separated and his wife disconnected from us, although there had been no falling out. We maintained our friendship with Daryl and his children. This was a really distressing evening. In my head I was no longer part of the present. I had been catapulted back to every abusive experience and although I was physically present, the longer the present day conversations carried on, the more disconnected I felt. It was like I was on the outside looking in and not really there at all. I couldn't understand that feeling at the time, the strangest feeling ever, to be physically in the present moment, but to feel like I was actually living and experiencing a time somewhere 35 years ago that felt so much more real.

Notes:

07.08.2015

I woke up feeling very sad and very shaky. I just wanted to cuddle myself in bed all day. I feel sad for myself and lonely and lost and afraid. I feel 10 years old in a 45 year old body. I hid it from the kids, I love them so much. My babies, they deserve better. Carol came this afternoon, she makes so much sense. To be angry at the bastards, to be determined not to let it dictate any more of my life. But I don't. I feel so terribly hurt and sad and lost and alone. I feel 10 years old. The television is on and I make all the right noises, I laugh and I comment, but in front of my eyes is 10 year old me. I remembered more stuff this afternoon, when he would get admitted to hospital with non-specific illness. He even had two operations out of three admissions. He used to be incredibly horny when he was discharged. Then he would rape me so violently. I remembered that today and then I carried on. I want to curl up into a ball and cry. Cry for me, cry for all my pain, my fear, my despair. I feel broken, I am so lost, I don't know who I am.

Reflection: When I first went off sick I didn't know what to expect. People told me I had had a breakdown. I don't know what that is. They said I would be off work for six months. How did they know? But as time was beginning to pass, whilst the flashbacks were violently hurried and loud and demanding of all my attention, it was like they were beginning to become more detailed, more in depth. It was beginning to become flashbacks about the detail instead of flashbacks about the events. This was getting really frightening.

Notes:

08.08.15

Shit, things are very bad. I have realised, before I can move on I need to process things. I need time to accept what has happened to me. For fucks sake, I was raped when I was a child. My God. It tried to tell Alan tonight, but Match of the Day started and he spotted his football team were playing, he is so absorbed. I need time, I need time to allow this to sink in. Then I can start to understand what was wrong and begin to heal. Everybody is away this weekend, Carol, Daryl and Melvyn. Now I am crying in bed on my own, because I hurt so much. I just want to be held. I just want to feel safe. I am so alone! I have always been so alone.

Reflection: And now I recognise it. Although I felt like I had lost all control, all sense of reality, in fact my core brain was still working. I could see what needed to happen. What I couldn't see then was how I was going to do it. Alan wasn't interested at all. Carol, she was a great colleague from work and became a very good friend. Daryl as I have explained was a mutual friend as well as Melvyn who I had known for many years. What I didn't have at that time though was any sense of who I was, any sense of myself. I needed those people to carry me. To hold on to me because I had no idea what was going on. I felt so alone because I really was alone. I didn't have me for comfort, I didn't have me to self soothe. I had lost that at a very young age. The age I first began to believe I was a bad person. If I didn't have anybody else, then I was an empty shell and I didn't know how to cope.

Notes:

09.08.15

A day feeling detached. Horrible thoughts right through my head. I just wanted to be alone to try and sort my head out. Shaking very badly. Melvyn told me I should tell Alan. So I did tonight, everything and I cried and I cried. He hugged me and told me none of it was my fault. He said he wants nothing more to do with my cousin. He said he knew exactly what he was doing. He looked shocked when I told him everything, but he really does need to know what's going on. I want to get well again, I want to feel strong. But strong because I feel it, not because I have to be.

Reflection: This was an interesting evening. This was an evening where I thought I was confiding in my ex-husband so that I could have an ally. In fact what I was doing was confiding in an abuser who would use all of my vulnerability to destroy me, but I didn't see it, not that night. I just wanted to be cared for and he did. Just like Jack, just like Stewart. A hug, an ear in exchange for my soul.

Notes:

10.08.15

I spent the whole day reflecting on what I had told Alan. I feel like I need to keep telling people. I am on my own with the kids today and tonight so need to keep distracting myself, shaking when it gets too much, so I focus on my assignment. Play badminton with Charlie. I desperately want to talk to somebody, but they are all too busy. I don't want to get on peoples nerves, but this is so overwhelming. I don't want to burden anybody. They tell me to keep talking, what should I do?

Reflection: Talking was releasing pressure for very short periods of time, I was lifting the lid off a pan that kept bubbling over and that's why I needed to keep telling people. The pressure was so strong, I would talk, it would abate for a short time, but then it would come back and I was constantly wanting to relieve that pressure.

Notes:

11.08.15

Silly me, I wish I could process things at the time, I got into a real state at lunchtime, panicking about counselling today. Carol came to babysit. I couldn't get money out of the machine, a reason not to go then. Then I would have no money to pay the counsellor, another reason not to go. I do go.... And we talk about how last week went. I talk about panicking and about coming today and how distressed I was last week. She said there was an urgency in what I told her, so before we begin to address what happened I need to develop positive coping strategies for when I think about this. God, how bad must this be if the thought of talking sends me into a panic. She said I had already developed them by staying in bed when I feel suicidal, also when I use my distraction techniques. Then I cried tonight because we didn't even get started on the stuff, the thought panicked me so badly. Carol is amazing. I know I can tell her anything and she really understands, but I feel I can't do this because of the extent of emotion it evokes. I am so overwhelmed. I feel like I might die, this is so massive. I have Carol, Daryl and Melvyn, so I will keep going. I will get better. I have to believe in me. Shit I feel so bad, still shaking.

Reflection: This was my second appointment with Vicky. I felt she was stifling me. She'd already told me there was an urgency and that's because these flashbacks were wanting to come out urgently. They had no more patience and they weren't prepared to come out calmly in any form. I didn't want to talk coping strategies, I didn't want to talk about techniques. I just wanted to verbally vomit it all out again because the pressure was so massive and she stopped me from doing that. When I left, I felt so much worse because I hadn't been able to release the pressure.

Notes:

12.08.2015

Today started off slow, then my mum called to say she was coming over 2-4pm, so we went to Daryls. He gave us lunch, it was very relaxed and easy, then my Manager text me from work and I was panicking. I'm going to see her on Friday. What the hell do I say? I didn't have too long to think because my mum came round and we went out. Daryl invited us back for a BBQ. We all went and I felt okay for a while and that felt so, so good. I will hang on to that. I won't worry about Friday until Friday. One day at a time.

Reflection: For whatever reason that day felt okay. I was already trying to practice living in the present. I had no insight to how I was actually coping when I really felt like I was falling apart. There was a core inside me that was very gently giving me direction, so subtle I couldn't see it at the time.

Notes:

13.08.15

Today I woke up shaking. Alan is off work and I have the day to myself. I go in to town and as I am walking through the car park I feel my legs shaking and wonder if I should go home. I decide to find the Meditation Café, then I go to the Very Bazaar and buy 2 beautiful rings. It is a very peaceful shop to go in, full of healing, peace and mindfulness. I have booked myself in for 3 meditation sessions starting Monday. I am still feeling anxious, but feel a sense of calm also. I go to the library, but the atmosphere is far from tranquil, so I leave and the bookshop I wanted to go to has closed down. I go back to the Very Bazaar and look round. Then randomly I go to Fenwicks Department store and I see things I like. I go to the counter and I feel I want to cry, because I have chosen things I like. I buy some ornaments, cushions, a throw and a teddy. This wasn't about material stuff, this was about things that make me feel good and they did. It made me feel calm. The textures I bought are all soft and that made me feel good. I bought moisturiser for my hands and found just stroking my hands soothing. I have never found anything I do for myself soothing. I had a bath and put on more moisturiser and I felt nice. I love looking at my soft textures in bed. I am meeting my Manager tomorrow and I feel sad, but not panicky. Today ended a better day.

Reflection: Wow! There it is. I had started my first tentative steps to self-care. Never before had I done anything like that and it did feel good. Who would have believed it, without any guidance or prompting I knew what to do. Looking back now I can't believe that I couldn't see it. I don't know how I knew what to do when all the time, on a conscious level I felt so broken.

Notes:

14.08.15

I wake feeling numb, I am going to see my Manager today at 11am. I get ready and leave, then I walk to the café where we are meeting and I start to panic. I go to the toilet and when I get back to the café I am really shaking. I get a coffee and we sit on the sofa. My Manager asks me how I am and suddenly I want to cry, so I tell her. She reassures me that I don't have to tell her anything, so we talk around the subject so she understands. She says "good for you" and "we'll get a new Paula back". She makes me feel okay about myself, she is very reassuring and my anxiety levels begin to drop. She tells me some really sad stuff about her life and the guilt and shame she has had to overcome, she helps me to understand the guilt and shame that I feel and assures me that I will overcome it. She also informs me that I will have to accept that some people will judge me, but I will be okay, because I will be okay! When I get home Alan is very flat. He is short with the kids and I asked him if it was to do with me. He said it was and said that he felt frustrated that he couldn't help, then he began to cry. For the first time ever in my life I can't afford this to be about somebody else. I can't allow him to punish me. I have a right to be whole, to be at peace, to be okay. That doesn't mean it hasn't affected me. I told him not to punish me. I can't cope with that. Carol came tonight and we talked it through. After yesterday and that little glint of looking after myself, I refuse to allow in thoughts of self-harm. Although I am biting me lip very hard.

Reflection: Talking is a brilliant healer, but sitting with somebody who can listen and empathise without even needing to know what is going on is utterly priceless. My Manager really did make me feel at ease. She had no idea why I was off sick and she was my Manager, yet she let me set the pace and she was calm and reassuring and that's all I needed. Although again I didn't consciously recognise what Alan was doing, I have written about it, so I could see it. In that broken world I had fallen into I still had insight. Perhaps even when you are broken, you are never truly broken. Perhaps no matter how destroyed the mind is, the soul is sitting quietly waiting and gently guiding, so subtly without intrusion. I don't know, maybe you do.

Notes:

15.08.15

I wake up feeling anxious. I didn't want to but I can't help it. Passive aggressive, Carol called Alans behaviour. Again, I kept myself distracted all day. My daughter Elizabeth went to a party. I went to my Mums with the boys, then I came home and the boys played whilst I did my assignment. Then Alan came home, he is still distant and quiet. I can't stand to watch television because I can't think about anything. I feel so very sad. I miss Elizabeth and I am biting my lip very hard. Not to hurt myself, but the pinch I get somehow makes me feel better. My boys are in bed and I miss my baby girl. Yesterday anxiety levels were very high, then dropped. Carol left at 2am today. I still don't feel tired, yet I think my anxiety levels are so up and down, I should be shattered. I'm sure sleep will come.

Reflection: Emotional abuse is so very damaging. I knew even then that I was on my own with this. I wanted the comfort of my baby girl. My children always loved me and whilst I felt useless to them at that time, they gave me comfort. They kept me going. Biting my lip, now that was becoming a thing. The sharp pain made me feel alive in the moment, it made me feel a physical pain that overtook the emotional pain and it made me punish myself for being bad and useless and weak and pathetic. It sharpened my senses.

Notes:

16.08.15

My baby girl came home last night at 11pm. She didn't want to stay. We snuggled up in bed together and she fell asleep whilst I stroked her back. Today she went back to her friends to collect her stuff and stayed all day. Alan still very quiet. I finished typing up my assignment and wanted to play badminton. Alan made it clear he didn't want to. He wouldn't smile at me. I feel like he's punishing me again. After the kids went to bed, I asked him what was wrong. Alan told me it was okay to do this on holiday, that is, not speak to me for five days. He got defensive about his behaviour, when that didn't work, he cried and started blaming himself. When that didn't work, he started verbally attacking me. Stating that I look too deeply into things, he feels I'm attacking him and he thinks it's only me who thinks that when you smile at somebody, they automatically smile back. I went to bed and cried. I don't understand anything. I don't know myself anymore, or what I thought was me, then I am all tied up in knots by Alan. He comes to bed and apologises. But for what?

Reflection: He wanted to take Elizabeth back to her own bed, but I told him I didn't want her disturbed. He didn't like it, but he left. I knew he was abusing me, but again not on a conscious level and I didn't have the strength on top of everything else to tackle him too. I needed to put a shield around myself, but I didn't have the strength. But being able to make him physically distant from me made all the difference. I didn't have to be punished any more. At least not that night.

Notes:

17.08.15

This morning I am very tired, I feel drained from last night. I am going to see the Occupational Health Doctor at 10.30am and I am very anxious. I leave the house and have a lump in my throat. I park at the Hospital and walk over to Occupational Health. I announce my arrival and sit in the waiting room. It is light and airy with lots of information on the walls. I am sat forward in the chair trying not to think. I start rubbing my thumb, then I begin to well up and tears run down my face. Dr Beckley greets me and takes me into her room. She asks me what's been happening and I start to cry. She is unaware of what has gone on. Eventually I begin to tell her bits of what happened. My Communication Course lifting the lid on my past sexual abuse. She listened and supported me. She said it's a good thing it happened now whilst I am young. She said it may not feel like it at the moment, but I will be better and stronger. She told me to take my time and not to rush. She asked me "did the police know? Was it close family?" I answered. She told me I would not be back at work in the next 3 months. She told me I may be better at my job, or choose not to return. She said Alan would also need support. She thanked me for telling her. I went home and Alan went to work. I had the GP tonight. I told him and Dr Beckley that I was no longer taking Sertraline. They both supported this. Tonight I went to my first meditation class and Carol came with me. I really didn't know what to expect. The Buddhist Monk walked in and sat at the front. We were in comfy red chairs facing him on a stage with a huge Buddha behind him. There appeared to be people from all walks of life there. I had a pre-conceived idea about hippie types, but I was wrong. Ordinary looking men and women, young and older, couples and friends. He talked about many things. He taught us how to meditate focusing on breathing and relaxing the body and clearing the mind. I was able to close my eyes for a short while, but kept opening them. I noticed I could not let my face and jaw to relax. He talked about receiving positive thoughts and feelings into the mind and transferring them to the heart and how to hold on to that emotion. Gradually altering you mind set with practice. He sang a prayer and I listened, but did not join in, it was okay. He talked about how our own emotions influence others, but also how we perceive others based on our own emotions. I really enjoyed it and Carol said she did too. I feel more attached to my feelings and I actually feel tired tonight.

Reflection: When I went to see Dr Beckley she made me feel so at ease. I had an owl handbag and she commented on it. She reminded me of how Martyn had spoken to me, calm and unhurried. I didn't feel like I was at an appointment, I felt like I was being listened to and she was confident I would get through it. I felt held again for a short while. When I got home and spoke to Alan, he told me he didn't want to talk to anybody, he said he didn't need to talk to anybody. I didn't want this to become about him, so I left it.

My first meditation class. When Kelsang Norpel walked down the aisle in his robes and sat cross legged, my instinct was to run. I keep thinking I can't do this. When he said we would be starting with a prayer, it was only the fact that the room was full of people and me and Carol were at the front that I didn't run. I sat trembling in my seat. Looking at the various statues of Buddha and the books and the flowers and the bowls with various things in. I became distracted with them and that made me feel warm and calm and safe. The prayer wasn't too bad either. I didn't understand it at first, but it kind of settled my mind. When Norpel started talking he was calm and unhurried and gentle sounding and I liked that. He was funny too. Real and not at all aloof, which was how I was expecting him to be. He talked about real life scenarios that people face in everyday life and talked about how we might think about how we respond to those scenarios differently. I liked having something to think about and although I couldn't meditate for very long, I was thinking about what he had said. The first thing I learned from Norpel was to look at things from all perspectives and to do this from an outside view point. In other words, not immersed in a situation, but emotionally standing back and observing a situation. Sort of on the outside looking in, instead of on the inside trying to see out. I loved it and I couldn't wait to go again. And I did for a good few years afterwards and I still meditate several times a day.

Notes:

18.08.15

Today was always going to be a busy day. Amica at 12.00, Martyn at 2pm and Quetzal at 5.30pm. I woke from what felt like a very deep sleep. I was actually looking forward to Amica to tell Kate what had been happening, and then I got there and I started feeling anxious, but I thought about last night and I thought about my breathing. I still felt anxious, but I was concentrating on my breathing and not my anxiety. I told Kate what had happened since I saw her last. I felt positive and arranged to see her again on 22.09.15. I saw Martyn about my assignment and that was very positive. I wished I could talk to him about stuff. Right at the end he asked me about my next module and I told him I was off work and would be for a while. He said if I wanted to talk to let him know. And I will, I had a message from Quetzal, my counsellor cancelled and to be honest I felt let down. It takes a lot for me to trust, but to cancel so early made me think she was avoiding me. Are my problems too big? I text Melvyn and told him my positive news and he was pleased. I text his wife Rachel about meeting at the weekend. Sadly they are busy, but she invited me and the kids for lunch on Monday. I was really pleased, but then I realised Monday is almost a week away. A week before seeing Carol, before meditation and before counselling. I got a lump in my throat and my eyes began to well up. Then Carol text and said "Monday is a long way off, shall we meet on Thursday". How the hell did she know that? I told her how I was feeling, going from high – I feel on top of this, to tearful, I don't think I can do this. Shit this is going to be an amazing read when I get through this. Another very emotional day.

Reflection: Because I was beginning to talk to people, I felt like I needed to hold on to them all the time. I never wanted to leave those I had begun to talk to, just in case I couldn't talk about things again. Everybody being away felt like I had been punched in the stomach. Felt like a shock. I had started to let these vile flashbacks and emotions out and I couldn't be left on my own with them. They felt much too big and frightening. I was beginning to lose faith in Vicky from Quetzal. I needed somebody professional to help me through this and not only did I feel frustrated at the end of every session, because she just sat and stared at me, I felt annoyed and anxious that she had cancelled. I really felt this was too big to handle on my own. Being let down so early on was too much to handle. I already had thoughts of trying to push everything back down again.

Notes:

19.08.15

Woke up at 06.00am today, got up, had a lovely time with Charlie giggling over breakfast. Tried to keep busy all day. Whenever I got a moment, I would look down and suddenly I felt at the bottom of a very deep pit. I saw Joelle tonight and told her about the last 3 weeks. I told her about Monday evening and how I managed to use it waiting to see Kate at Amica. I stared at a wooden knot in the door, focused on it to calm my breathing and then focused on my breathing. I was aware of the knot in my stomach and realised it's there for a reason. I remembered Alan saying he was worried I would set myself on fire when I told him I was going to light a candle when I had a bath on Thursday after my shopping trip. I felt so sad. I felt so alone. Today I feel tired, I just want to sit for a while with my head in my hands because I can't deal with anyone else's emotions. I took some paracetamol for a headache and thought shall I take a load and end it all now. I thought about submitting my communication assignment that triggered all this. The scenario where the midwife had to gather information from a teenager who had been sexually abused and had tried to kill herself. I thought about how I felt then and how I feel now and thought my conclusion would end with, "two days after submitting the assignment the midwife committed suicide". Why? Why do I want to write that? Because this massive bubble my head is stuck in, full of memories seems impossible to pop. I have locked everything away for so long, it's like a plague has broken out and it is going to kill everything in it's path in the bubble and my head is in the bubble and the plague is my memories. Happening sudden and fast I lurch from shock to panic, back to shock. I feel like I am going mad with the massive contradiction of emotions smacking me in the face. When you have a nightmare and you scream stop and you suddenly wake up and it's gone. When I am in the middle of the swarm, the plague, I just want it gone and in an instant I could make it be gone. And that's why I think about suicide. Because I want it gone. I want the swarm to stop flying round my head and writing that ending in my assignment would tell everyone that that midwife could not make it stop and the swarm got too much and the plague killed her. I want to let people know how I find It all too much. But I am in bed and I will stay in bed because it is safe, for now.

Reflection: Mocking me for lighting a candle in the bath. Now that made me feel like the lowest form of scum. Alan had such a damaging impact on me at that time. Every time after that when I had a bath, he would mock me and tell me not to set myself on fire. I believed he was using this to put thoughts into my head. I believed he wanted me to completely shatter. Break into a million pieces. He would make these and other comments many, many times. Passive aggressive, subliminal messages. He knew I was struggling and he was enjoying it, he was getting power from it and at that time, it only made me sad and feel incredibly bad about myself to think he had such a low opinion of me, gave me an even lower opinion of myself. Now however, I can see how damaged he really is and why he needed to do that to me for his own emotional gain.

Notes:

20.08.15

Today I woke at 0400am, feeling very low. Had a nightmare about the old school and the Head teacher and nobody listening to me. Felt low all day, the pressure is rising because I have to be okay for the kids and if I am not distracting myself the memories and feelings are there. It is when I stop, the kids ask me if I am okay. It is so, so hard when I just want the chance to sit with my head I my hands and get my thoughts and feelings together, but in a sense I am still having to block it so I can stay okay It is then that I start to think I can't do this. I have to wait until Tuesday. It would be so easy to give up. Today is not a good day. Today has been a very hard day.

Reflection: It was like torture. Overwhelmingly powerful flashbacks and emotions were constantly vying for my attention and I wasn't allowed to just let them flow. I couldn't sit with my head in my hands, I couldn't cry it out. Not because the children were around, I could manage that, but because even though I was off work, my emotions weren't allowed to be exposed or I would be mocked for being mad, crazy, or criticized for 'not getting over it'. I had to leave the house to talk, I had to behave 'normally' at home all of the time. I don't know to this day how I didn't completely breakdown. The pressure from within and around me was incredible.

Notes:

21.08.15

Big lightbulb moment today. I am sleeping badly and having nightmares, I'm trapped and I am not being listened to. The pressure is really building. I have fleeting suicidal and self-harm thoughts. Then I realise why. I am constantly putting others thoughts and feelings first. I have always neglected my own. If ever I do something for myself I am wracked with guilt and wonder what others think. Always doing for others I crave acknowledgement, attention, self-worth. I have been a good girl haven't I? When I don't get that and the good I do is not acknowledged, appreciated or criticised, I feel bad, so bad about myself. I'm worthless, I'm rubbish, I'm no good. I'm a mug. Why am I not good enough? Why am I so bad? Why don't people want to be nice to me? Why don't people love me? I tolerate everybody's emotions, but I have to hide mine because people don't like it. Why? The answer is I don't. I don't have to be any of those things. I just have to love me and stop giving myself away to everyone in return for love and affection. I was going to become a street worker, make men pay to abuse me, instead of taking me for nothing. All of me has been taken, I have been destroyed physically, emotionally, sexually and spiritually. I have no idea who I am. I ache so much inside. I'm tormented every day with what happened, who I was and who I am trying to find.......Me! I think it's too much. I am lost and scared and so very vulnerable. Do I have the strength to carry on? I'm tired of protecting everybody else, I just can't do this anymore. Please somebody help me hold on.

Reflection: Look at that already. It's there I know the answers. But I was two separate people. I knew I needed to become whole and wanted to love myself, because deep down I did. But I didn't have that connection at that time. I still felt that I needed to be validated by everybody else in order to love myself. I can see it now on the page. If it was a quiz, I'd be screaming "look the answer is right there, you have written the answer right there". I did know exactly who I was, I just couldn't see it. I didn't have faith in me, I didn't have the confidence in me. I was all there, but totally lost. I knew the answer so early on. Once I loved myself and validated myself, I would be more than half way there. But I hadn't made that connection, I couldn't see it. I really wanted to love myself, but only if everybody else did first. Oh my goodness, so near, yet so far.

Notes:

22.08.15

Crying uncontrollably last night. Why, why, why do I keep remembering things. Nightmares for the past few nights. Last night it was my father-in-law, he used to touch me inappropriately and kiss my neck when nobody was looking, he would come up behind me and do it. Why? My mother-in-law walked into the bedroom at her house when we stayed and I was naked. When I protested she ignored me. Whenever I protested about anything I didn't like I was ignored, or they would get angry with me and I was made to feel wrong, bad, and abnormal. But if it was wrong why did it keep happening? I can't stop crying. My appointment on Tuesday – I needed it. I am having massive rush of emotions and memories and I am overwhelmed. I will wait until Alan goes to sleep. I will sit at the bottom of the garden with the red knife and try to work out why all this stuff happened to me, why it wasn't my fault. It kept happening, I kept feeling bad, I did nothing, so it happened again. I hope I fall asleep before Alan. I don't feel safe. I am in bed, but I am waiting until he goes to sleep. I don't feel safe. I will text someone!

Reflection: I desperately wanted to self-harm that night. So many questions. My mind was spinning and the physical pressure in my head was enormous. Every muscle in my body was tense. I had to relieve that tension. The longer I was awake, the more the pressure increased. I felt if I cut myself the pressure would be released. Like opening a flood gate. I needed to relieve the pressure. I was also really angry and frustrated with myself because I was so ignored, even my voice wasn't enough to stop people. I really despised myself that night. I wanted to feel the physical pain that matched the emotional pain and I wanted to open myself right up to release the pressure. Even reading this I can feel that pressure. With the will inside me that I still didn't recognise, I didn't do it.

Notes:

23.08.15

I fell asleep before Alan came to bed. Woke up feeling very drained. It's the raw emotion that overwhelms me. I feel sick when the memory floods in. Just as I did at the time. Carol called me and I went to see her. I told her It's like a constant nagging. It begins to do your head in and you will do anything to make it stop. I have to learn how to stop what happened last night. It is a pressure that builds and builds until I can't take it anymore and that's when I want to end it all. I don't even think I want to die. I love my children so much, but when I feel like I did last night I can only feel pain and all I can think is I will do anything to make it stop. Anything at all. Last night all the stuff I had done to help myself meant nothing. I'm just beginning to care for myself and I love the feeling it gives me. But the ***BAD*** stuff is so much bigger, it's massive and it blows all that way when the pressure gets too much. I love the good stuff. I love how it makes me feel inside. I want the good stuff to carry on, to get bigger. I am still so much on guard. We talked about music and wearing headphones. I can't do that because when I wear headphones I am not alert to everything going on around me. I still have to be alert. I have always loved music because music has been what I related to my emotions. Certain songs resonated with me and I expressed, no the music expressed my emotions for me. Now I can't stand the radio being on because those emotions are real and raw now and hearing the songs intensifies those emotions. I used to have the radio on all the time so there was background music and chatter. This stopped me listening to my own thoughts. But now I am listening. Now my thoughts are very much with me and as shit as they are, they are mine and I am truly listening. There will be no hidden demons left and I love the thought of that. Thirty five years of sickening thoughts and feelings invading my conscious whenever I was off guard. Thirty five years of battling to control it all. Containing it, hiding it, ignoring it, but feeling it constantly picking, chipping away until I was caught off guard. I can tell Carol anything, she understands me. She laughs with me and she makes me feel okay. She makes me realise I am going to be okay. She walks alongside me, when I feel shit, she feels shit with me, when I want to cry she wells up with me and when we laugh it's just the best feeling ever. Today ended better an any other so far and to congratulate myself tomorrow I am going to buy myself some flowers. Tonight I am in bed smiling. I feel warm, excited, yet calm. I feel I know, or am beginning to understand where my problems lie.

1. Learning to be good to myself.
2. Learning to love myself.
3. Learning not to be afraid to deal with the past, suck it up, go with the shit and clear it up.
4. Learning to recognise when I am feeling the pressure begin to build up, listen to my feelings, not ignore them so that it doesn't reach a point where the urge to harm outweighs the urge to protect.

I will do that. I will. I want to and I will forgive myself along the way.

Reflection: Wow! I amaze myself reading that. I'm already identifying the connections I need to make, I just didn't know I was making connections, so I had no concept of what I needed to connect them to, to make them work and I didn't have anybody around me who was either aware that that needed to happen, or who knew how to make it happen. Not at that stage anyway.

Notes:

24.08.15

Busy day today went to mediation with Carol. It was very powerful. He got us to look at compassion. Feeling compassion for ourselves and thinking about people who worry. He got us to feel about how we feel and then how that person must feel. I got stuck and started to feel agitated because I haven't yet learned how to make myself stop feeling anxious. I am learning to think about things before I get anxious, how to calm myself. I felt irritated for a while, then we had peppermint tea. Carol and I talked and talked all the way home and I felt very positive. It is so good to talk feelings out.

Reflection: If you are reading this and you have never meditated, then I would very strongly recommend it. To go to a guided meditation class anyway. Why? Because it gives you a break from what you are trying to deal with, but it also, in a safe environment allows you to look at scenarios that you can probably relate to which subtly gives you the tools you need to help you to deal with what you are going through. It is absolutely incredible. But that is only my opinion.

Notes:

25.08.15

I usually only write at the end of the day, but it's morning and the clarity I am feeling is immense. I want to remember this so I am writing at midday. We saw Rachel, Melvyn's wife yesterday and I talked a bit about what was happening. She told me a bit about her anxiety and suddenly I felt equal to her. This morning I text her because I have anxiety about food and cooking. I asked her if she would help me to prepare a meal that we can all share. I told her the reason I didn't cook for them was because I was too anxious. She is braver than me, but she is anxious about the same but cooks for us anyway. She said she will help me and that makes me feel so good. So good I don't have to pretend or hide anymore. It is so liberating not to have to divert to give the illusion of coping. Not trying to control everything by hiding insecurities. This really is all about me and how I see things, feel things and respond to things. This morning the kids began bickering whilst I was doing something elsewhere. Normally I would feel compelled to complete my task whilst getting more and more wound up by what I was hearing. This morning I stopped what I was doing as soon as I began to feel myself tense. I went to the children and asked them calmly to stop what they were doing and they did. I was calm and they were calm and I got back on with my task. I think I am beginning to understand what it feels like to be in control. Being in control of my thoughts, feelings and emotions and not controlling what I am doing or what is going on around me.

It's amazing how things can change in a day. I was due to see my tutor tomorrow, but late this afternoon he had to re-arrange. Completely understandable, but my pressure relief has gone. Then my counsellor told me she is unable to see me for the next 2 sessions. I spent the time I had telling her what had been happening and now I can't talk for 2 weeks. I feel so flat, so flat. I want to deal with this stuff, I don't want it bottled up anymore. I spoke to Carol and she made me feel better. She always makes me feel better. But the pressure to thinks gets more and more powerful and when I have to keep a lid on it, it becomes too much and I become suicidal again.

Reflection: This isn't selfish. Reliability and stability is so crucial when somebody is dealing with a mental health crisis. Being let down by counsellors is so damaging. Of course situations arise in everybody's life, but to commit to supporting and holding clients is more than a job, it's a real responsibility. It can be a real life saving responsibility. Finding the right counsellor can be really difficult and when somebody is so vulnerable like I was then any counsellor, even a bad counsellor will do and that can be very, very dangerous. Also be aware of dishonourable friends. Rachel who said she was happy to help me prepare a meal, later told Melvyn that she didn't feel comfortable about it and he said she didn't know what it was all about. Opening up to people when you are really vulnerable is also risky. A risk you have to take and with no resilience it can also be very dangerous at the time. Now it has made me more self-reliant, more resilient, but I am healed now. But then I was very much broken and this could have gone either way for me.

Notes:

26.08.15

Alan is giving me time to myself today, but I feel so flat, so empty. I feel stuck, unable to move forward. The pressure is building again. The Quetzal called and instead of cancelling my 2 appointments they are being moved to a Thursday for the next couple of weeks. The relief is immense and I feel dizzy following the call and thought I was going to faint. I have no appetite, I am eating very little since this all started really and I am not sleeping. For the past week it is probably 2 hours a night. My eyes are tired, but nothing else is. The only time I sleep well if following my meditation class. When I get better at doing it, it might work at home. I am incredibly jumpy. I am still hyper alert. I am not relaxed. I need help.

Reflection: I'm really just holding on here. I have no direction, no focus, nothing to aim for except my next opportunity to talk. This was such a solitary place to be and there were many more times like that.

Notes:

27.08.15

I spoke to Melvyn today. I told him about all the abuse. I didn't cry but I wanted to. I told him that I had tried to look up the man who abused me and I had thoughts of confronting him. I also said I was thinking of texting my cousin and reminding him. I told Alan tonight and he helped me look. He found them on Facebook. I feel really sick. I don't know what I want to do. It was good to talk to Melvyn about how I had been feeling and my suicidal thoughts. The pressure lifted for a while and now I feel so, so anxious and I don't know why. Maybe because I have just seen a photo of the man who sexually abused me. I want to cry.

Reflection: Now here is the beginning of a focus, a direction. I couldn't see it at that time, but it was a tiny seedling of strength and the beginnings of taking back some control. I still couldn't see it though.

Notes:

28.08.15

I feel so subdued. The impact of seeing him has really hit home. I spoke with Carol this morning and was really excited and felt powerful. I will write him a letter and we will go to Liverpool together and post it, or even hand deliver it to him. He will know I know where he is and I can come for him. He will never be sure when it will happen. This isn't about revenge, it's about making me turn this huge monster, this huge memory around. Picturing a frightened man is far less scary than picturing a monster. But as the day went on, I got lower and lower. I spoke to Melvyn and he told me Rachel does not want to allow him to meet me on my own. I felt sad because our friendship means more to me than anything. But also feel so wrong, so bad. Men have wanted to abuse me for as long as I can remember and women feel threatened by me. What is it I do that makes this happen? I have lost friendships because of it. Liz felt threatened, so did Elaine, so did Caroline and now Rachel. Why can I not just be without someone seeing me as a target? Kim fancied me and became aggressive when I didn't respond. She would touch me and stroke me and because I didn't like it, she said I was cold. I didn't like men, I didn't like women what was wrong with me she said. Jane said the same because she tried to control me and I couldn't handle it. If I self-harm nobody will be attracted to me and maybe I will be left alone. But I don't want to be left alone, I just want to be accepted. I haven't done anything wrong but why do I have to be punished? I don't want to be abused, I don't want to be seen as a threat. That's why I wanted to die when I was little because I have always been seen as a target. I wasn't a boy, I wasn't disabled, I couldn't be loved without abuse. And I couldn't find safety without being viewed as a threat. What then, - if I shouldn't kill myself, what am I supposed to do? I think I should be in hospital because I just want to rest. I just want to be cared for and accepted for who I am, because if I can't then I really, really shouldn't be here.

Reflection: So, there I was looking for answers. All those questions I had about my failings, my inadequacies. I had no idea that if I just looked at them and their behaviour then the answers once again were all there. Put very simply and I mean simply. Abusers seek out vulnerable people. I was vulnerable. The women that felt threatened, felt threatened because they knew their partners would prey on vulnerable women. People who tried to control me were incredibly insecure. Parents who reject their children are deeply damaged by something inside of them. None of it takes away the horror of being abused, neglected and rejected, none of it was my fault. It's just so sad that all of that lead to a life of self-loathing, self-harm and self-neglect. I just hope that somebody who reads this can understand that before they destroy themselves in the way that I did.

Notes:

29.08.15

Suicidal thoughts are a weekly occurrence. I have felt desperate all day. Carol came. We talked about how I feel guilty. I took myself to that family. He abused me. I was willing to have sex age 11, so it gave him permission to finger me later when I didn't want him to. I went with that lad when I was 13. I went to be raped, I allowed myself to be taken. I hated being violated, but I thought that's what happened, so when I was raped when I was 16! Hey this is life, so I married a man I confided in and he used that knowledge to rape me, tear me, humiliate me and violate me. He tore my mind and body apart. The guilt is massive. I have been judged, I am seen as a threat. I am fucking manipulated for merely existing. The only reason I am here in this very dark moment is my kids. They love me unconditionally, they don't judge me, they don't feel threatened by me. My own husband has turned his back on me when I am torn apart by self-loathing and guilt. For fucks sake when will I be accepted. I was sexualised as a child and as an adult I am being judged, punished and I don't know how the fuck I can make it stop.

Reflection: I think this goes on to illustrate exactly what happens when children are abused. This is what happened in my case anyway. I didn't really stand a chance. Reflecting on this I can see absolutely why I felt the way I did, but I still didn't have the right person in my life to help me break that cycle. To make it stop.

Notes:

30.08.15

After I had finished writing yesterday I went back downstairs. I was crying as I was writing so I went into the dining room and cried painful, gut wrenching tears. The whole time I was crying I was crying for me. I cried for my loneliness as a child. I cried for the mummy and daddy I wanted to scoop me in their arms. I cried for my sister, I cried for the scared, confused and frightened me. I cried for the sickness I felt in my gut every single day as the abuse was repeated and I cried and cried for me because I didn't know. I didn't know being molested and raped was the wrong thing to do, the wrong thing to happen to me. And when I cried that bit, I got a flash of anger. I didn't know it was wrong, but all those abusers did. The took me and they used me and the violated me. They destroyed my body and my mind. Then I cried and cried for all those lost years, but I stayed angry. Today when I woke up I felt very tearful, but still angry and I do still feel angry. I didn't get back to bed until 02.30am and I was shattered. I emailed my tutor in the night saying how disappointed I am that I can't get my brain to think straight and I know I am capable of better. I was very surprised that he responded and I have been given an extension on my assignment. I don't need to be disappointed in myself. He has no idea what that means to me. I have the opportunity to be proud of myself. I have felt so tired all day, subdued and tearful, but in a positive way. Charlie played badminton with me and I was kept distracted all day. But today that was okay because for the first time properly last night and this morning it came out and I didn't try to stop it. I couldn't wait until the kids went back to school to let it out and why should I have to? I also feel angry at all those who judge me. It matters to me. I have to try and work that out. Today feels very, very different. But this is today and my journal doesn't judge me.

Reflection: There! I'm back. I knew what I needed to do and I did it. I still couldn't see it though. I couldn't see that I was getting stronger. There is so much determination in that journal entry. So much strength and I couldn't see it.

Notes:

31.08.15

Today I felt on edge, unsettled. I am thinking a lot about suicide. How I can turn my back on it, how I can stop feeling so bad that I want to die, then so high I feel I can take on the world. I spoke to Daryl today about contacting that paedophile. Just writing the word makes it hit home. He was concerned about me making contact with him in case there are repercussions for me and my family. I had never thought of that. He said he may have abused others, or maybe not. It was thinking about him being a sick individual that drove it home today. Sick people abuse kids. I remember him as a family man who sexually abused me because he didn't like me. To think of him objectively as a pervert, a sick individual makes it worse and all the more tangible. I saw Carol tonight, we went to meditation and she told me she had the same concerns about how he might react if I made contact. I was sexually abused when I was a child and raped. I cannot comprehend the severity of it. The impact has not hit home. I was shocked by it, I was terrified of the memories, but the impact, that feeling is beginning to become so very real. I am so scared of what might happen when the impact hits me hard.

Reflection: I was still being overwhelmed by the enormity of the abuse at that stage. It was like the reality was getting deeper and deeper, bigger and bigger. I articulated my feelings in the last sentence and yet again within that entry I am beginning to see the experiences for what they were. This was a battle that went on in my mind for a very long time. It's really scary when you begin to develop insight. Sometimes it made me feel strong, really strong, but then sometimes it made me loath myself even more because I would be angry with myself for not seeing what was really happening and effectively then 'allowing' it to happen. Insight can be a real tipping point and a really crucial time for in depth support. At that time I didn't have that support and thankfully I had no insight. I had two minds.

Notes:

01.09.15 12.30pm

Today is the first day on my own and I am panicking. Only I know how hard I have supressed the feelings and memories I have right now. I decide to go on my exercise bike. My skin is crawling, crawling with the feeling of somebody's hands all over me, abusing me, using me for their pleasure. The feeling is right there. I'm feeling it physically and I start to feel sick. That cock, that filthy rapists cock shoved in my mouth and I think I am going to vomit. I keep telling myself it's just a memory, it's just a memory, but I can't bear the images and I feel more and more disgusting, dirty and sick. I need to scrub myself hard in the shower, HARD to get rid of the feeing. I can feel the bile rise in my stomach. I want to scrub HARD to get rid of feeling those hands all over me. I want to vomit to get rid of that filthy bastard out of my mouth. I come upstairs and start crying, I don't want to hurt myself, I just want the feeling to go away. I curl up on the bed wrapped in a towel and start rocking and whispering to myself, "It's okay, no more, no more". I am crying and rocking and whispering to myself and stay curled up in a ball until I feel safe again.

I only had her for 7 years. When she died, I missed her desperately. She was my right arm. I was her legs. She was a pain in the arse and she always got me into trouble, but I loved her so much. I felt so safe when she was alive. I was safe when she was alive, I just didn't realise it at the time. I was so lonely when she died. I wanted to feel part of something again. I wanted to be loved. I really didn't mean to do the wrong thing, I didn't mean for him to do that to me. I just wanted to be wanted, I just wanted to fit again. I'm so very, very sorry I did the wrong thing. I didn't know fear and dread before she died, although I do remember one night my mum and dad went out, we didn't have a babysitter, so my mum told me they were going and not to tell her because she would be scared. I was scared and I didn't like that much at all.

22.21pm. Today is the first day since all this began that I have been alone and my thoughts have been allowed to surface. I was right to be scared. I stopped myself from self-harming today JUST! I looked after myself, but it was so fucking hard. Feeling the skin crawling, the abuse and feeling that tight knot and nausea was almost too much. I wanted a hand to hold when I was 10 years old. Just like I wanted a hand to hold today, but it's not there. I need a hand to hold, I need something to hold on to because I don't know if I can hold on much longer. I'm so frightened.

Reflection: So at that point the physical sensations had kicked in. Not only was my mind tormented, but now physically my body was beginning to react to sensations. Curling up in a ball really helped because the physical sensations were so strong, curling up meant I was defending myself against them. Just like you would if somebody was attacking you. Being wrapped in a towel felt like I could stop anything from touching my bare skin. Crying stopped anything going in my mouth. Grieving for my Sister was also something I had never been allowed to do. She wasn't talked about, referred to hardly ever. I can still smell her now, see her face. She really was a part of me. Jack sexually abusing me I believed was all my fault, because I had taken myself to that family, because I was so scared and lonely after my Sister died. Why at 10 years old would I ever think that something bad happening to me, that I instigated wouldn't be my fault? Because, of course I was 10 years old when it happened and that part of my physical 35 year old brain was still emotionally 10 years old and I couldn't comprehend it being anything other than my fault.

Notes:

02.09.15

Woke up feeling very scared, I feel dirty. I want to change the sheets, but I feel too dirty to be in clean sheets. I will soil them with my filthy mauled body. I shower without scrubbing, but I still feel dirty. I wish I could rip my skin off and let new skin grow. I still feel sick. The sensation, the taste in my mouth I want to vomit. I spoke to Carol today and she is worried. I spoke to Melvyn and told him about yesterday and how I feel today. He told me I am feeling anxiety. I didn't self-harm yesterday, I just have to ride the feeling out. He reassured me I am not going mad, or falling apart. It's okay to feel it, as awful as it is, because it will pass. So I allowed myself to be distracted to have a break from the sensation, the nausea. As soon as I was not distracted, it came back. The image, the sensation, the nausea. It's so awful, so fucking awful, I can't see past this, but I have to believe it won't last. I have to ride it out. I am so tired, I just want to sleep to block it all out. I am shaking again.

Reflection: I think this explains itself really. The physical sensations felt like they were ravaging my body and I couldn't do anything to stop it, except sit tight and ride it out. I've learned that the important thing about any emotion, however uncomfortable or distressing it is, is that it does pass. In fact, the more you try to avoid it, the more it invades your thoughts and feelings. Facing an emotion however difficult, diffuses it, gives it its own voice. Allows it to be expressed so it can leave when ready. I wanted to be heard. I wanted my voice to be heard, yet I didn't want my emotions to be heard. I still had two very separate minds.

Notes:

03.09.15

Managed to be distracted today. Got up at 06.00am following a disturbed night with flashbacks. Counselling tonight, very anxious about disclosure, but decided had to take the step and talk about images, sensations. She asked me if I could describe them. Mouth taste, sensation being forced to perform oral sex. Skin sensation, talked about him sat opposite me in his dressing gown with his legs open exposing himself to me, then coming and sitting next to me, putting his arm round me and asking me if I can see. I look hard at the television and tell him "No" as the arm of the chair is in the way. He pushes my head round to look at his exposed penis and tells me I know what he means. He starts to tickle my stomach and asks me to do the same to him. I tell him I don't want to so he carries on moving his fingers further down until he is touching my privates. I sit forward and tell him I don't want him to do it anymore. He sniggers. The next time I am sitting on my front door step. My dinner is nearly ready and I am asked not to go away. I am so lonely, I go back to the flat. I am on my own with him again. He sits next to me and tells me we are going to play a game. He tells me he is going to tickle me and I am to tickle him in the same place. I'm scared, he tickles my tummy again and I tickle his. He moves his hand down and starts to tickle me in my knickers. I tell him I don't want to do it, but he makes me carry on, I start just touching his tummy and thighs with my fingers. He tells me there is one place I haven't touched, but I don't touch it. His legs are open, but I won't touch his penis. I tell him I don't want to play anymore. He just sniggers and tells me he will carry on then. He carries on touching me, his fingers in my knickers, he only stops when she walks back in the room. I tell them I have to go and race home. My mum tells me off, she shouts at me for going away. I am crying and shaking and she shouts at me for crying and shaking.

I talk about being willing to have sex with my cousin following this. I was about 11 now and he is 15. He was about to penetrate me when my mum, dad, auntie and nan came home. A few months later he fingered me as I was coming down the ladder in my Nan's back yard. I had been too scared to climb across on to the air raid shelter. I was angry because I couldn't get down without him fingering me. And that sick feeling that there was nothing I could do about it. The male I met in the field who I allowed to lead me away. He mauled and raped me, I was 13. I feel so guilty allowing all this to happen' my skin is crawling and I feel sick with the physical sensation. I talked about not knowing how I felt to be scared until my sister died, apart from one occasion when they couldn't get a babysitter and my mum told me not to tell her because she would be scared. I didn't like that. After she died my mum and dad went away for 2 weeks and left me with relatives. They were getting on with their life and I was lost. I remember one afternoon there was a storm. It went really dark, really early, so I got ready for bed. It was the middle of the afternoon, but I wanted to go to bed, because I wanted my mum and dad to come back tomorrow. When they did come back and took me home my sisters bed had gone. My room was decorated. It was like she never existed. I felt like my soul mate had gone. I was left on my own after that whilst my mum and dad went out drinking. They said I didn't need a babysitter anymore because I was a big girl. I was 7 years old and terrified, left with a can of coke and a bag of crisps. They would come home

very drunk and have violent rows and violent sex. The headboard banging against the wall, my dad growling. I was terrified. My mum always did and still does flinch when he touches her. When my ex-husband raped me I just believed it was normal and I was the one who was wrong because I didn't like it. I had no boundaries. One night, during this marriage I cleared a whole table of glasses and drinks as I swiped my hand across the large round table I was sat at, at his works do. My adrenaline was high. I had no sense of consequence because I knew I was going to get worse when I got home. I am consumed with guilt. I allowed all of this to happen except the rape when I was 16. I am overwhelmed with new memories and trying to process that it wasn't my fault, all in one go. I felt really high at the thought of contacting him, writing to him to let him know I know where he is and I will be coming for him when I am ready. I felt amazingly powerful. Then I was made to consider that a man who sexually abuses children may be dangerous and if I tell him I have found him he may come for me and suddenly he is a monster all over again. I am fluctuating from very high to very low. I have lost all sense of who I am and I am scared. Finally, I talked about wanting to set fire to my mum and dad's bed when I was little. To burn my dad for hurting my mum. My counsellor recognised how frightening that was for me. I talked about strategies for getting rid of the sensations and using self-harm as a coping strategy. Self-induced vomiting to get rid of the taste, to clean my insides. Maybe reverse psychology, because when I left my appointment I thought why would I self-harm because of an extreme flashback/memory. She said self-harm is viewed as a coping strategy and is better if the only other option is suicide. I have decided looking after myself and being kind to myself is a better option than self-harm or suicide.
I am shattered tonight, but fearful of sleep because of the flashbacks.

Reflection: So, big disclosures went on that night. I was allowing myself to express all of my emotions. That's why I was so tired. Feeling very high and very low were common for a long time. I would develop some insight and feel very high, but then I didn't know how to use that insight to my advantage and would come crashing down to a very low point. This was when I felt unpredictable. I felt I could easily self-harm, or worse attempt to end my life. I began to recognise when I was high and dreaded how I would feel because I knew the low meant I would come crashing down. There was no stability in my mood at that time. It was like my inner compass was spinning all over the place. There was no level.

Notes:

04.09.15

I was restless in bed last night again. Alan said I was kicking out. No wonder I am tired today. I am walking to see my tutor Martyn and I start thinking about what the counsellor said yesterday. The difference between before and now is; before I was self-harming. I was anorexic, trying to drink myself to death, running to lose weight quicker. Now I am doing none of those things, but instead I am talking about it. I see my tutor and try to reassure him that what I am talking about is what my counsellor, GP and Occupational Health Doctor are aware of. I apologise for when I said he had broken me. He hadn't of course, it was the course. I thanked him for not doing the wrong thing when he was told that I was suicidal. I read to him the awful stuff that was going through my mind and asked him to read about my needle phobia. I told him if he had done the wrong thing I would have killed myself, because I couldn't cope anymore. If he had told somebody else at that time, I would have continued to say it was about work. I would have continued to feel worse inside when I was already not coping. I would have tried to commit suicide. If he had not allowed me to read out what I was feeling it would never have come out. I told him what I read to him was just the tip of the iceberg and that I had remembered a whole lot more once I had read that stuff out. I told him I went to see my GP on his advice, told him I was suicidal and he prescribed medication.

The medication made my world a fog, but the abuse and emotions were very clear. It reminded me of when I finally realised that my ex-husband had been raping me. I drank so much to blot it out, but it didn't. It blocked my world around me and made the rape crystal clear. So I stopped taking the medication and my world has become clearer again. My essay of my scenario is so difficult to write. I am drawn all the time to how I am feeling, focusing on the impact of sexual abuse and the risks of suicide. He understood what I was saying. I told him I had concluded the essay by writing "2 days after submitting the essay, the midwife committed suicide". Because I was so caught up in the scenario I wanted to make it clear how really bad it feels. He told me he would help me and I felt safe talking to him. I told him I don't think I want to die, I just want the overwhelming pain to stop. I talked about the sensations and images that are affecting me now and how frightening they are. That I have lost a sense of who I am. I am either really high and on top of the world, or very low. It feels very, very frightening. It was good to talk to release the pressure.

I met Alan afterwards, we spent time together and I felt calm and tenderness towards him. I kissed him softly and at first he laughed. He did stop and kiss me back. I had a bath and lit a candle, but when he found out he again said it was dangerous and what if I set fire to myself. When he realised his comment upset me he tried to make a joke out of it, but I felt very low again. I moved on and kissed him tenderly and I dressed in my new nightie and gown. I felt feminine and pretty. Alan brought me a drink, put the television on, he had a drink, ate some crisps and fell asleep. He doesn't want me. He sees me as damaged, he doesn't know what to do with me. I feel rejected, punished, as dirty as the sensations are making me feel, I feel very, very bad. So bad I want to harm myself. I hate myself, but I am trying so hard to love myself. I want to punish myself, so I feel worse than he can make me feel, but he is in bed next to me, so I can't text anyone and I can't make a fuss. Guilt sex would be as bad as prostitution or rape. Doing it out of a sense of duty, to feel wanted or accepting what I no longer want. My adrenaline is going mad, I am so, so scared.

Reflection: This was a repeat pattern of behaviour I was embarking on. Sacrificing my body and mind to be accepted and when it was rejected the self-revulsion was there to confirm what a dreadful person I believed I was. It confirmed all the reasons I needed to hate myself. I had absolutely no self-worth. Absence of self-worth is what fuelled my belief and validated the belief of all my abusers.

Notes:

05.09.15

I woke today feeling very low. Completely lost, nothing fits anymore. I am on my exercise bike and I am crying. I feel revolting. I hate myself and I feel I am being punished. I want to cut myself, I want to cut myself so badly. I want to hurt myself so I can't feel the pain of being punished by anybody else again. My counsellor suggested self-harm can be viewed as a coping mechanism. I don't know what to do, my head is everywhere, I am so confused. I told Martyn I talk about feelings of self-harm instead of doing it. Talking about it with people who are safe helps to relieve the pressure, so I message Carol. I talk to her about what I want to do and she talks to me about why I am feeling like this. She talks to me about my qualities. She never judges or makes me feel guilty. My adrenaline is high and I want to go for a run after an hour on my bike, but she keeps messaging me and I gradually calm down and the conversation changes. The kids are up, I go and have a hot bath, put my dressing gown on, have a warm drink and snuggle up with the kids. I got through it, this time. I felt lost, irritable all day. Carol came round and we talked about what happened. We talked about sex and my view of sex. I never realised until we talked that I viewed sex as a task. A beginning, a middle and an end. A process to be got through. She talked to me about how it could be, how it should be. Fun, loving, exploring and being with someone, truly with them. Intimate, personal and loving. She suggested maybe I talk to Alan about how things have been and how we could talk about how they could be. I have always seen it as a function – sex. Something to be tolerated, irrespective of my feelings for that person. Something to be achieved with as little fuss as possible and no active input on my part for fear of causing myself harm from the other person and definitely no resistance in case it became forced.

Reflection: The pressure to self-harm was growing. No longer were the small windows I had to talk, enough to relieve the pressure, enough to make it lessen. If anything it was forcing it to become much more powerful. Talking to Alan about sex was very uncomfortable. There was no empathy or understanding and I felt like I was behaving like a whore. It felt like another sense of duty and I hated it. I needed to deal with the feelings around sexual abuse, before I could address any loving relationship and at that time I didn't believe it was possible.

Notes:

06.09.15

Today has mostly been a calm day. Distracted by being busy. I'm beginning to feel tired. Incredibly tired. I feel that if I stop I will fall into the deepest sleep. Tonight when Alan was settling the kids at bedtime I started googling ways to overcome suicidal feelings, self-harm and thoughts of self-harm. I started pinching my skin, but the feeling is not the same as I get when biting my lip. The release is phenomenal. I am reading this because what I am trying with Alan is brand new, but will it carry on? The urge to self-harm yesterday morning was so massive. I am scared that if something goes wrong I will act spontaneously. The urge has never felt so strong as it did yesterday morning. I am trying to find a safety net in case it happens again. I think this is a good not a bad thing. I'm not reading because I'm likely to do it, I am reading about it because the urge was so strong I'm afraid next time I might do it. Whilst I am calm now I am trying to develop a plan for myself and reading some of the websites, this is exactly what they advise you to do. Call or contact someone you trust, rub ice or pen on your arm. Eat a chilly to make your mouth burn. Basically try something that give you the release you need without causing harm. I am so very tired.

Reflection: The pressure to self-harm when there is nothing else to relieve it only heightens the need. My arms were beginning to ache, an ache that made me want to cut them with a knife to ease the pain. Not only was the pain emotional, but it was becoming physical too. Like a scratch that needed to be itched. Incredibly powerful and all consuming.

Notes:

07.09.15
Woke feeling very tired, but another busy distracting day. Had nightmares last night, I'm calling for help but either nobody can hear me, or they don't come. Went to meditation tonight. A different teacher and the room was very hot and uncomfortable. Talked about patience with the monk following this session. Practising patience sounds easy, putting into practise by accepting it is what it is, very difficult. Had big flashbacks tonight of period pain when being raped, being dragged around the bed, feeling angry, but powerless to make it stop. Experiencing that tearing pain when being raped and that brief second of terror when he takes it out, then forces it back in, that ripping pain. The second of terror, knowing the pain is about to come. I feel so tired.

Reflection: I'm not sure this needs any particular reflection. It's quite direct and explicit and was all consuming. The emotional pain, though was beginning to become physical pain. Such as the period pain. Not only could I not control my waking thoughts, but sleep was also a frightening prospect. I couldn't control what I would 'dream' about. I was so frightened to go to sleep. And that in itself brought back associations with being 10 years old when I was frightened to go to sleep in case Jack climbed into my bedroom. Flashback upon flashback, now that's epic.

Notes:

08.09.15
No plans today except rest and sleep, but Charlie off sick from school so busy again. Getting frustrated again with the lack of time for my own thoughts. I fell asleep briefly twice today and twice got woken up. Had more nightmares last night and today when I dozed off. Always calling for help and people just looking and not helping. Becoming more frustrated as the day went on. Desperately wanting both time with my own thoughts and time to sleep. I changed the bed sheets today and had a bath in the evening to try and get clean before getting into bed, but even that was interrupted. Today was a very difficult day. I had flashes of self-harm as I fear Alan will be distant because I allowed him to have sex with me, but I didn't even get chance to sort it out in my own head because I have been a caring mum all day. Alan was very reassuring when I told him and that helped, but I am feeling very frustrated and so very tired. I feel dizzy.

Reflection: Not having time to process thoughts was really difficult. The flashbacks invaded whenever they wanted to, but everything felt like it was rushing all the time in my mind and I just craved time to sit with my head in my hands and allow the thoughts in so they could slow down. But constantly being forced to put on a brave face and appear to function throughout the day made those thoughts stack up, so when they did overwhelm me it was always violent and hurried.

Notes:

09.09.15

Today I still feel tired. Kept quite busy to keep distracted, when I stopped I felt the anxiety that I have always felt about this so I wrote down all of my thoughts and feelings on paper to take to the counsellor. I wrote and wrote and wrote until I didn't have another thought in my head. The past two days I have been so, so hungry and so, so tired. I am not shaking, I feel calmer and more focused. I keep trying to meditate, but as soon as I close my eyes all the thoughts and feelings of abuse come back. That's why I have decided to write it down. I scrubbed my arm with a flannel in the bath last night, the immediate feeling of scraping felt good, but seconds later it began to burn and I didn't like that. I wish I could find something that gave my skin that scraped clean feeling without the burn afterwards. I hope writing my thoughts and feelings down for the counsellor helps my mind to calm down.

Reflection: I was making tentative attempts to find out what it might feel like to self-harm. I was heading towards a fall.

Notes:

10.09.15

Counselling went really well tonight. I shared my paper with her, the thoughts and feelings. I am so tired and so hungry all the time. Positives that came out from today's counselling.

1. My starting again relationship with Alan.
2. Taking control of how I want my counselling to go. Talking about the feelings by getting the counsellor to ask me questions.
3. Asking the counsellor to tell me when we are nearing the end of our time.
4. Talking about how meditation is helping my mind to think calmly and more focused, even if I can't yet clear my mind.
5. Recognising through meditation that my mums behaviour is about her. Even if I can't yet accept that what was happening when I was little, but I can talk about it objectively and not as if it is about me. She really is cruel, self-oriented. Heartless and cold. She is demonstrating that by her behaviour towards my Dad.
6. Recognising that I need to think about how to deal with feelings of self harm when I am calm. So far texting trusted friends is my only strategy.
7. Recognising I am impatient and acknowledging it and trusting the counsellor with this information.
8. Recognising 2 steps forward and 1 step back is a blip.
9. Recognising that I feel writing to the man who abused me when I was 10years old is enough to satisfy me, that making him feel anxious will be enough. Or is it?
10. Recognising that I am very high and that I could easily crash back down. Being aware of the risk.

Daryl looked after and fed the kids tonight whilst I went to my appointment. We got talking and he showed me a cookery book and encouraged me to give it a go. He gave me a stock pot. He gave my confidence that I could give it a go. Carol, Daryl and Melvyn are incredible friends.

Reflection: This was exhausting. It was good to be focused on 'recognising', but they were all quite superficial. There was nothing about me and how utterly broken I was. It was all about practical, objective solutions and nothing about comfort and nurturing and holding and being allowed to be vulnerable. Being allowed to feel destroyed and battered and utterly, utterly broken.

Notes:

11.09.15
Continuing to have dreams where I am asking for, but can't get help. Busy distracting day today as my son's 9th Birthday. Spoke to my Dad's CPN this morning about how cruel my mum is to my Dad. When I finished the long conversation I felt very tearful. Both for my Dad, but also because it was a reminder that it is about her and not about me, but why? She is cruel to my Dad because his is now vulnerable, in the clutches of Alzheimer's, she was cruel to me because I was not vulnerable. Why couldn't she just love me for who I am? I hope I find a way of looking after me without being so harsh. I plan to work on it.

Reflection: It's there again. I wanted to look after myself, but I didn't even know where to start.

Notes:

12.09.15

I feel very low today. I woke up feeling low. I dreamt I couldn't get home. Every time I tried something blocked my way. A concrete screen, a water fountain. I keep dreaming of asking for help and nobody listening, or as last night, being blocked in every direction. I am still very tired and very hungry all the time. I had a missed call from a friend, a friend who I had tried to talk to in the past, but she had told me to focus on the now, what I have now and leave the past where it is. The missed call was last night and Alan asked me why I don't call her back. He asked me again today. I told him I didn't want to have to explain to her how I was feeling. I don't want to have to justify myself to her when I know she doesn't understand. I feel bad enough without allowing somebody else to make me feel worse. More guilty, more inadequate and weak. That is the thought that already goes through my mind. Why can't I just get on with my life? Why am I letting it get to me? Because it does and I am weak and ashamed and embarrassed and maybe that's why I feel so low today. On the positive side, yesterday and today I did a ten minute meditation before starting work on my essay. Yesterday my mind was buzzing with my cruel mum and my vulnerable Dad, but after meditating, I was totally focused and energised. Today, until now I didn't know why I feel so low, but ten minutes of meditation again and I was ready to focus. I was talking very loud in my head "breath in – breath out", but it blocked out the other distractions and all I was concentrating on was my lungs inflating and deflating pumping oxygenated blood to my brain to allow it to focus on my essay. The more the distractions tried to be heard, the louder I became – and it worked. I have a terrible headache and I am so hungry and tired and now I know why I feel very, very low, but I didn't call my friend back. I protected myself from feeing worse

Reflection: For a very long time I had recurring dreams about asking for help and not being heard. I still find it difficult to not be listened to. It doesn't bother me if people don't agree with me, but not being listened to is so very damaging. It damaged me until I believed I was damaged beyond repair.

Notes:

13.09.15

I have had a screaming headache since yesterday morning. Tablets aren't working and it kept waking me in the night. Feeling very flat following another nightmare. Being married to a violent man who is locked up in a hospital. I have to go and see him and sleep with him. We have a 3 year old daughter who sees him being violent towards me. When I leave with my daughter the next day, people are telling me I married him, I have to stay with him and what do I know at twenty five years old. I keep telling people I am forty five, but they won't listen. It's been a really difficult day feeling flat and low with the bad headache. I realised also the self-loathing is still here and the only reason I am okay is because nothing has happened to make anything go wrong. Thoughts of why I am not calling my friend back are running through my head. If I felt okay about myself and what's happening, I would call her back, because it wouldn't matter what she thought. But I don't because I am living in the past and I feel disappointed in myself for not being able to cope. I feel low.

Reflection: This really was a very exhausting time. I was looking for answers and I didn't know where to find them. I'm not surprised I had bad headaches around that time. I did protect myself though by not calling my friend, even if I still had the self-loathing for feeling a disappointment. One connection was definitely there, but it still had nothing to connect to.

Notes:

14.09.15

Tonight it is very hard to write. I don't want to - why? Because I feel lost. My crippling headache won't go, I am still having nightmares about being trapped in places and unable to get out. I saw Carol tonight and it is so good to talk. Before I came out I had been talking to Alan and we had a disagreement. He thought it was because he has been spoiling Charlie and he said I was jealous. The truth is I love him spoiling the kids and he couldn't spoil them enough. He problem is I am seeking attention and I want a reward just to feel good enough. I hate myself for saying to Alan "maybe one day someone will think I'm special". I hate it that he knows now that I feel worthless he knows I feel worthless and he won't give me a treat. So I must be worthless and he thinks I'm worthless. I hate myself. Why am I not good enough? We went to meditation tonight and we talked about the difference between practising patience and suppressing anger. We talked about how to cope when others hurt us. Norpel talked about pushing the abuser to one side and just focusing on your own emotion. By either practising forgiveness, or realising the emotion is only hurting yourself and not the abuser, so refusing to give the emotion any of your time and thought. He did not advocate revenge, but believes in Karma. We talked about the time and energy and stress the emotion causes us and that it only affects us and nobody else. I know it all makes sense, but I feel so lost that I can't do any of those things because I feel so bad. It hurts me so much and I have wasted half of my life being affected by this abuse, but trying not to be. I so desperately want it to go away, but I can't ever imagine it not being so awful. I feel so low, I can't see a way forward.

Reflection: This was a time of turmoil. I did understand what was being said to me. I did understand how it could be different, but I hated myself so much and I had nobody to help me to explore why I did. I had more punishment inflicted on me instead, which validated my reason to hate myself.

Notes:

15.09.15

You only get one life – your own. I heard that today. Saw my counsellor today, she told me, or reminded me it's okay to be up and down. I need to stop trying to focus on other people. Stop thinking I am letting people down if I am not okay. I am entitled to my feelings. I want to hold on to that. Stop looking at the goal. So I'm not going to. Say my Dad today, he told me he punched my mum yesterday. She was humiliating him, degrading him for being filthy and having dirty clothes. I felt so sad for him, but I also realised she is intolerant of him as she was of me as a child and I realised suddenly it never was about me. It has always been about her. I told her (the counsellor) I feel guilty for feeling sorry for myself, for never having the opportunity to grow, develop and explore my own identity. Never enjoyed having a young attractive body, always trying to hide it as I felt it was my body, my whole being that attracted unwanted attention. She reassured me it is not feeling sorry for myself, it is grief I am experiencing and perfectly acceptable. I am going to try hard not to be what everyone expects me to be. I am going to try hard to be me, because I really want to be me, whoever that is. Maybe I can stop being so high and so low and maybe I will stop putting demands on myself like I have just done. I want to just be. I don't want to just focus on not letting everybody down. I almost cried tonight at that lightbulb moment. I want to feel how it feels to be me. And I will.

Reflection: I'm finding it astonishing that I have the answers right there. I am writing down exactly what I want and it's being left to just hang there. It's how I imagine recovering from a brain injury might be like. Having a concept, an idea, but then a blank screen with no suggestions, or ideas. Nothing, just completely blank. Half of my mind was completely switched off. Disconnected.

Notes:

16.09.15

Okay I had to stop myself from distracting how I feel. I sat on the settee, closed my eyes and my first thought was I love learning. I loved learning and then I was sexually abused and I learned no more. I began to cry and almost got up to do something else, but I reminded myself to say with it and the tears came. I didn't learn and I wanted to be a nurse, not a shit shovelling nurse as my mum called it. A nurse. My earliest memory of caring was helping my Sister out of bed and helping her on to the potty. When she finished I emptied the potty in the toilet. My mum would say years later that she heard me doing this. My Sister was heavy to me. She would get to the edge of the bed and I would help her down. I was worried she might fall, she never did. I didn't see it as helping or caring. She is my Sister and I just did it because she was part of me. I just wanted to get married and have babies. That was wrong too My mum controlled everything and not learning at school meant my choices were limited. I cry so hard for that lost time, the chance to develop my own identity was robbed. I only ever remember having a voice at school before I was abused. Being part of everything. After I was sexually abused I became aware of the whole of me and I was standing on the outside looking in. And I cried for no longer ever being able to fit in ever again. I started to cry for my lost innocence, my lost body, but I couldn't cope with it any longer. Have been so tired since then, but quiet, so quiet and I lit a joss stick and attempted to meditate. Today I really felt something.

Reflection: Grief is amazing when it's allowed to happen. Yes it's very sad, sometimes devastatingly sad, but I think grief sits right next to your soul. When I was allowed to grieve I was able to sit and think about how what had happened made me feel. Then I was able to feel it and that felt like such a relief and I felt just a little bit connected to me for that short time.

Notes:

17.09.15
Quiet day today. I kept myself distracted all day because yesterday felt quite a thing. I stayed out all day and busied myself with the kids when they got home. Feeling stuff is harder than I thought. It's like there is another layer of me, a layer that I haven't explored. I don't know why it feels hard. I thought it would be good, refreshing and healing, but it feels like I'm intruding on my private thoughts. Yet these private thoughts are what have niggled me for as long as I can remember. I guess I will get used to it. I need to persevere with it so I become comfortable with my thoughts and feelings. That's what I want.

Reflection: How incredible that I found a layer, a layer that was anything other than the superficial mask I was showing to the world. I did find it hard and now I do find it good, refreshing and healing. You can't 'intrude' on your own private thoughts, because they are you. I still saw myself as two separate minds, even separate beings. The one I portrayed to the world, the one I knew and the one I hadn't been in touch with for a very long time. Like a long lost relative.

Notes:

18.09.15

Today did not turn out as planned, I was having a quiet day. Dropped the kids off at school then stayed at my mums longer than necessary due to anxiety of allowing myself not to be distracted. But soon after I got home Alan told me he was coming home. I had an hour. I tried my best to meditate and I did feel calm and peaceful. I allowed my thoughts not to be distracted and feelings of deep loneliness began to emerge. And fear, fear of losing everybody. My Sister had died, my right arm. My mum and Dad went away and left me. For a week I was told, but at the end of that week I was told it would be another week. I was very frightened inside. I was staying with relatives I barely knew. I had at that point never ever felt so lonely in my whole life. I had a knot in my stomach, I was lonely and scared. I didn't know if there were ever going to come back for me. My safety, security and sense of not having to think will everything be okay, was gone. And it never came back.

Reflection: So a day of being with my thoughts the day before had been enough to cause me some anxiety, but I persevered and insight began to emerge.

Notes:

19.09.15

Feeling very angry tonight. Fell for it again for the last time. I went out last night with my mum and talked about how she was coping. She really opened up, or so I thought. She said she feels sorry for my Dad and she makes him do things to keep him active. So we talked about not doing that and she agreed. Then today my Dad came round to my house very confused and wanting to talk. *"Yeah where were you when I was scared and on my own? You were off down the Legion with my mum getting pissed whilst I was scared at home on my own, or at Jack and Emilys watching horror films on video. They gave me nightmares for years. I was 7 years old when my Sister died, where the fuck were you then?"* When I took my Dad home tonight my mum asked me if he had told me what had happened. She was very aggressive towards him and I could see he didn't have the words to defend himself. I told her he hadn't because he was very confused. She was venomous in her reply *"He isn't confused"* she spat at me. Last nights conversation meant nothing. She played me. She is a fucking bitch. They are both playing me! Elizabeth came in to me tonight crying, she'd had a nightmare about Dr Who. I rubbed her itchy legs with cream and told her when I was little I had nightmares about scary programmes. I used to imagine the camera man sipping coffee in their jeans and T-Shirts yawning and burping and hoping nobody got their lines wrong so they could go home early. I told her all the monsters and Daleks and scary people climbed out of their costumes and were excited to go home to read their kids bed time stories. Elizabeth said *" I bet Nana just said to you, get back to bed"*. I want to cry, because Nana wasn't even there. She was out getting pissed with grandad, or else I was in bed at Jack and Emilys in Sarah-Jaynes' room. So being in a room with a baby felt less scary, but it was all so scary, because after the first time Jack Sexually abused me, I was really scared he would come into the bedroom. I have lived my life being scared and now I am expected to be there for everyone else. I want to be there for my children, but nobody was ever there for me and now I am an adult wanting somebody to be there for me as a child. This is so bad. I can't stop crying.

Reflection: These are the times I needed to share with a good counsellor. This was the time I was beginning to really connect with my feelings, but there was nobody to help me to process these feelings, so I turned them inwards.

Notes:

20.09.15

I thought I was calm this morning, but I feel very angry inside. I can't remember things, or where I have put things and I get very angry with my stupid brain. I couldn't find some chocolate for a dessert and I got angry. I couldn't find a receipt and I got angry and then got even angrier when a large order we made is incorrect. I know it will be sorted, but why am I angry? I had terrible nightmares again last night and I am angry about believing the good in my mum and it was all shit. And I am angry with my brain because I can't remember stuff. And I know why. Because I was neglected, sexually abused and raped when I was a child. So I shouldn't be angry with myself, but I am VERY, VERY angry! I just want to be on my own. I am angry because I trusted her again and she let me down again. And when will I learn? I am so angry I don't know what to do with myself. I hate being like this, I hate behaving like this, I know I shouldn't I could pretend not to be angry, but I am. So FUCKING ANGRY.

Reflection: Excellent, I had found anger, but it was with myself, at myself and I had nobody to help me to direct it where it belonged. This was never going to end well.

Notes:

21.09.15

I can't remember the last time I didn't have a nightmare. I am so tired of it happening. Always the same. Either I can't get home to the children, or nobody will listen to me. My manager text me today asking me how I am feeling and that opened the flood gates. I told her I feel very low. I am crying for what I have lost, angry because I have lost it and really, really sad because everything could have been so different. The grief I am struggling with is being neglected, sexually abused a number of times and raped when I was a child. Then emotionally abused and raped throughout my marriage. I have been dead inside for 35 years. Existing only in survival mode. If not that, then attempting suicide, or having feelings of suicide or self-harm.. Now it has all come out and I don't have to try and survive it anymore. Instead I am feeling it and trying to get my head around it. I was crying when I sent the text and cried even harder when I read it and the enormity of it was staring me in the face. How do I get my head around all of that? At the moment I can't see a future. This feels massive. My body has been violated and my mind ripped apart. How the hell do I manage to put it all back together? I went to mediation tonight and the lady Buddhist said, *"no matter how huge our troubles might me, our mind is bigger. Our troubles are only ever a thunder cloud within a big blue sky. The blue sky is infinitely bigger than any cloud."* I can't find my blue sky. I am suffocating in a thick black cloud and I can't find my way out. How do I start again? Half of my life gone. Half of my life damaged emotionally, physically and psychologically. I just want to be well, but my soul has been ripped out. I don't know how to carry on. I am so scared. I can't see a way out. I am so tired. I've been destroyed and I feel very weak. I can't go on. I don't know how to do it. I can't go on.

Reflection: Although I couldn't find it at that time, I have held that thought ever since. I understand and believe that there is always hope. Even in the darkest of days, the largest of thunder clouds, there is always blue sky waiting for the clouds to go. I was never going to see it at that point though. I was being tossed around in a huge thunder storm and I was completely disorientated with my thoughts.

Notes:

22.09.15
Counselling today at AMICA. I talked about feeling overwhelmed. I can't get my head around the enormity of it. Kate tried to help me put some jigsaws into place. I have a narcissistic mother that made me look for love elsewhere. Of course I would look for love, where I was accepted as part of a family. I didn't go looking for sexual abuse. Every child wants love. Every child wants to be accepted. No child deserves to be sexually abused. I didn't deserve to be sexually abused. Have my life torn inside out. I can't stop crying. I feel so sad.

Reflection: I had it, I knew it, but I still couldn't process it. I felt sad, I was grieving, but it was too soon to move forwards. I needed that time to sit with being really sad. I was beginning to have my own feelings.

Notes:

23.09.15
I feel revolting, I don't know why I just feel revolting. Emotionally and sexually torn apart I feel like I want to scrape myself inside out. I have tried so hard not to give in to this. But some people commit suicide because they cannot cope with what's happened to them. I feel like I am letting everybody down, but the pressure is too much to bear. I need somebody to hold me, to stop me, but there isn't anybody. Everybody tells me I am doing so well, I am getting there, but I'm really not. I'm really not coping and I am trying so hard to get it right, but now I've let everybody down because I have cut myself. I have scraped my arm so hard with a knife and the relief was so huge, the feeling of tension going was so big I didn't want it to stop. And now I feel so bad because I am letting down everybody who believes in me. I have let myself down, I have let everybody down, but I tried so hard. So very, very hard. I am so sorry. I just want it to go away. I want it all to go away. I am so, so sorry. I am trying to make my mind calm and peaceful I am trying so hard. Trying so hard to make everything okay again. Trying so, so hard to make my mind calm and peaceful, but it isn't It isn't calm and peaceful it's tormented. Tormented to death. I am so frightened, I don't know what to do.

Reflection: I remember that day so very clearly. I was calm. Really, really calm. I was sat in the conservatory and my mind went blank. I got up, walked to the knife rack and I picked the knife out and I stood looking out of the kitchen window and I hacked at my arm. I scraped it and I stabbed at it and the more I did it, the deeper I wanted to go. My arm started bleeding and I knew I should stop, but I really didn't want to and I moved to another place and I picked and picked into my skin with the knife. It felt incredible. I felt no pain, only incredible relief. All the tension left my body and I could have carried on, but I stopped. I didn't feel the slightest bit guilty, I felt like I had finally done something for myself. I had released the tension that nobody else could. I had to release it myself and it felt great.

When I did manage to put the knife down, reality kicked in and I looked at the mess I had made of my arm and I thought about everybody else and how they would feel about me and the self-hatred was back. I was absolutely devastated. My arm is aching now as I write this reflection. Self-harm is incredibly powerful from an emotional point of view. It opens the floodgates, quite literally sometimes. I am so fortunate to have not been left with any scars, but I didn't believe that at the time. I wanted those scars, I wanted everybody to see the scars, so they could see how much emotional pain I was in and how much physical pain I had been in. Self-harm is very, very powerful and incredibly dangerous. I needed to be seen, I needed to be heard and I needed to feel again and self-harming did all of that for me.

Notes:

24.09.15
I feel disconnected. I feel as if I am falling further away from reality. I think I am asking for help. I think I am, but maybe I am not. I don't know. I am beginning to think I shouldn't talk to anybody. I am beginning to think I can't be helped and I am really losing my way. I need to hold on to something. I need to keep thinking of a reason to stay. When I cut myself yesterday I wasn't scared, I wasn't panicking, I just knew I needed to do it. I don't want to fall away, I want somebody to talk to me. I want somebody to help me through this really, really rough bit. I can't do this on my own. I've text somebody. I can't do any more than that. I just don't want to let anybody down. I don't want to let myself down; This is unbearable. I feel dizzy, I am having a panic attack, but it will pass. I have text somebody how I really feel. I don't feel as though I've ever been so scared in my life ever. EVER.

Reflection: Feeling disconnected is a frightening place to be, until you feel even more disconnected and then you feel nothing. I didn't feel like I was living in the real world at that point. I was on the outside looking in, like watching a film. I wasn't experiencing any emotion for anything that was going on around me and I felt out of control of the emotions that were raging inside me. I felt like my body had been taken over. I was physically present because my body was there, but I couldn't make myself heard, I was feeling worse because the flashbacks and nightmares had worn me out and I couldn't function in the present. Beginning to think I shouldn't talk to anybody was beginning to let go. To question whether I should even be here at all. That's why I was scared. I was contemplating my future and it wasn't the future that belonged here. I was scared because I didn't know what was going to happen to me, or how it would feel to die. I was thinking it was time to make a decision. Fear that I was being pushed towards dying, but only because I was too exhausted to live.

Notes:

25.09.15

I can't articulate how low I am. I called Martyn today and talked and talked. I told him I have cut myself. How I feel more and more disconnected from people. He was kind. He talked to me about how feeling better in the short term was not the reason to cut myself. He said I am harming myself. I told him I was afraid to tell anyone because I feel like I am letting everyone down. I told him how I can't just release how I feel for just one hour a week. It's too massive. I have suppressed this for so long that all the emotion has hit hard in one go. I am so sorry that I am not stronger than I am. Martyn explained that it will take a long time. That I have learned to think in a particular way for a long time and changing that will take time. I should not put pressure on myself. I told Melvyn, he did not respond. I told Carol and she was brilliant. She actually said she was amazed that I had not done anything before. Then I plucked up the courage to tell Alan. He hugged me. He told me he wanted me to talk to him because we were now on another level. He told me he loved me. All of my fear and nobody judged me. The urge to cut myself is so strong. I just want to feel something else. The relief was amazing. If I didn't have my children I don't think I could do this. I am so tired now. I realised why I feel everyone will be disappointed in me. Because my mum and Dad were always disappointed in me. When I failed at school, when my marriage failed, when I told them I was training to be a midwife. When I told them I had been sexually abused when I was 10 years old. They actually told me they were disappointed in me because I hadn't been strong enough to tell them. Now I know where my ongoing fear of being a disappointment and having to be strong has come from. Another lesson learned. I remember before I had children I was obsessed with suicide. Now I have children.

Reflection: Alan only allowed me to talk because he said I had reached "another level". That angered me for a long time. Why don't people listen when you have strength and resilience? Why do people only listen when all your strength, resilience and hope has left your body? Because by then for some people it is too late. My children saved me in those early months and they have no idea, unless they read this. I felt at that time though that even my children would be better off without me. I felt an absolute failure and I was convincing myself that they deserved a better Mum. A Mum who could function.

Notes:

26.09.15
Saw Melvyn and Rachel today. Talked to Melvyn about cutting and talking to Alan. He asked me why I haven't been talking to people. I explained I thought I had, but I would try, so I spoke to Alan tonight. I now understand why I went looking for love elsewhere. I was neglected. I now understand why my mum was the way she was towards me. She is narcissistic. It starts from here. I went to a family I was loved and accepted in. Then he sexually abused me by putting his fingers on my fanny, playing a tickling game. TWICE. He took my body away from me. He took that love and acceptance away from me. He made me scared and I stopped living. I agreed to have sex with my cousin when I was 11 years old. He was 15years old. We almost did it. He said he was scared he might hurt me, but I said it's okay do it. My Mum, Dad, Auntie and Nan came home then so we didn't. A short while later at my Nanas we were daring each other to climb the ladder in the back yard and step onto the air raid shelter. I lost my nerve and started to climb back down the ladder. Nick put his fingers up and started fiddling with me. So I yelled at him to stop. He laughed, just like that man did when I told him to stop. And he told me the only way to get down was down the ladder. So I had to climb down the ladder whilst he fingered me all the way down. I felt angry and guilty because I had agreed to have sex with him. Then when I was 13 I was walking to my friends when a man approached me. He started talking to me and I went with him to a field where he started kissing me and fondling me, then he lead me to another field further away and he raped me. I allowed myself to go with him, because I thought that's what was expected. I hated what he was doing every second, but thought it was normal, so I allowed it to happen. Then when I was 16 years old I went to a disco with a friend. A YTS disco. Two lads wanted to walk us home and I didn't want them to, but my friend said it would be okay. She walked home with a boy and this boy walked me back. He started to kiss me, then he pushed me into the bushes and he raped me so violently. I was torn, I was bleeding and in a lot of pain. I could feel him inside me for days afterwards. When I got home I saw all the blood, but I had to go to bed because my mum and Dad were in bed. I told my friend what had happened and she said she should tell someone, but I said no. I felt so guilty for allowing him to walk me home. I felt sick, I felt violated. I believed that men did what they wanted to you, even if you didn't want them to. My ex-husband asked me to describe what happened just before he raped me. And I allowed it to happen. I tried to explain to Alan that I cut myself because I feel totally destroyed by everything that has happened, but people keep telling me "I'm getting there". But I am feeling more and more devastated by what has happened. I don't know if he understands, but I have told him. Just like Martyn advised me to do. I have never cried so much in my life.

Reflection: Repeatedly writing what I had experienced also helped to relieve some pressure. It wasn't relieved for long, but I needed to be as explicit as possible, to get the horrifying flashbacks out of my head and on to paper.

Notes:

27.09.15
I feel shattered today. I feel tearful, but calm. I went to see Carol. I tried to explain why I cut myself, because I wanted to feel something other than what I am feeling and I don't feel what everyone else is feeling. I talked about Martyn and him saying I am hurting myself. I don't believe I am hurting myself, I am relieving a pain. Carol pointed out that that is exactly what is wrong with it. That I don't see it as self-harm, I see it as a way of helping me to cope with the pain. I know it's wrong because it leaves scars and it can cause infection and it is addictive, but it feels so good. It really feels like a release albeit short lived. Although I feel calm today, I couldn't bring myself to repeat the conversation with Carol. I have been numb to it today. Carol told me she is scared that I am going to die. I am scared because I cut myself when I wasn't panicking, I didn't feel I needed to tell anyone to make me stop. I just needed to do it and I just did it. I wasn't nervous, I wasn't hesitant, I just did it. My brain has taken to own it's own. That scares me. I don't want to die, I want to get better. I want to be able to talk about the irrational feelings that I have. Because right or wrong, they are my feelings. I want to hold somebody's hand and be able to talk. It all feels so hopeless. It just seems too big, too overwhelming. Too awful, too devastating to comprehend. Too sick and completely violating. I was physically and mentally destroyed and feeling how that happened feels as if it is destroying me now. This kills people. People do not survive this and I am battling and I am losing this battle.

Reflection: When Carol told me she was afraid I was going to die, that scared me inside. I remember getting a knot in my stomach. I began to believe I was going to die. If she was scared then there was a real possibility. Another example I think, like the earlier one I have mentioned that when somebody reflects something back to you in real words, rather than emotional feeling, it is really powerful and can be very dangerous. This happened again a few years later, documented in this book. It is so, very dangerous. I started to believe that the only option was to die.

Notes:

28.09.15

I had a missed call from my cousin today. I got home and had a panic attack. I text Melvyn, told Alan and my GP. All said not to contact. Good idea I think. I can't cope with talking to him. I spoke to Carol today. I told her going to that house made me feel part of a family. I belonged, I was accepted. When he started tickling me and then fingering me I was petrified, I was trapped. I was confused. When I told him I didn't like it he laughed. I was so careful not to be on my own with him, but then I was. He started tickling me and made me tickle him. Then his hand wandered lower and lower and he was fingering me again. He said I had to touch him where he was touching me. When he was touching my fanny, I didn't touch his willy. I was scared. Scared of what he might do. He kept saying *"there is one place you haven't touched me."* I felt trapped, petrified, and scared to touch his willy in case he shouted at me, or jumped on me. I didn't know what to do. I jumped up and escaped out of the house. He took that all away from me. He took a family I belonged to, accepted by, loved by. He took that all away, all away with my body and left me with fear, emptiness and loneliness. I was prepared to have sex with my cousin, because I wanted to know what it really felt like. We almost did it too, but my mum, dad, Auntie and Nan all came back. But then a short while later, he fingered me coming down the ladder and I couldn't do anything about it, I was angry, disgusted, trapped, powerless and he laughed too. When I was going to my friend's house I was approached by a man who befriended me. He held my hand and took me to a field. He mauled me, slobbered all over me and then he took me further away and he raped me. By the time I was 13 years old I had had enough. A girl was attracted to me who I played hockey with. She would push herself up against me, touch me and when I resisted she said there was something wrong with me because I didn't like boys and I didn't like girls. And so I believed it. Then when I was 16 years old I was made to walk home with a boy against my wishes. He pushed me into the bushes and raped me so violently. It took my breath away. I was torn and bleeding and felt him inside me for days afterwards. I had to go to bed with blood soaked legs. Then my ex-husband would ask me to describe what had happened to me when I was 10 years old. He would tell me it was my fault it was painful. I was always torn and bleeding. Was desperate for it to heal before he raped me again, but it never did. I have never known pain like it. He emotionally abused me and sometimes physically. I can't get my head around all this. Why did it have to get worse and worse? Why did I have to be taught a lesson and why did I allow all of it to happen? I can't cope with these feelings. It's as though I am living them all again, but for the first time. The abuse took place over 16 years, but my head is trying to make sense of it all in one go. It's too big. I can't cope. I told the Occupational Health Doctor and GP that I cut myself last week. Neither were surprised. Didn't condone it, but not surprised. I cut myself to feel something other than the massive overwhelming feeling I have got right now. Some people die because they can never get their heads around it. I am hanging on by the skin of my teeth. I can't cope this is so massive, I really can't cope. I am hanging on. I can't take this anymore. When I told Carol tonight she said it is too big for her to get her head around. Maybe this is too big for me. Maybe I can't survive. Maybe that is the lesson I am being taught. I can't go on I am so tired.

Reflection: I can still feel how close I was to completely giving up. Carol telling me it was too big for her was another indication that I should end my life. If it's too big for her and she didn't experience my abuse, then how could I possibly survive. I was no longer scared, but I was getting increasingly worn down.

Notes:

29.09.15
I am desperate. I have suicidal thoughts, but not intention. I feel like I can't hold on anymore. The counsellor I am seeing is just not working for me. I need somebody alongside me who will listen to me, but also help me. Help me to see a way through this. How to make sense of this. It is devastating my mind. I am trying so hard not to let it, but I am struggling so much. There has to be a way, there has to be before I give up. I come out of counselling more frustrated than when I go in. It's destroying me, it really is destroying me and I am finding it harder and harder to hold on. I feel like I can't breathe.

Reflection: I was no longer considering other options. I was starting to really believe there was no way out of this alive for me. The hopelessness was all consuming.

Notes:

30.09.15
Numb. What I do know is I can't cope anymore with my counsellor. I keep disclosing stuff, keep feeling worse and she looks at me and smiles. She changes the subject; she keeps saying we don't have to talk about anything. Well I need to or it is going to kill me. I have contacted a new psychotherapy service and I have an appointment on Friday.

Reflection: It's quite scary to see how this deteriorated. I went from Angry, scared and hopeless, to numb. The wrong counsellor can be more damaging than no counsellor at all.

That morning I was sat on my bed and flicking through google looking for private counsellors. This was my last ditched attempt to sort myself out. I had decided in my head that I wouldn't be alive to see out another week. Rutland House Counselling and Psychotherapy kept coming up first. It was irritating me, I remember, but why I don't know. Because if began with 'R', but kept coming up. I kept googling and it kept coming up. I rang in the morning and it rang and rang and rang. I kept ringing. Around lunchtime somebody answered the 'phone and I was a bit rude to the person on the other end, who I now know to be called Rhema. I told her I had been ringing all morning and nobody had answered. She was really apologetic and calm. I explained that I needed to talk to somebody and she offered me an appointment the following Tuesday. I blurted out to her that I couldn't wait that long (because I knew I wouldn't be here). Without any question she offered me Friday the same week.

Notes:

01.10.15

AM: Thoughts of self-harm are getting stronger. I feel as though my mind is ripping apart. I am scared beyond comprehension that tomorrow they will tell me I can't be helped. I keep having a vision, I walk out of the building and straight under a bus. I need it to stop now. I need it to stop getting worse and I am so scared. I don't want to die. I just want to be able to cope. I have let my guard down. Allowed myself to stop avoiding it. Now I need help before it kills me. Living a normal life has been a lie for me. This is how I really feel. Sad, isolated, alone, trapped with memories and feelings. Hopeless, empty, nothing left. Destroyed, defeated.

PM: It's nearly 10pm. I am unbelievably anxious. I have no reserves left. I know I can't cope with this anymore. Tomorrow can't go wrong, it just can't. I've got nothing else left.

Reflection: I was so unbelievably frightened that night. I knew that tomorrow was the absolute last time I was going to try and overcome this. I was so tired, so very tired. The place where the counselling took place was about a quarter of the way up a street. At the end of that street the buses drove down into the town. I kept having this image over and over again of the bus coming round the corner and me stepping straight in front of it, I knew it would have no time to stop. It wouldn't be going fast, but it was fast enough if I stepped right out just before it got level with me. I knew exactly how it was going to happen. I had rehearsed it dozens of times in my head and I was absolutely terrified that it was going to be happening in real life. I was so frightened of that tomorrow.

Notes:

02.10.15
I met my new Counsellor today. Her name is Jayne. The place is so welcoming. Everybody smiles and talked to me in reception. It was a packed 50 minutes. Talking about what had happened with my old counsellor, briefly what happened to me. She gave me her text number and she said it is big and there is a lot to get through, but she said she will walk by me all the way and take as long as it takes. She also said she will always make sure I feel safe and grounded before I leave each appointment. I left and had a panic attack, but went to the Buddhist Café for peppermint tea. I calmed down, then came right down. Now the anxiety of the Counsellor has dropped, the reality of dealing with it came forward. I think a lot of my panic and anxiety have been about disclosing and then being left with it. I am exhausted. I am so, so tired and it feels like an uphill climb. I am mentally shattered, I have no reserve left.

Reflection: I remember walking into the building and waiting for Jayne. The therapists were sat waiting for their clients in the reception. How amazing is that. They sat amongst us. I didn't feel on the outside, I didn't feel like a patient, I didn't feel judged. I felt like a human person, sitting with other human people. There was gentle music playing in the background and that made me feel calm and everything started to slow down. There was also a calm fragrance from a freshener in the room. I wanted to sit there forever.
Jayne came down and collected me and we went upstairs to her room. She began by introducing herself and I talked about what had led me to seeing her that day and she told me she was a person centred counsellor. I looked at her and I felt disgusted. I had just spent two months with a 'person centred counsellor' and that meant sitting, staring at me whilst I wrung myself out for 50 minutes and then left in a worse state than when I arrived. But Jayne didn't sit and stare at me. She talked to me, she listened to me, she smiled at me. She definitely didn't look scared of me. She appeared calm, spoke steadily, quietly and in an unhurried manner and after the shocking blow of telling me she was a person centred counsellor, she went on to say she would walk by my side all the way for as long as it takes. I couldn't believe it! She didn't tell me I'd been horrifically abused, she didn't tell me it was too much. She told me she was going to be by my side for as long as it takes. That meant she absolutely believed I would recover at some point and she was going to be with me. I felt held for the first time in thirty five years. Somebody had hold of me. Somebody was about to hold me whilst I let go and they wouldn't let me fall. Saying there was a lot to get through suggested it could be got through. I believed right then that I could get better. I could conquer this. I had no idea how and I had no strength left, but I had somebody. I finally had somebody. Giving me her text number also made me feel like she respected me. I felt treated as an equal. She normalised me. In that 50 minutes, Jayne was already right by my side. I was no longer inferior to the rest of the world. Jayne met me completely at my level and I felt safe. I did not walk out in front of that bus, nor did I want to. I had hope!

Notes:

03.10.15

I woke with a very strong urge to cut myself. I have had nightmares all night and I just want to feel different. I messaged Melvyn and Jayne. Seven weeks of not being heard by a counsellor and all the time thoughts and feelings becoming more and more intense, becoming overwhelming and totally consumed. I actually feel physically sick. I distracted myself and made a promise that I would not cut as long as I can vent. Then I slept most of the afternoon to escape it. I have just had a 10 minute meditation on compassion as I found I was hugging myself tight. I meditated on all the young people who have been abused, or feel like I do and felt true compassion for them. Not one of them is to blame. So whilst I can hang on to that I will try to practice compassion for myself until I believe I was not to blame. I will try hard. My head aches and my gut feels wretched, but I have to hang on. To believe it will pass.

Reflection: The urge to cut came because I had been talking about my experiences. It gave the flashbacks a surge of power. It was almost like I had a demon inside me, the more I talked about my experiences, trying to exorcise them, the angrier and more aggressive they appeared to present. It was like they were angry with me and wanted me to keep quiet. The more I was exposing them memories and flashbacks, the angrier they got. They were angry with me because they needed to hold on to the power they had over me. They still had more power over me than I could conquer, but that wasn't going to last. It was a really strange feeling. I still felt like I had two minds, but I also felt like I was two people. There was me that wanted to heal, to recover and live and there was another me that wanted me to stay a victim, hurt and traumatised. Recovering me was tiny, injured me was massive and very, very angry because it was being challenged for the first time ever.

Notes:

04.10.15

Although this is not happening now, I am feeling it for the first time NOW. I can't shake it off. I get up, get dressed, interact with family, but all the time I feel shit inside. All the time I keep going I feel shit inside. Today I told Charlie off for being lazy. Alan verbally attacked me. "That is the old you", meaning you are bad, very bad. "You are over reacting, you are talking out of context". BAD, BAD ME! I was crying and he kept attacking. I knew I shouldn't have trusted him. He has thrown my vulnerable self-back in my face. BAD ME! BAD, BAD ME! I want to cut myself so I can feel worse than he can ever make me feel. I slept all afternoon to block everything out. I have no strength left to defend myself. I opened up to him and he has used it against me. BASTARD!!!

Reflection: I was completely unaware on a conscious level that he was emotionally abusing me, but this was what he did. He humiliated me, he put me down and he was trying to keep me as a vulnerable victim. This was happening more and more and my familiar pattern of behaviour to hate myself, to berate myself was far too strong. But then the last word I wrote, in capital letters. That was me, that healing me who could see what he was doing, healing me that did on some tiny level value me. I wrote it down, so I did feel it, but it was still so much smaller than injured me. But it was there, that little kindle of light was definitely there.

Notes:

05.10.15
I have to do something to change my mind-set. I got up at 6am and spent an hour on my exercise bike. I got ready, took the kids to school then went swimming. I was properly shattered, but getting angrier as the day went on. I went to meditation and learned about impermanence. Is this it for me and Alan? By the time I got home I was boiling with rage. I tell him I can't understand why he shows no compassion, no understanding, why he wants to humiliate me and put me down. He tells me he didn't mean it and he apologised. He said he doesn't know what to do. How can you not know how to feel compassionate when someone you love is in emotional pain? I can understand he doesn't know what to say or do, but how can he not know how to love me if he claims to love me? I really don't understand and I fear for our future together. Does he even care about me?

Reflection: That day was a day for recovering me. I knew he didn't love me, or care for me on a subconscious level, I wrote it and sometimes when I wrote it was almost like my hand was writing and I just let the words flow onto the page. It came directly from my soul, straight onto the paper. I was definitely not consciously thinking these things. However, I wasn't quite there with it at that stage. I was still asking questions about his feelings for me, I wasn't making statements about what I really understood his feelings were for me.

Notes:

06.10.15

Had a very bad night's sleep. Nightmares, woke up shattered. So I feel down again. Alan is meeting Melvyn today. When he gets home he doesn't want to talk about it. But he is more attentive. I feel so down. I am very, very tired, but I just want a peaceful sleep. I try to meditate every day, but as soon as I sit quiet all the thoughts rush into my head. I try not to get frustrated. I try not to push them away, but acknowledge them in order to let them go. The problem is I acknowledge them and they stay and grow. When is it going to ease off? This is ripping my mind apart. I keep being told it won't be like this forever, it will get better. But how the hell will it ever get better when it never leaves my thoughts? HELP HELP HELP HELP me!!!

Reflection: There was a lot of determination inside of me at that point. I'd stopped saying I can't do it and I was screaming for help. Jayne had offered me a lifeline and I didn't want to take it delicately, I wanted to grab it to stop myself from drowning. I had some energy that day, but that was not always a good thing when I was feeling really down. That energy could be used to move forward positively, or to very aggressively punish myself. When I was feeling very negative and I had a lot of energy I felt very spontaneous and that scared me.

Notes:

07.10.15

Met with my Manager today. She talked about a Duty of Care to report the abuse. She asked me to consider that he may have, or still be abusing others. I told her I don't feel strong enough, but she said all I have to do is report it and the police will do the rest. I can't bare to be judged by anyone who doesn't know me. To challenge me. Now I feel like a very bad person. If I don't report it I am failing to protect other children. I really can't live with that burden. I can't take much more.

Reflection: My Manager was supportive, she was also very direct. The conversation that day added to the pressure I felt. I was trying to get my head around what I had experienced, I was trying to recover and then to add to the guilt I loaded myself with the responsibility of every other child who may or may not have been abused. I have noticed whilst writing these reflections, that it is when people directed a statement at me that it intensified the abuse I had been subjected to or exacerbated my emotions. It made everything very real. Like I was being told I had been abused for the first time. But it was the first time every time.

Notes:

08.10.15
I talked to Jayne on the 'phone. Talked about what happened with Alan and my manager and always wanting to be asleep. She tried to reassure me that I am not responsible for what happens to anyone else. I only need to think about me. We talked about coping strategies and writing down the images and thoughts and feelings. It took ages to buy a notebook. Too big was scary, because the thoughts are out there. Pretty was wrong because of the filth inside. I wrote "My thoughts scare me". The image of his mocking sniggering face scare me because I was trapped and revolted by the images. Those gut wrenching fear.
I saw Martyn today. It was the first time I said out loud *"the thoughts and images scare me."* I told him I don't want my cutting wound to heal because it's a visual for me to see the pain I am feeling. I talked through everything that has happened and he was very supportive. He tried to help me see that I am not responsible for everybody else who might have been abused. I told him I couldn't understand why he didn't have an affair if he wasn't 'getting it' from his wife. It was pointed out to me that he was 'getting it' from his wife, but he wanted to abuse a kid. I told Martyn I'm remembering it as an adult. He said "yes" and not the 10 year old child. That was a very stark reminder. I almost cried. Shit, it was me age 10, not me the adult. Ten is so tiny. That makes what he did even worse. Ten years old. What the hell ever interest would a man have in a 10 year old child. ME! That's a big reality check. How young was I! Oh shit! That is so sad, that is so disgustingly overwhelming. I just want to scream.

Reflection: It was interesting buying that notebook. I didn't want to buy a pretty note book. I wanted to buy an ugly looking book, because ugly, disgusting, dirty things were going to be written in it.
Jayne and Martyn only ever talked about me and how I could try to support me. They never spoke about what I should do, they never told me to behave in a way that was acceptable to other people. They accepted me exactly how I was and they were by my side whatever I talked about.
Even pointing out to me that I was abused by a man and I was a kid, was a savage smack in the stomach. A loud hard statement that screamed at me that I had been abused. Every time I was told I had been abused it destroyed me, it shattered me, it shocked me. But at that time I had Jayne and I had Martyn and they never told me I had been abused. They never TOLD me anything, they listened and they responded and I never felt threatened, or attacked, or like I was being abused all over again like the others did when they made those savage statements.

Notes:

09.10.15
Today was a numb day. Until........I had a dream about him last night. I was looking after his twin boys, Christopher and Daniel. I don't know why because he didn't have twin boys. I was looking after them and I didn't want to. I didn't want to because of what he had done to me, but I tolerated it. Did it because I got on with it. Just like I got on with what all of them did. Why? Because they all made out it was normal, that it was me who was strange for not liking it or making a big deal out of it.
Then I saw my mum today and she was all about me! Me! Me! How her life is affected by everything and I remembered then. I did have thoughts and feelings, but she would constantly tell me what I was thinking, what I was feeling and if it wasn't what she was thinking – I was wrong. And so because none of them thought what they were doing was wrong, then it must have been my fault. All of it must have been my fault and I can't live with knowing I allowed it all to happen. It's driving me mad. I just can't bare it. What a bad person am I.

Reflection: I was blaming myself and that was really destructive, but I had grown up with a Mother who blamed me for everything. Everything I did, said, or felt, she would tell me how it made her feel. She would mock how I spoke, so I became self-conscious about talking, she mocked how I walked, she mocked me when I ate. She controlled me by denying any desires or needs I had that she disagreed with. I grew up with being forced to be absent from my own thoughts and feelings, so much so even I grew to resent my own thoughts, feelings and desires. So when I was abused and my thoughts and feelings were not taken into account and my voice, my dreadful voice went unheard, then I could only feel revulsion towards myself. I had been conditioned to do so.

Some examples to explain what I meant:
If I felt hungry and it wasn't a meal time, I would get angry with myself for having that thought and then I would deny myself food.
If I felt cold and I was told it wasn't cold I would deny myself the comfort I needed from gloves and scarves, or cardigans and jumpers. I would instead be angry at myself for feeling cold. I would wash my freezing cold hands in boiling hot water as a punishment for them being cold. I would stay in wet clothes when I'd played out in the snow to deny my feelings of being cold. I would be angry with myself for being cold and feeling uncomfortable, so I wouldn't do anything to rectify it.
When my periods started I was angry with my body because they lasted longer than I was told they should, so when I ran out of sanitary pads, I would use toilet paper instead.
Much later I denied my feelings altogether, because I believed I didn't have the right to feel. My boundaries were shattered and if I was physically, emotionally, or sexually abused I would be angry with myself and punish myself much more than anybody else could. Just so I could reinforce what a disgusting, revolting person I was for feeling anything. I believed I had to allow whatever happened to me to happen and how dare I voice any objection, or feeling. My soul was destroyed.

I was a very aggressive person, so when I was hit I knew I deserved it. I created behavior's to justify the punishment.

Notes:

10.10.15

I had a nightmare last night. I'm not aware of it. Alan said I was whimpering in my sleep. So now what's happening? The first time I write my nightmare down to share with the psychotherapist Jayne, the next night I am unaware of it. I has gone deeper. Is that a good thing or bad? I saw Carol today and we talked a lot. I told her I want to let go of the control I hold over myself. Body image and food. I text it to Jayne so she knows I want to talk about it. That's 35 years of control and very exciting, but equally scary to make a decision to let go. I have a very heavy heart this afternoon and I feel very subdued, but not conscious of why. I talked today about always worrying about what other people might be thinking and that's because I know if I was unhappy with something I would go along with it, but feel unhappy, so I think others do the same. I want to stop that too. To do what feels right for me and be confident in my decisions without putting the feelings of others before my own. I want to do that. So three positive things, so why do I have a heavy heart?

Reflection: There are a few things I could reflect on here, but the one that strikes me most is the nightmare. It fascinated me that something I had no control of, or even existed in any physical form appeared to have taken on a life of it's own. Flashbacks and nightmares loved to torment me. But when I started to talk about the flashbacks, they became more violent, more aggressive, like they were angry with me for exposing them. Then I talk about nightmares and they present so deeply that I am unaware of the content. It really felt like I was possessed by a demon that I had woken inside me and it was doing everything in its power to stay in control of me. Either by becoming more aggressive, or burying itself so it stayed inside, so I couldn't find it. It was becoming so desperate to stay in control. I felt like I'd been invaded.

Notes:

11.10.15

I feel so very low. Nightmare about trying to get home, but being stopped at a service station which turned out to be Shopping City. I cannot escape this, I am totally ground down. Why, why, why won't it stop? I've no anger left, no fear. I just despair. I cannot see a future like this. I am always on the outside looking in because everything is wrong. I am going through the motions. I need someone to reach into me. To make something click.

Reflection: My little demon was playing havoc with me. My internal compass was spinning all over the place and I couldn't connect with anything. I couldn't interpret my nightmares and I felt possessed.

Notes:

12.10.15
I can't remember the last time I had a peaceful night's sleep. I want to cut myself, the urge is so strong because I just want to feel something different. Just like the day I did it last time. I am going mad inside. When is this going to stop?

Reflection: I felt stuck. Nothing appeared to be shifting and I was exhausted, absolutely tormented.

Notes:

13.10.15

Feeling very anxious about being on my own today, so kept busy. I went swimming and swam 100 lengths in an hour. Not bad hey! I swam 1800 metres. I looked this afternoon at images of where I grew up. It really is a dismal, grim concrete wall of habitation. It looks, ugly, dirty and hostile and it was. It truly was. My old school Comprehensive has been demolished. It feels really weird and frustrating that my past where I experienced massive negative emotions does not exist anymore. For some reason it makes how I feel even worse because a massive part of my life, my memories no longer physically exists. The flat where he abused me still exists I think, the bungalow I grew up in is still there, but the place I spent most of my time engulfed in deep emotion has gone. I cried tonight because I made a promise not to cut, but I desperately want to feel something else.

Please somebody help me. If I knew what to do I would do it. I really would do it. Whatever I have done wrong, to whoever, I am so sorry, please let me get past this, please take this guttural nausea and ache and tension away. Please, please I will do anything - PLEASE!!

Reflection: It was very difficult to not be able to return to those places I had grown up in. I needed to see those places so it would validate the pain and hurt that I was feeling. When I saw that my old school had been demolished, it was like a large part of what I was feeling then had no substance. I couldn't pin it to anything because it no longer existed. For a long time I would google and look back at where I grew up and grow increasingly frustrated when those places had either been demolished, or regenerated and unrecognisable. The images in my head, needed to pin the real images to them, but they couldn't.

Notes:

14.10.15

I feel calm today. I think my brain is allowing me some rest. I had a good meditation about compassion and tried to carefully steer it towards me. The compassion image was of a little girl, I couldn't quite connect to me, but I left it there. Jason, my cousin, called my mum this afternoon and my anxiety levels have grown. I can't keep avoiding him. Avoidance increases anxiety I read, but that was to do with lifts, planes and driving. Does it equate to sexual abuse? I read about the process of contacting the police and making a statement. Would that give me some peace? I don't know what I am doing any more. I've lost my core. I know what my gut feelings are, but I don't know if they are rational. I just feel like I'm losing my mind. ☹

Reflection: I was beginning to gain some direction again. I couldn't see it, but I was focusing a little bit more. Trying to find answers, trying to work out what to do next. That last but one sentence illustrates that I did know what to do, but I had too much self-doubt to realise it.

Notes:

15.10.15
I feel physically sick tonight. I was retching in the bath. Charlie asked me what was the scariest thing that ever happened to me, even as a child. My anxiety levels are very high. The image in my head, being raped when I was 13. Being taken to a field away from houses, whilst his hands roamed all over my body and he pushed his fingers inside me. His tongue was in my mouth, his breath, his taste. My whole body tense and trapped. I was so trapped. I feel very sick. I feel like I can't breathe. I can feel his hands all over me , I feel so sick.

Reflection: A simple question and it overwhelmed me physically and emotionally. The flashbacks, the memories, the images, they were all vying for my attention, they were still really powerful. This is what thirty five years of suppression amounts to.

Notes:

16.10.15 – First major breakthrough

Saw Jayne today talked about images I had written about in my book. Talked about how my mum dictated every emotion and feeling. So *"You are not hungry", "you are not cold"* etc. I was in the wrong place at the wrong time. Doing what any child would do looking for love. My gut instinct told me all the abuse was wrong, but my gut instinct had been stripped away from me by my mum and my abusers who behaved normally after the abuse, leaving me feeling I was wrong to feel what I did, but also to blame for "allowing" it to happen. In fact I didn't "allow" it. I was a child and I put my trust in adults who led me to what happened and then behaved normally afterwards. My gut feeling was always spot on. My physical reaction was "I froze" I didn't run away, or stop it, because my brain was confused by the normalisation of it all. That man sniggering because I didn't like it, then behaving normally afterwards. My Cousin laughing because I was angry that he was fiddling with me, but I was trapped. That stranger talking nicely to me, so I walked with him, then he mauled and raped me, then asked me to meet him the next day. Not being listened to when I didn't want to be walked home, then being raped. All compounding that my thoughts and feelings don't matter.

Then my ex-husband ignoring me, my feelings and my pain, behaving normally towards me. No wonder I believed I was to blame, but I wasn't! The guilt has gone and I am now seeing it as an adult. God – so much, that's why I feel sick. I am feeling it now as the adult and Jayne explained there is fight, flight and freeze and that is the reason I froze and perceived it that I "allowed" it to happen. Because of how mentally I had been groomed by everybody. How fucking sad!! This is what I meant about making sense of it all. She told me that often physical and emotional responses can conflict with each other. For example, gut feeling of revulsion, but not stopping what's happening. Sympathetic and parasympathetic response. God she's good! I want to learn to trust and act on my gut feeling instead of waiting to deal with how I feel about something afterwards.

Reflection: Jayne is brilliant. I don't think I need to say more than this is what happens when you have a great Counsellor. For the first time ever, something made sense to me. I understood what she meant and I could relate to it completely. For the first time in my life on that day in that counselling room I recognised that what had happened to me was not my fault.

Notes:

17.10.15 – My voice is heard for the first time.

What a massive emotional ride. Elation because I now truly understand and believe I was not responsible for what happened to me. I froze. My true gut feelings stripped away. Now overwhelming terror looking at the adult perspective. The adult that I am. Looking at all that abuse as an adult. No child to hide behind, to focus on blame, shame and guilt. All of that gone now. Anxiety levels very high thinking about living as an adult, taking responsibility. My Cousin appears to be getting closer. He called my mum and I don't have my child to hide behind, but I have to take responsibility as an adult. I had a panic attack in the bath just thinking about it.

But I did it! I text him reminding him what he had done, how it had made me feel all my life and told him I had never forgotten.

I always felt when I saw him that there was "something" unsaid between us, I told him how he was part of something that screwed my whole life up. I told him I didn't want to talk to him because I don't want confrontation. My anxiety levels very high. What's going to happen next? He did text but I didn't read it. I didn't need to. Alan read it and told me he denied it and was not going to contact me again. To me that was validation. Anybody I believe who is accused of sexual abuse, if they didn't do it would not accept any allegation without a fight. Anxiety levels still massively high. What have I done? This is massive, I have made my voice heard.

I dreamt my mum found out and questioned me. "What are you doing?" And in my dream I said "I am tidying up". And then my anxiety levels started to drop. I am having a voice. I am tidying up the shitty mess in my head. I finally have a voice. I took adult responsibility and told him I hated what he did and it contributed to screwing my life up. I feel like an adult. For the first time in my life I feel like an adult. I did a very adult thing. I responded as an adult to something that happened to me as a child. I feel so different. I have always tried to keep myself small. Child-like, not look grown-up, because I have always felt like a child and I don't anymore. For the first time EVER. I feel like an adult.

Reflection: I'm not sure I can add to this. Other than to say that Alan read the text message and deleted it and told me to switch my brain off. I was absolutely elated and I couldn't express it. I was scared, excited and I felt very powerful and very emotionally high. Brilliant from an epiphany perspective, but when I took an acute emotional high, there was only one way that could go and it came down just as hard and just as fast as it went up. This was the start of an incredible journey with huge peaks and troughs.

Notes:

18.10.15

Feeling very uneasy and restless all day today. I did something massive yesterday. The world didn't stop turning, time didn't stop. Everything carried on the same, yet I feel completely different. I feel like I don't know who I am. I am new, different, a weight has lifted, I have had my voice heard. But I feel very shaky inside and very, very vulnerable. When the thoughts of being sexually abused enters my head, I want to scream and cry. So much happened to me, my head won't let it in. I have a tight feeling in the pit of my stomach. I feel as though I am avoiding looking at it because the lump in my gut tells me something big will happen if I do. The picture has become hazy. I can't even write down what happened because I will see it for real. For what it really if and just writing about it makes me want to cry. I don't think I can do this. Help me please. Somebody help, I am panicking. Oh God, I am shaking so badly, I don't want to be on my own. Help!

Reflection: I had spent up until this point viewing the abuse I had been subjected to as a child. Even the rape I was subjected to by my ex-husband I experienced as a child, even though I was an adult. Now, suddenly I was thrown into another camp and I was suddenly experiencing what had happened from the perspective of being an adult. That was what was making me shake. That was what was frightening me so much. I had been ten years old all this time, now I as seeing it through my adult eyes and once again I was experiencing it all for the first time. I was very frightened.

Notes:

19.10.15
Today has been very hard. I just want to sit with my head in my hands. I saw Carol and told her about my cousin and the text message. She asked me how I felt, I said I just wanted to let out a guttural cry because his response made it real. She said it is real and I felt a punch in my stomach. I talked to Alan tonight and started retching. I tried to explain that I have always felt to blame, always felt it was my fault, then upon realising it isn't my fault, wanting to somehow be mistaken. But I'm not and I panic thinking about it. It's like when people are told shocking news and disbelieve what they are told. It is so hard to write this down because I can't comprehend all the sexual abuse that happened to me! I can't deal with this. It is too massive. I am not going to be able to cope. I'm so scared, I can't do it. HELP!

Reflection: Now I was starting to grow up, now I was going to have to do the real work and yes, I was really scared. I hadn't done anything up until that point as a grown up. I had always been that ten year old child. Every experience I had had in my life I had experienced it from the perception of a ten year old child. I felt like I had been catapulted into an adults body and mind and I didn't know how to handle that.

Notes:

20.10.15

I'm feeling very shaky, very vulnerable. The emotion I want to express has to be suppressed because the kids are off school for half term. I saw Carol today, talked about my issue with food, how my mum ate soup and an apple for lunch and dinner for years and still she was fat. So how can I possibly eat normally. I want to and I am going to. I will be what I will be, but at least I will be healthy. I talked about not being able to cope with looking at this as an adult. It's like the page is open on a book and I can't look at it. Then tonight watching television I start to think why hasn't Jason text me to say I'm mistaken, why has he not done that? The thought intruded into my mind and my throat started to get tight and I could feel I was going to retch. Then I wanted to cry. I can't believe what has happened to me. There is so much, I feel if I look at it I might scream, I might become so hysterical that I totally lose control. This is bad news on a huge scale, I can't comprehend and that has caused my anxiety levels to sore. I can't do this, I'm terrified what might happen. Please help me someone, I'm so scared, somebody please hold me, keep me safe.

Reflection: The reality of every that has happened to me was beginning to really kick in. I was really feeling it as the adult I had become and it was very overwhelming. It felt like I was constantly being dealt these blows. Hearing everything for the first time and at times it felt too much. Too much of a mountain to climb.

Notes:

21.10.15
Very difficult day, wanted to cry all day, but kids at home. Felt like screaming. Feeling that I have to face something so painful is so totally overwhelming. I don't want to face it, I don't want to look at what happened to me but I know I am going to have to, to be able to move forward. I don't know if I am strong enough. I don't know. Will this kill me? I tried to talk to Alan, but then I started retching again. I'm in so much pain and so very alone. I can't make my mind calm and peaceful. I have got to face this, but I can't, I'm just not strong enough. I am so worn down I just want it all to stop.

Reflection: I felt very exposed. Like a wound had been ripped open and I was staring into it and there was nobody to put a plaster on it. Only this time there wasn't going to be a plaster. This time the wound was going to be cleared out before it could heal. The pain was unbearable. I felt so trapped.

Notes:

22.10.15
Today my mind has given me a break. I have felt spookily calm. I took the kids to the cinema, I began to cry during the trailers. I don't know why. Twenty minutes in I fell asleep, a voice in my head telling me it was okay to fall asleep, I am safe and around people and for a few minutes I was totally gone. I didn't feel tense or anxious. I feel very down. So down I don't know if anyone can reach me. Tomorrow I get to talk to Jayne.

Reflection: This happened on a number of occasions and I don't know what happens inside. But I would be tormented for many days, I would feel every emotion intently and then occasionally, very occasionally I would wake up and I would feel either numb, or calm. Perhaps you know what was happening during those quiet times.

Notes:

23.10.15
Saw Jayne today explained to her how the penny dropped and how I realised none of what happened was my fault. Explained how Jason had validated the abuse in his denial and refusing to contact me ever again. I became very emotional, over-wrought about having to see what happened as an adult. See it for what it is. She talked to me about dealing with it in manageable chunks. So it's okay to block out parts just until we are ready to deal with it.
I went to see Norpel and I told him my mind is tormented. He explained when you try to protect yourself, your heart becomes stone, but the problem with that is you don't experience any emotion. Once you allow emotions in you can become whole. He said the rush of emotion you feel can be very frightening because you are dealing with such powerful emotion from painful experience. He said *"Don't be scared, don't be afraid of it because it will calm down. Look at it, face it and gradually the intensity will ease"*. He talked to me about how to meditate when there is so much going on in the mind. To count the breaths to 10 and start again. Until eventually the space between the breaths and intrusive thoughts widens. He said it took him 2 years, but it works. He said when they pop up just look at them and say *"It's you again – go away"*. He told me not to be scared, that they will ease and gradually be able to let go. I did feel calmer after talking to Norpel. He said it was okay to be tearful during meditation and said he sometimes gets tearful. He said sitting and meditating in front of a Buddha is a very powerful emotional thing.
I slept for a while this afternoon, just to have a break from the pain. Today has been a painful day. I am hurting so much inside. I told Jayne I am scared to be an adult in case people say I'm getting there when I feel so bad inside. She rubbished the idea of 'getting there'. Where the hell am I supposed to be going? I told her my child had gone now I had realised it wasn't my fault and I felt lost, alone and very scared. She said maybe my child didn't have to go just yet, but she could stay for a while and hold my hand. I like that very much. I have been so alone for most of my life. She is smiling at me now because she is not in pain anymore and she is happy to hold my hand until I am ready to let her go and she can be at peace.
That gives me a very strong inner comfort. I have a hand to hold.

Reflection: I think this entry really explains itself. It explains itself because Jayne was supporting me. She was by my side and responding exactly to the things I was talking about. Norpel did exactly the same. All I had ever wanted was a hand to hold and I felt like I had it in Jayne, Norpel and my little child. Somebody on my side who didn't judge, didn't direct, but just met me at my level, the level I could work from.

Notes:

24.10.15
Numb most of the day, trying to work out what part of my mind hasn't been destroyed. What part of my mind isn't just going through the motions? If I had a broken leg it would heal. Then if in the future I got residual pain I could talk about it. I have been sexually abused and raped in every way imaginable. I am facing it all for the first time now. Alan says *"you will get over it"*. Carol says *"you will get there"*. It's like they are waiting for me to fixed then I can never refer to it again. Tonight when I said this to Alan he said *"Where did that suddenly come from?"* My mind is with me all the time. Just like a healed arthritic arm or leg, that gets commented on. This is why I feel so alone. This is why I am terrified to face it. It's now or never, or now than never. But I can't do that. I can't.
Committing suicide would end the pain. Committing suicide would be me thinking of me, putting me first. Nobody chooses to be in pain. People do anything they can to get rid of pain, so why should I have to not only live with it, but keep it to myself? I have thought about suicide most of my life. I have used it as my comfort blanket, if things get too hard. I want to talk about suicide, explore it, just like other people talk about the best pain relief for them. But I don't want my pain relief to be suicide. I don't know what else it could be. I can't talk about it, I can't take pain relief. What can I do? I am so alone and I feel so down. I don't think I can do this. Please help me. Please somebody hold on to me.

Reflection: I found it very difficult to understand that people expected me to recover from this and never speak about it again. I have since learned that I can talk about it whenever I want to. Even if the receiver doesn't want to hear it. I don't have to be silenced by anybody, but back then I believed I did. I believed I could only talk when permitted and then not again. I wanted to recover, but I didn't want to recover enough so that I wasn't allowed to speak about it again. I put myself under a lot of pressure, but only because I still didn't understand.
Suicide had very much been my comfort blanket for a long time. My 'go to' should the going get too tough. Because it was all I had, I didn't have any other coping mechanism. I believed it was my only pain relief because I still hadn't recognised that I can talk whenever I want to. My soul still belonged to everybody else and their needs.

Notes:

25.10.15

A lot of the time I want somebody to talk to me to ask me how I am, just so I can talk. Talk about the fear of suicidal thoughts, talk through the fear of getting through day to day. I wish my mind was calm and peaceful. Alan said it was good to see me get into my reading again. I have dragged my mind back to my Kindle just like I did at the start, because I don't trust myself to be alone with my thoughts. Norpel said *"Don't be afraid"*, but I am very afraid. I just want to get the kids to school tomorrow so I can call the Samaritans and talk about how desperate I am feeling. How I feel like I don't belong on this earth. Alan, my children, they fit so happily into their life and I'm on the outside and I am trying to get in, but I can't, I keep trying, but I have this constant tension around me and in my head and I can't shake it off. I want it to go away. I want to be at peace.

Please somebody, please!

Reflection: I was talking about peace in terms of suicide. My fear came from being inquisitive that actually I might recover, there might be something else beyond my torment. I was beginning to reach out. My fear was if I did it and yet there might be a better life for me. My fear was good for keeping me alive. Jayne had made me feel inquisitive about life. Those last three words. I was reaching out again. It was a good sign, I just couldn't see it because it was absolute torment.

Notes:

26.10.15
I broke down tonight. I talked to Alan. I told him I am too afraid to face up to all the abuse because I will have nothing left of me. I told him that suicide was always my option if I had to admit I have been totally physically and emotionally destroyed. Alan was brilliant and he helped me to look at what had got me where I am today despite all the abuse. It turns out I have always had my spirit. I have never lost my care and compassion. I have never lost my determination. I didn't learn anything at school, but I was determined to achieve and I did. I achieved 'A' Levels, a diploma, a degree and I'm now working towards a Master's Degree. I am intelligent after all! I was determined to become a Mum and I did it with my first born, who transformed my life. I was determined to meet and marry and expand my family and I have. Nobody has destroyed my spirit. I am determined to work through this and get back to work, get my soul back, get me back and live my life fully. Sadly I have been determined to hold on to suicidal thoughts and now I am determined to let it go. Suicidal thoughts hold me back. I want to learn to deal with pain in a more positive way. I want a life and I want me back and panic attacks, or no panic attacks, I am going to face this now head on. I refuse to be scared of a memory any more.

Reflection: Reaching out more, determination kicking in. Another good sign.

Notes:

27.10.15

That didn't last long. I had counselling at AMICA today. Told her events leading up until now. I couldn't hang on to my self-belief. I talked about cutting myself and suicidal thoughts. I talked about how I didn't want to have suicidal thoughts anymore, but explained that I'd made a pact with myself that if I was ever raped I would kill myself because there was nothing of me left not violated. She asked me to visualise what I thought would happen if I face it. I said I'm frightened of what I might do because it's too big. When I drove home I had a panic attack and when I got home I thought I was going to faint. I messaged Carol and Daryl that I had urges to cut myself. I called the Samaritans. The person on the 'phone helped me to understand what I am feeling. She said I had spent a long time viewing this as a child who had allowed it to happen, guilty and self-loathing. I only understood less than 2 weeks ago that that isn't true. Was never true. She said viewing now as an adult for what it actually was after 35 years is looking at it for the first time and seeing the truly awful abuse it was. She said if I had realised at the time it was wrong, then I wouldn't have gotten over it in 2 weeks. And she said that I'm not going to come to terms with abuse spanning 16 years in 2 weeks. She said I was right at the beginning and it would take time. I wish I could have hugged her down the 'phone. She understood exactly how I am feeling. I understand now why I feel frightened. Because I am so frightened, I know the memory can't hurt me, but the realisation is very painful, overwhelming and frightening. I feel like I am going mad. She told me not to hurt myself, but to look after myself. I am trying to look after myself, but feel guilty all the time because I think people expect more of me. I am going to try really hard to accept myself, look after myself and be kind to my hurting mind. I can't help being overwhelmed by it, so I will try and accept it. Not accepting it will not make it go away. But I can make it easier by accepting it. My throat feels so tight.

Reflection: I wish I knew who that person was who spoke to me on the 'phone. She was another person who could step into my emotions, understand what I was saying from my perspective and make things make absolute sense. Thank you unknown person, you will never know it but you made an incredible impact on me.
Still holding me back though was my constant reference to other people and my perception of what they expected of me.

Notes:

28.10.15
Saw GP today. He is not happy that I have rejected the idea of anti-depressants and the idea of a psychiatrist when I talked about troubling images. I was very anxious when I arrived home. Why do I feel like this? Very, very panicky. I called the Samaritans, Jennifer was so kind. She said it wasn't uncommon to feel overwhelmed, particularly as there has been a shift in focus from child perception to adult. She told me I was very brave to call, to keep talking. She said I was a super woman to have come through all that and get married and have 3 children. That made me feel good. I talked about the urge I have to cut myself when I feel wrong for feeling a certain way. She told me it wasn't wrong and many people find it to be a useful way of coping, but it is addictive. I explained I have been anorexic in the past and that I have an addictive personality and I would cut to cope, rather than look for positive coping strategies. She praised me for my intellect and analytical abilities. That made me feel better too. She asked me about suicidal thoughts and I told her it frightened me because sometimes I think it would be less trouble for everybody if I was no longer here. She said that wouldn't be the case and said she doesn't want me to die. How lovely for somebody who doesn't even know me to say that. She helped me to feel less afraid, but made me realise I need to believe in me and not worry about how I feel or how other people think I should feel.
I want self-belief. It is so hard to just go through the motions of the day. I get up, get the kids sorted and to school, go on my exercise bike, have a shower, lunch, meditate, get kids, do dinner, when every sinew in my body wants to be curled up in a ball and I want to put my head down and hide. Every single day.
I talked about Jason and what happened and said not only did he do what he did, which violated a boundary, but he is my Cousin, FAMILY!! No wonder I am so fucked up. Jennifer told me I can call the Samaritans any time to talk through how I feel and that has taken the pressure off my head. Knowing when the images become too distressing, I can call and I don't have to wait for my counselling appointment. I might feel like I am losing my mind, but I'm not. I believe what the Samaritans have told me. I'm common in my thinking and that is reassuring enough not to make me think I am falling apart. At least not today. Also realised this surge of emotion is a rebound from the kids being off at half term. Just like the summer holidays and when they went back to school.

Reflection: Another amazing person who spoke to me on my level. It's incredible that the most simple conversations are the most healing. I'm not saying the conversation Jennifer had with me was easy in any sense, but she talked to me about my feelings and normalised the conversation. Again she didn't judge, direct, or put me under any pressure at all. She simply had a conversation and because she did that I could open up more because she made me feel safe, normal and not going mad. Although deep down I knew I wasn't, but my thoughts were a little 'out there' even for me in my vulnerable state. Because Jennifer gave no hint that the conversation was in anyway difficult, I could talk my feelings through and even find some answers myself.

Notes:

29.10.15

I had a nightmare last night. I took the kids to see an acrobatic performer at the seaside. He was stood on his hands with his penis hanging out. Why? Why do I have to have constant nightmares about this? When will my head be left alone? Today my brain gave me a rest. I watched a You Tube video with Tara Brach which looked at exploring who you really are inside. When external influences and emotions cause us to behave in a particular manner, stop and look into them to who we really are and not what society and experiences groom us to be. It actually made me feel so very peaceful, more peaceful than I can ever remember. I was almost falling asleep. I fell asleep again this evening so I am going to practice just looking right into my sprit as I fall asleep to find that peaceful place again. Today was a truly peaceful day and a day that re-affirmed I should not only believe in myself, but to be confident believing in myself irrespective of what anybody else's opinion of me might be.

Reflection: What's this? Looks like a bit of healing and insight to me.

Notes:

30.10.15

Saw Jayne today. Talked about the week. Told her my mind is numb and I have to read my notes to prompt me. She thinks I'm in denial. I do too. I want to feel safe before I start talking about what happened. I need to feel safe in myself. I decided to go and do a bit of Christmas shopping after my appointment. I was looking for slippers for my Dad. I saw a pair of Moccasins and I was right back there in his living room. I felt dizzy, but I was meeting Alan so I was distracted by his chatter. After I got home I look online for Christmas presents. I looked for slippers for my Dad. More moccasins. My chest felt tight. I had to leave to go to school. I felt dizzy, my chest felt tight and I was right there in that living room again. With him and his family. A parent in the school playground approached me, she said I appeared to be miles away. We talked and I could feel the tremble in my voice, I felt weak and I wanted to cry. I felt very subdued and as the evening went on, I felt lower and lower. I felt okay this morning. The impact I keep saying is massive. Moccasin slippers brought on such a powerful response. I am so frightened. This feels too big. Just writing this I am getting a tickle in my throat. This hurts so much and feels endless. Alan said he was worried because I was biting my lip tonight. He says that's when I appear troubled, but he didn't ask me, so I didn't tell him in case he says *"Where has that suddenly come from?"*

I want this to go away more than ever, but slippers for goodness sake. If I can't cope with slippers how am I ever going to cope with this!

Reflection: So, this particular style of slippers are the same as Jack wore. So when I saw the slippers I was catapulted back to the flat and sitting in the living room where Jack sexually abused me.

In relation to the notes I wrote. I bought a note book because when I went to see Jayne I couldn't think of what to say that was on any deep level that was troubling me. My mind would go blank. So what I did, was I bought a notebook and when a thought came in I would write it down. When I referred to the book when I saw Jayne, I could recall the emotion, or the flashback, or the memory. It was like I was catching it before it hid away inside me. Really, the only way I can describe this is like a little demon would attack me, frighten me, torment me and as soon as I was able to talk about it, it would hide. It would even squeeze my throat so I couldn't talk about it. An incredible physical response when I reflect on it, but it happened a lot. My throat would either become tight, or I would get a tickle and I couldn't talk. I felt processed by this evil demon inside me. It was controlling everything about me.

Notes:

31.10.15
Spent the afternoon with Rachel and Melvyn. It was great to talk about what happened over the past 2 weeks. I also realised again how much self-doubt I have and my default to blame myself. Two things I am going to work on. I felt very panicky in the evening and I don't know why. I hate feeling panicky inside. I wanted a glass of wine to relax, but I found it only makes me more anxious. This reminds me of when I drank so heavily after I separated from my ex-husband. I drank to blot the abuse out. What actually happened was the abuse became crystal clear and the rest of my life became a fog. Just like the anti-depressants the GP prescribed a couple of months ago.

Reflection: I drank very heavily when I was growing up. I began to drink alcohol when I was about 12 years old and I would drink before school. My friend Karen would call for me and fill an old medicine bottle with Martini and I found that after I had drunk it, I would feel a little lighter inside and my head would feel floaty. I enjoyed that feeling. When I was being raped by my ex-husband I would drink myself into oblivion to block out as much pain as possible and then later I was using it in an attempt to kill myself. I would drink a bottle of wine, washed down with vodkas and anything else I could get down my throat before I passed out, hopefully for good. When I drank to block out the rape after my ex-husband left, it blocked everything out except the flashbacks and they became very vivid and very aggressive. When the GP prescribed me Sertraline it had exactly the same effect. The world became a blur and the flashbacks intensified and became very clear.

Notes:

01.11.15

Felt very anxious all day today. I don't consciously know why. I hate feeling anxious about everything. I can't stop it, but it compounds everything, consumes me. I feel paralysed. Paralysed with a fear I know not what of . Met with Carol for Meditation tonight. It wasn't on. It starts next week. We went for a coffee. It was good to talk again and hear her news. When I left her I felt panicky, very panicky about my job. I just want to be. I just want to roll with the waves. I am sick of living everything twice. Once in my head and then again in real life. The stress I feel is enormous. I'm so frustrated, I just want to take life as it comes. I just want to live in the day. Please, please let my mind relax. Whatever I have done wrong in a previous life I am sincerely sorry. I really am. Please give me some peace.

Reflection: What I am describing here is severe anxiety. What I would do was anticipate every single action and play it out in my head. But not only every action, I would play out every day. I would anticipate all the different variables, how things might turn out and what the alternatives might be. It was so exhausting. I was living every day twice. Once in my head and then in real time. The panic came from the what ifs. It was very exhausting, but once again I have written the answer. I just didn't know how to get there.

Notes:

02.11.15
Alan has gone away until Thursday. That's 4 days away. I took him to town, stayed for a while. Went to my mums, then had to pick up a prescription for my Son. Daryl came in the evening to discuss a problem with bullying. All in all a very busy day. No time to think about anything, but all the time a nagging feeling in the pit of my stomach.

Reflection: It was a relief when Alan went away. I didn't have to pretend. I didn't have to be 'normal'. I could just be quiet, I could be calm and allow my thoughts to settle.

Notes:

03.11.15
I slept well last night. Kept busy again today, my mum and dad called over at 5pm and stayed until 7.30pm. Watched TV with the kids, then bed. Eizabeth was with me last night and tonight in bed. Still a nagging feeling in the pit of my stomach. Suddenly felt very low this evening and like I wanted to cry. I feel like nothing fits any more. I don't know what I am feeling or thinking. I am just trying to stay okay whilst I am on my own with the kids. I saw a programme advertised that wanted to explore rape last night and I turned the channel over so quickly I was panicking and shaking. I feel like there is a volcano inside me. It's rumbling and when I let my guard down its' going to explode. This feels endless, it's like something is coming, but I don't know when. I wish I was okay. I just want to be okay, but I am frightened because I don't know who I am any more.

Reflection: I felt like I was in limbo. I no longer belonged to the victim, because I knew it wasn't my fault any more. I was no longer the 10 year old child. But I had been catapulted to an adult and I didn't know what to do, or how to do it. Not only that, but the enormity of taking responsibility for processing this as an adult was feeling too much. I had lost my security blanket.

Notes:

04.11.15

Kept myself busy all day washing, ironing and watching the TV. Have to keep going, can't stop, must banish all thoughts. Then tonight started biting my lip. Bit it hard because I am so anxious, so very anxious. Why did it have to happen to me?

Reflection: Now of course avoiding thoughts is not the healthiest way to deal with something. You can't deal with something by avoiding it, but I didn't know what was coming and I was on my own, so I did the next best thing. I avoided it until I knew it was safe to let it, whatever it was, out. So I'll take that entry as a positive on reflection.

Notes:

05.11.15
Kept busy again today. Blocking out all thoughts except those that are caring and self-nurturing. I turned the heat down on my hairdryer so I didn't burn my head. I took tablets for a headache and lay down to try and relieve it. I haven't been on my bike for a week now because I have a pain in my back, hip and legs. Trying to ease the pain by resting it. Alan home tonight. He thinks I'm on drugs I am so calm. All week I have been trying to be mindful of me and look after me. I really like it too. Tomorrow I will talk a bit more. I just need to be sure that I am safe before I talk. Make sure I can cope with what I unravel. Tonight as every night this week I will take me into a dream. A dream where I want to go. A place that makes me feel safe and happy.

Reflection: I had started meditating myself to sleep. That's what I meant by taking me into a dream. Falling asleep during meditation is incredibly uplifting. I would recommend it to anybody. My meditation techniques were clearly beginning to work as Alan believed I was on drugs, I was that calm. Thanks Norpel, meditation is the best drug I've ever taken.

Notes:

06.11.15 He really isn't interested.

I spoke to Jayne today. We talked about her seeing me twice a week and she suggested I may hang on to emotions, rather than cope if I see her more often. She is right. Just like cutting. I would cut instead of cope, so yes I would hang on instead and look for coping strategies. Shitty, shit, shit. I have realised that by coping whilst Alan was away the rebound reaction is going to hit and hit hard. Now Tuesdays counselling offer has gone, that terrifies me. Alan said I looked sad, he blew me a kiss as he carried on watching whatever on his tablet. He later said I looked sad, so I told him what we had been talking about in counselling. He then kissed me on the head and left the room. He came back in and started playing with a football with Elizabeth. I thought when she went to bed he would ask me, but no. He gave me wine. He knows it's my weak spot, I told him last week I drink to feel different, but it doesn't make me feel good different. It didn't tonight either. We watched tele, he fell asleep and is asleep in bed now. I feel so disconnected from him. So sad, so unloved and uncared for. He says he loves me, but saying it is easy. I feel like nobody truly cares. It's all conditional. No - my kids love me unconditionally, but they have their own lives. I felt so alone when I was abused, molested, raped, so alone with all the dreadful feelings. That's still how I feel. I talked about how I truly cared for myself this week. I rested from my bike because my back was hurting. I took painkillers for my headache. I even turned the temperature down on the hairdryer so I didn't burn my head. I recognise I need to be kind to myself, I should never have hurt myself all this time. I need to feel safe in myself to be able to talk and Jayne understands that too. But I feel so very, very alone and I have never ever gotten used to that ever since my sister died. That loneliness has stayed with me. She loved me unconditionally. Now nobody does.
My children do not walk alongside me, nor should they. The hardest part is people being with me because *they* want to be, but when they have had enough they back off. Just like Carol, Daryl, Melvyn and Alan have done. And I am on my own with me. Alone, I feel so sad and so very, very alone.

Reflection: It did feel sad to think all of those people backed away. But they backed away because they were wrong for me and not because I was wrong for them. I didn't realise it at the time and I didn't for a long time after, but I was developing a sense of me and with Jayne's encouragement I stuck with it, but it was hard. It was hard to lose the abusers, they were all I had ever had. But I didn't want the abuse any more.

Notes:

07.11.15
Felt very tearful today. Explained to Alan how I felt sad that he didn't talk to me anymore. He apologised then went out to football. He took us all out for dinner tonight.
I have never felt so lonely in my life.

Reflection: I'll give myself a pat on the back for being honest with him, even though I felt lonely. He didn't have an honest bone in his body I was later to discover.

Notes:

08.11.15
Woke late we all went swimming. Alan paid and paid for a drink afterwards. Carol text to say she wasn't coming to meditation due to bad weather, long weekend and work tomorrow. I asked her if she was really okay. She replied *"busy and tired"*. Now here's the thing. I went into meltdown and started crying. It's all about me. I trusted her, told her such personal intimate stuff and I feel she has taken it away. Then something kicked in. There is nothing wrong with me trusting her and confiding in her. If she is avoiding me then it's about her, not me. I have done nothing wrong and have nothing to feel bad about. I was tearful this morning. It is remembrance Sunday and my Sister's birthday. Nothing odd about that, except I had a true emotional gut feeling. Nothing I have experienced before, so I allowed it to happen. It only lasted a few minutes and I felt compassion towards my mum. I went to meditation tonight. Norpel talked about painful emotion and how it can feel like a tsunami. He said it's okay to accept our own suffering, because the intensity won't last. That had me in tears. Also he talked about our minds being like a lake and when the water is calm, we can see clearly to the bottom and all the slurry, but when the water becomes turbulent we can't see because the water becomes foggy and the bottom of the lake gets churned up and we can't see properly, just like our mind being turbulent and we can't think properly. To calm the mind is like calming the waters. As it calms we can begin to see clearly again and then we can see what needs to be cleared up. Tonight I feel a real connection with what Norpel was saying. Carol did me a favour. Not coming made me panic. I wouldn't be able to get her take on things. I have realised I have to have my own take on things in order to clear up the mess in my mind. That's why I have been so frightened, frightened to accept, acknowledge or even recognise my very own personal feelings. I have to be true to myself. Connect with myself and I feel I am beginning to recognise what those feelings are and I understand now why I am so tearful, because what happened to me was so very, very sad. Alan asked me if I wanted to talk tonight so I did.

Reflection: It's so lovely to see me beginning to work stuff out for myself by myself. Even though I still felt wretched.

Notes:

09.11.15
I slept badly last night because Alan didn't and he kept disturbing me. But today was a good day. A proper good day all round. I got up, showered, got ready, took the kids to school. I went to in to town with Alan and we looked at Christmas stuff for the kids. He bought me coffee. He went to work for an hour whilst I had my eyebrows waxed and bought some stuff for my face. More looking after myself. Then he met me, took me for lunch and we came home just before getting the kids from school. I felt cared for, looked after, loved. Alan actually wanted to be with me. I don't remember a good day without anxiety of some sort in like forever. I got a bit wound up because I couldn't find a poppy for Charlie, but then the school receptionist had a spare one that she gave to me. Today was a good day I am in bed now feeling slightly apprehensive about tomorrow, but I am going to contain that by falling asleep during a meditation and I am going to take somebody into my dream with me. I have started doing this last week and it really works. I take the kids into my dream with me and we do something nice and then I am gone. Fingers crossed for tonight. Goodnight 😊 I am going to sleep with a warm feeling in my heart and my gut.

Reflection: Another good day, not much more to say, except I am still looking to be loved in order to make myself feel good and I did do that for a good while longer. But the meditation was all me, by me and for me, so I'll accept baby steps.

Notes:

10.11.15

I kept a bit busy today, I think I was scared to be on my own, but I was okay in the end. I raked up the leaves in the garden for a couple of hours and allowed my thoughts to intrude. I reflected on Sundays meditation thinking hard about not being afraid of the surge of emotions. I do feel calmer, the thoughts and how I feel is horrible, but I am not panicking. I thought about Carol and how she did me a favour in the end on Sunday. She made me think about how I truly feel about everything and for me to be able to move forward I have to talk truly about how I feel, I can't use her as a buffer to my deepest emotions. So I text Jayne and I told her I was ready to begin talking when I see her next. Then for the rest of the day I felt very subdued and my throat was hurting because it was very tight. My throat has gone tight again now just writing about it. But I have to do this, because I don't want this to dominate my thoughts like it has done for the past three months and dictated how my personality has developed over the past 35 years. I don't want it to catch me off guard and shock me ever again.

Reflection: I was beginning to develop some resilience.

Notes:

11.11.15

Starting to feel anxious about Friday, but that's okay. I will feel anxious because it's difficult to talk about. I am doing different exercises to try and get my tummy smaller (body image). I looked after myself this afternoon. My legs are really hurting so I got myself a few biscuits and my cuddle blanket and curled up on the settee to watch television. My mum came over and that was okay. I'd had an hour to myself after Alan went out and I was beginning to feel a bit wobbly about Friday. She, (my mum) needed to talk about my Dad and that was okay, it distracted me and she came to school and the kids liked that. I messaged Melvyn about how I am going to deal with things and I had a very positive response. That made me feel good. "Recover", I like that word. Jayne had talked to me about going back to work. I said I didn't like the word 'better', or 'getting there'. We decided on 'together' or 'whole', but I like recover. When I go back to work it will be because I have recovered, from my breakdown, from the torment the abuse held over me since I was 10 years old. 'Better' suggests I have improved because I was not as good before. Recovered means I have returned to a normal state of mind and regained possession of something stolen and lost. That suits me, because that describes to me what has happened. My body and mind have been both lost and stolen and I am getting them back. I saw Joelle last night and I didn't talk about any of this because it is personal to me. My stuff, my recovery.

Reflection: I appeared to be getting a lot stronger quite quickly and reconnecting with my thoughts and feelings.

Notes:

12.11.15

I dreamt about looking for a new house last night, it was a really lovely dream. I am feeling nervous about tomorrow, but it's okay. It feels good to be able to feel anxious without panicking, to need to talk to someone to make it go away. I know why I am anxious and without predicting what might happen if I cry it's okay because I am expressing and allowing my true emotions to be expressed. I have permission to do it. I give myself permission to do it, so I will. I have not done my exercise today because my legs are hurting and I need to let them recover.

My appointment tomorrow got cancelled this afternoon. Nobody can imagine the intensity of emotion that throws up. Allowing painful memories to come to the surface ready to talk about, then another week has to pass. Containing that is so hard. My mind used everything it had to rationalise. There is nothing I can do, but wait until next week. My body though is behaving differently. Panic, tension, biting my lip, but it's okay. I have to own this to be able to deal with it. I can't keep being rescued to buffer how I feel. But this is hard, allowing painful memories to come to the surface ready to talk. This is so hard. I know I can't do anything about it until next week. I have to look after myself, cry if I want to. I will call the Samaritans if I need to. But I have to feel this pain to be able to learn to manage it. I don't want to hurt myself, I want to look after myself. I don't want to offload my emotion, but I need help to manage it.

Okay, I don't need to panic. Take one day at a time. Allow emotions to flow and look after myself. Not to be hard on myself. I will do what I need to, to help me cope. I was thinking about my new exercises and that actually made me feel calmer. Focus on positives, that's what I need to do, because there is nothing I can do until next week. Focus on myself and care for myself. The harder it feels, the more I will care for myself.

Reflection: This was the most difficult day ever. My Counselling appointment had been cancelled and I had let the emotions, the flashbacks, the memories all bubble to the surface, I had psyched myself up to let it all out and suddenly that opportunity was gone. I was devastated. I didn't know how to hold on for another week. The emotions were up and I didn't know how to squash them back down for another week. I was seriously panicked.

Notes:

13.11.15

Last night was distressing. It was a bad night. The recovering side of my mind was saying *"it's you again negative thoughts, go away"*. Norpel talked about looking at emotional pain and choosing time to just look at it, hold it, or send it away. I kept trying to reason with myself. There is nothing I can do until next Friday. My time will come to talk, I can spend time looking after myself. Box my feelings, recognise they are there until it's time to let them out. The damaged side of my mind was telling me "next Friday is too far away. I have allowed my emotions out of the box, they won't go back in, next Friday is too long to wait, cut yourself one more time to make yourself feel better, give yourself a lift to help you get through to next week." The damaged side of my mind is still so much bigger and I knew cutting would make me feel so much better, but a tiny voice was saying *"no"*. God I was tormented. I lay in bed with my eyes closed tight, I have a small teddy and I had hold of it and rubbed it's ear and rubbed and rubbed, trying to focus on the ear until I fell asleep. I was panicking so much, I was so afraid I would give in before I fell asleep, but sleep came and I don't remember going.

Why did this happen? Because I was already feeling stressed and I had a glass of wine. A couple of weeks ago I told Alan, even though I only have one or two glasses on a Friday, I was looking to it to make me feel better, but it wasn't, it was making me feel how it did before, more focused on what's on my mind. I told him I didn't want to drink any more. At least not whilst I feel like this.

Last night he told me to pour us some wine and my resolve being low, I did. I was desperate to feel relaxed. Just to feel some distance between me and my mind. But of course it didn't work. Today I felt like I had been run over by a bus. I feel so tense, tearful, heart palpitations. I don't have enough reserves to hold on to. Next Friday feels such a long way away. I am desperate, I am so lonely, why won't my mind do what I want it to do? I can't change anything. I know I have to wait, but my body won't relax. I am trying so hard through meditation and positive thinking, I am trying so hard. I feel like a huge war is raging inside me. I know I want peace, to face my fears, to recover, but a huge part of me wants a quick fix. Cut, drink, get off my face, just get away from all of it. End it all now because I can't live with this torment.

No! No! No! I hate these thoughts. I HATE THEM. I NEED HELP!!! IF EVER I NEEDED HELP IT'S NOW!!!

Reflection: Okay, so now you get the picture, it was hard! I don't think I can reflect any better than the original journal entry for that day. I'm sure there could be a lesson learned here somewhere. I have always stored things up until I feel ready to talk, but when I'm ready, I am literally about to burst. Not the best strategy.

Notes:

14.11.15

I woke up panicking and then heard there had been an atrocity overnight in Paris. It shook me out of it for a while. I took my mum Christmas shopping and at times during the day just wanted to run home. I messaged Carol to ask if she was going to meditation tomorrow, she replied that she's going to a concert. I feel let down. Did she not feel the need to tell me? She asked me how I am, I told her, no reply. I feel terrible and I don't want to. I opened up to Carol, trusted her, talked to her. She has been a massive support, then gone. I don't want to make myself vulnerable to her, but she asks how I am and then I tell her, then nothing. I don't understand. I feel anxious and vulnerable. I'm not pathetic, but I trusted her, now I feel she has just walked away. Picked me up, then dropped me. A very, very bitter pill to swallow. My chest is tight, I am panicking. I hate feeling like this, I can't make it stop. I think something bad is going to happen. I'm really scared.

Reflection: I can see this now as panic because Jayne wasn't available and Carol had gone. I felt very vulnerable and alone, but also vulnerable because I had exposed my deepest feelings and I felt they had been taken away by Carol. I know now that I don't share anything with anybody unless I am okay to take responsibility for my own feelings. If I'm not, then I hold my own counsel. But that is now and was most definitely not then.

Notes:

15.11.15
I woke feeling tormented. I can't wait until Friday. I am going to go out of my mind. I went to meditation on my own again tonight. No tears, positive. I had a good meditation, I managed not only to clear my mind, but lost all sense of my body too. I felt as though I was going to fall. Norpel talked about clarity of mind. The blue sky, lake, even fish tank when explaining how to calm the mind. I still like the lake analogy. I held it all the way home. A short respite from torment. I don't know what to do. My emotions are fierce and I have contained them all weekend. I feel as if my mind will explode. Too much, much too much.

Reflection: The pressure inside me was immense. I thought I was going to have a stroke. I had forgotten I could have rung the Samaritans to get some release. I could have rung any helpline, but I was heavily relying on those I had come to trust.

Notes:

16.11.15
It is so hard to write tonight, my mind is tortured. I saw Dr Beckley today. I told her that now I have allowed my emotions to the surface, the urge to self-harm is so intense. She said it will get more powerful because my emotions are more powerful. She said I had to be strong. Dig deep (my words, not hers) and use everything I have to keep myself safe. I got home, I cried, distracted myself all day and on occasion it surged so strong. I was drying the knife after I'd washed up and thought *"just do it"*. I was lying on the bed and thought *"just do it"*. The urge surging through my body was enormous. I have a headache. Dr Beckley said it will be okay. I will get through it, but if feel trapped. Trapped in a mind of torment. I really need help.

Reflection: Dr Beckley made perfect sense, I just didn't know what to do. Look at the strength I had by not self-harming. Brilliant!

Notes:

17.11.15

Had nightmares last night. I was being told I as worthless, pathetic, not good enough to be loved unconditionally. Woke up this morning feeling all of those things. The urge to cut myself is so high. All those who sexually abused me gave me attention, but being abused didn't give me unconditional love, they took my body, gave me attention then left me, or abused me more violently. My Mum and Dad never gave me unconditional love. I was never good enough for anybody, not even Alan. He didn't want to marry me and I begged him. How humiliating and pathetic is that. My deluded mind is telling me I am worthless, but my recovering mind is trying so hard to keep me safe, but it is so new and this is so hard. Today came and went with waves of despair. I feel like shit. I look like shit, but I have to if I am to recover. I just don't know if I am strong enough. Jayne text me a reassuring message this evening as I have been texting her these thoughts. 3 days to go.

Reflection: I can still feel that pressure as I reflect on that incredible week. Obviously I was stronger than I believed. Something inside me on an unconscious level was keeping me safe.

Notes:

18.11.15

Today has been hard. Alan worked from home so I couldn't relax. I went for a walk and had to sit down to fend off tears. I slept for an hour, just to have a break from it all. Then the urge to cut became stronger and stronger, for my mind cannot cope with feeling this bad. I wanted to call the Samaritans but Alan was working and the kids were still awake. I messaged Rachel and we messaged for about an hour. It calmed me down and I felt absolutely shattered afterwards. I always do. I have an appointment with Amica tomorrow. My last appointment, I don't think I can cope any longer. I have buried these feelings for 35 years and felt bad. Now they are not buried and are unmanageable. I can't live with them. I can't cope, I am trying so hard to fight this urge to cut, but it has to go soon, because I really can't cope and I don't want to let anybody down. Ever! I don't want anybody to be disappointed in me. Ever! I need help. I really need help. COME ON!!!

Reflection: My shoulders are tight just reading this. But I didn't break.

Notes:

19.11.15

Saw Kate at Amica. She thinks I need medication. I felt so weak, I called the surgery for a telephone appointment. I went and sat in my car. I thought 'fuck this' I have been raped and sexually abused, I have been suicidal in the past, I am not re-traumatising myself, I am not here to live it all again. I am here to clear it away so I can get on with my life. I rang and cancelled the Doctor. I cried and cried when it dawned on me that I have done all this before. Now is the time to say bye bye. I don't want to talk to people any more to diffuse it. It's time to accept what happened in the sense that I can't make it all go away. I have to learn not to let it dictate my future. I am so tired.

Reflection: That comment from Kate made me feel like she had stopped believing in my ability to deal with this myself. I'm not saying there is anything wrong with medication, but for me and my situation I didn't want anything to mask what I was going through. I wanted it dealt with and cleared out completely. I didn't want anything to linger inside me so that it could overwhelm me again. I was determined to do this. Her lack of faith in me gave me the nudge I needed. The determination. How dare she not believe in me.

Notes:

20.11.15
I saw Jayne this morning. She'd had a family bereavement and was in intensive care all night. Her relative died on Friday morning. I felt so sad for her. I told her everything that has happened over the last 2 weeks. I began by telling her about my birth. I was born the week before Christmas, in an ambulance under an angel attached to a street light. The story has been told to me many times. The ambulance driver wasn't keen to wrap me in his jacket seeing me covered in gunk and neither was my Mother. She and the ambulance driver left me naked and by the time I arrived at the hospital I was blue, put in an incubator and placed wrapped in blankets to warm up. The Doctors told my Mother to have me christened because they believed I was going to die. They asked my Mum to name me, but she wouldn't because she had wanted a boy and said she couldn't think of a name. The nurse looking after me was called Anne. So I was christened Anne. Paula came later after my Auntie Wendy. (Her name is actually Paula Wendy).
My Sister had Spina Bifida and she was a year older than me. Stephanie was her name, but everyone called her Stevie in the family. She was the other half of me. She was just everything to me. I would help her out of bed and on to the potty in the middle of the night, then I would empty the potty in the toilet. I can remember that. I remember also the week before she died, we pledged to be friends no matter what. But the day she died she got angry with me because I told my Mother that she felt unwell. She went to sleep on the settee and never woke up again.
I opened the door to my mother and father when they returned from the hospital. My Mother told me *"Stevie's died"*. I cried so hard I thought my heart would rip. I wasn't allowed to go to the funeral afterwards, instead I was sent to a relatives and my Mum and Dad left me. I have never felt so alone in my life. My sister died, my Mum and Dad gone. I didn't know when they were coming back. Whey they eventually returned to take me home, everything had gone. They had decorated our bedroom and they never spoke to me about her. Half of me had gone. I had an emptiness inside, a hole where something had been before. I was lost. I was seven years old. The attention went. I was told nothing was special any more. It wasn't the last time she said this to me. I wandered and roamed, empty inside. My Mother and Father would go out and leave me at home by myself. I was so frightened. I was too frightened to go to the toilet. They would come home very drunk and have very violent arguments. I had never been so scared, so lonely in my life. Everything changed when Stevie died.
When I was 10 years old I was out playing in the car park near my house. A couple were sat on the grass in the sun with their baby. Jack and Emily and their baby Sarah-Jayne. I started to play with the baby and talk to Jack and Emily and before long my whole world was transformed. I would go round whenever I possibly could, take Sarah-Jayne out in the pram to get her to sleep, even carry her upstairs and put her in her cot. I stayed over at weekends, helped feed and get Sarah-Jayne ready for bed, they took me swimming, I stayed for Sunday dinner, they even took me to London to say with relative. I felt complete again. I belonged.
One day I went to Emily and Sarah-Jayne were in bed. I sat with Jack in the living room, he was sat opposite me, sat wearing a dressing gown. He had his legs open and he asked me if I could see. I leaned forward to look at the tele and told him the

arm of the char was in the way. He said "you know what I mean". He came and sat next to me. He told me to look. I said I didn't want to, but he put his arm around my shoulder and insisted I look. I looked quickly and looked away. He laughed and tickled my stomach. He commented on me being ticklish and moved his hand down until he was tickling me between my legs. I told him I didn't want to play, but he carried on with his fingers in my knickers. I got up and told him I was going home. He laughed. Nothing happened for a while and I thought I must have been mistaken. Then both Emily and Sarah-Jayne went for a sleep. Emily was pregnant. Jack told me we were going to play the tickling game and I had to tickle him where he tickled me. He started off tickling my stomach and then his hand moved down like before. He had his legs apart and his flies open. He said I had to tickle him exactly where he was tickling me. I told him I didn't want to touch him, I told him I didn't want to pay anymore. He carried on sexually abusing me until I told him I had to go home. He laughed, I ran all the way home and was told off by my mother because she had told me not to go away. I felt I'd been so bad, so naughty. My Mum and Dad didn't want me and now they didn't want me either.

I was so frightened, I was shaking, I was so upset. I was terrified he was going to come to the house and get me. I stopped sleeping, I stopped learning. I had, up until then been so bright at school. I started drinking before school, a friend would bring it round. He took everything away from me. A family, belonging, love. I was so desperately lonely and so very frightened.

I feel that's what all my abusers have done. Used me, laughed at me, then discarded me. I have never been good enough and felt more and more worthless. My feelings have never counted and that's where suicide came into play. I believed it would be better off if I wasn't here anymore. I wasn't good enough for anyone. My Mother and Father disappointed in me. My Sister was the only person who ever gave me unconditional love.

I went to meditation after my appointment and cried silently throughout. I'd told Jayne the self-harm and suicide threats were almost a way of keeping me silenced. I became aware that I was going round in circles, focusing on the suicide instead of talking. Telling Jayne all of this was a huge release. Yes I cried and at times I could hardly speak, but I ploughed on relentlessly. I couldn't let it keep me silenced.

When I got home, I began to look up when the films, the horrors I watched were released. I realised some of them I had mentioned were released a bit later, then realised I had seen them when I went back.

A couple of years later my Mum bumped into Emily in town. She told my Mother they had moved and she had just had another baby. She now had Sarah-Jayne, Jack and Joe. One day when we were in the Old Town my Mum suggested we go. I told her I didn't want to go, but she told me she lived opposite a church, so she took me to where she believed Emily lived and we knocked on the door - and she answered. It began all over again. I would get the bus down and stay on a Saturday night. I would stay up and watch video's with Jack and Emily and I belonged all over again. I began to think I had been mistaken, but Jack would often be stood in the corridor upstairs looking at me in bed. I would close my eyes and when I opened them he was gone.

Then one night I woke up. Sarah-Jayne and little Jack were in Jack and Emilys bed and Jack was in bed next to me. I remember lying staring at the ceiling and I remember him getting up and going back to bed. He whispered that he needed to get back before everyone woke up. I never went again. Then the shame kicked in. I feel disgustingly ashamed. I didn't want to go back, but I was so happy again. I couldn't look Alan or the kids in the eye. I could hardly speak and when Alan asked me if I wanted to talk I just cried. I feel so, so ashamed.

Reflection: I don't think this entry needs any more information. The outpouring speaks for itself.

Notes:

21.11.15
I just want to be invisible. I feel so bad. Guilty, ashamed, anxious because I can't remember. This is the event I buried so hard. I feel like Alan and the kids can see what I have done. I went for a run to try and clear my head. It didn't work. I went to sleep for a while this afternoon, to block it out for a short time. I felt embarrassed going back downstairs having to face everyone. I am trying to remember why it's not my fault, but I loved being there, I went back and kept going back, but I didn't want it to happen again. But it did and I can't help feeling it's all my fault. I feel so ashamed.

Reflection: I needed to go through this. I had forgotten that I had realised none of this was my fault. I needed to start again with the full disclosure so I could work through it. I understood the responses of flight, fright, freeze. I just needed to learn to attach that to my experience. I had to go through it to get back to that point. I had to learn by example and not just theory. The theory I understood on a logical level. The experience I needed to understand on an emotional level.

Notes:

22.11.15

I don't know what I dreamt of last night, but I woke today feeling better and thinking this is all about responsibility. Not in the sense of blame, but taking responsibility for my life. What happened when I went back to that house happened. It's what I do with it now that matters. I can't remember, it can't make me feel any worse, so I can't dwell on it. It's not an additional trauma. I don't like my body, flabby bits etc. There is nothing I can do about it, but I can take responsibility for what I eat, how I take care of it and keeping myself fit. These thoughts I had this morning were very liberating. I found myself smiling. Instead of being afraid of everything I do, I need to think about why I am doing it and take responsibility for anything that might happen. Elizabeth is seven years old and she is very tearful at the moment and I think she wants my time. I asked her if she would like to go to the park and her face lit up. I am waking up to my children. Charlie came too and we had a lovely time. It's not about money or possessions, it's about time and love.

I went to meditation tonight and learned more about compassion for others. Elizabeth was tearful in bed again, so I took a risk and asked her if she felt frightened and alone at bed time. She nodded and started crying. We hugged and talked and she said she wanted me and had nobody to talk to. She was better when I left her, I told her it would pass and everything would be okay. My terrible experiences have helped my little girl. I felt worthwhile and told her never to feel lonely or alone ever, because I would always be there.

I never want my children to experience one single second of the fear and loneliness I grew up with. Norpel talked about possessions we think will make us happy, but they don't and we very quickly realise. He taught us that being truly happy comes from the feeling we get inside when thinking about other people. It's true. I made the possessions to be happy mistake for the last time. I felt a little more anxious again at the end of the day marking time passing, but it was fleeting and I felt better after meditation and so much better after talking to Elizabeth from my heart. My feelings towards my children is changing.

I have always loved them dearly, but I am beginning to feel something deeper. Their emotions are beginning to pull on mine. I feel deeply when they are upset, angry or vexed. It's so hard to describe. Almost a burning feeling inside, a clenching in my gut. I feel as though my mind is beginning to alter, reform, recover. The lump of tension inside has gone, it feels wide open and the tight feeling around my body has gone. It's like something has let go of me. Something has left me. And this deep feeling, burning feeling has replaced it. Almost like a blockage has gone.

Reflection: I was becoming a real, person. I was learning to feel from my soul. I was becoming whole, but I didn't see that for a long time to come.

Notes:

23.11.15

Still feeling better with occasional snatches of anxiety. The images have gone. Thirty five years of a nagging ache has gone. I feel lighter, empty, but a bit wobbly. Afraid to take my eye off the ball, in case it hits hard. I feel vulnerable. If somebody should have a go at me I wouldn't know what to do because that guarded, get ready to fight feeling has gone. When I felt anxious today I meditated and the anxiety quickly left me. I meditated on thinking about others. I feel empty, somehow exposed, but in a good way. Very difficult to articulate. I sorted Elizabeths bedroom today with a real passion and intention. I felt I could feel her mood. When she saw her room she was so appreciative. She hugged and kissed me and said her room being messy is what had made her feel tearful. How could I be that intuitive?

Reflection: The best feeling ever was when I suddenly felt a warm glow inside and I don't remember having it before. Something was replacing that hole that had lived in my core for longer than I could remember and if felt warm and glowing.

Notes:

24.11.15
A bit of a mixed day today. My mind felt quiet for the most part. Then at dinner time I felt very irritated. The kitchen was a mess, Melvyn had said we would be able to catch up this week and I've heard nothing. When I really wanted to tell him how I was feeling, but I didn't want to be selfish and text in case there was something wrong, so instead I felt irritable. What I should have done was either be direct and ask, or concentrate on the fact that he may have had something on and not think about myself. I just don't like being messed around, people being vague. Then to-night I started to feel really anxious about what might happen about money, my job, etc. I felt anxious to be on my own. I asked Alan to be with me and he did. The anxiety passed and I feel okay now. The images are still gone, I guess I feel out of control. The thought of going Christmas shopping scares me and I don't know why. I just want to be at home where I feel safe. The only time I don't want to be at home is after my counselling appointment. I don't want to be alone with my thoughts, I like to wander aimlessly, processing stuff, feeling calm and then I go home. Funny day today, Not good, not bad, just very mixed.

Reflection: When everything is changing it's really difficult to feel settled about anything. I felt everything was changing in my mind and I felt mixed up I think is the best way to describe it. Everything was in a jumble. Thought processes were changing.

Notes:

25.11.15
My mind felt quiet today. A couple of flashes of anxiety, but very self-limiting. I seemed to be able to rationalise what's going on and relax my body. Also to accept the situation I have felt anxious about. I still don't want to go out. I feel safe at home. I just want to be at home, I don't know why, but I am accepting it. I'm not afraid to be out, agoraphobia or anything like that. I just want to be at home and I want to be quiet. I have started watching television though and concentrating a little more. Menial tasks feel like such an effort. I have to be patient. I am just delighted to be feeling different. Relieved. Like a huge burden, lump, tension, it's hard to describe, has been removed.

Reflection: I will never underestimate the power of communication again. The difference inside of me since my outpouring to Jayne. I do still like to be at home, I do still like quiet and if I have things on my mind I will turn off the television or radio. I don't like lots of mental chatter and most importantly I do still meditate.

Notes:

26.11.15
My mind is quiet.

Reflection: Ooh bonus!

Notes:

27.11.15
I saw Jayne today. A reflective appointment explaining how I have felt all week. Still not feeling rested after a nights sleep. Not really sure why. No nightmares, no flashbacks. Still not keen to be out of the house, safe at home.

Reflection: Home felt like a retreat. It was warm and quiet in the main and after a very busy, very loud, overloaded mind all I craved was warmth, peace and quiet.

Notes:

28.11.15
My mind is quiet. Still not sleeping great. Feeling better.

Reflection: Sleep disturbance, now that was suggestive that something was still lurking. Consciously I felt a whole lot calmer, but everything hadn't come out and it was the calm before another storm. Thankfully I had no concept of that at that time.

Notes:

29.11.15
My mind is quiet. Still not relaxed sleep. Feeling better. A little anxious about work, but went to meditation and that always helps to bring me back in to the moment.

Reflection: Meditation, my best decision amongst all the wrong ones.

Notes:

30.11.15
I talked to Alan tonight. I saw my GP and he was really pleased I am feeling better. I text Melvyn and Carol and they are both pleased that I am feeling better. Jayne is pleased that I am feeling better. Alan has said nothing! I spoke to him about it and told him I felt unloved and uncherished. I told him I am worth more than that. He didn't want to know what was going on at the beginning and he shows no emotion now. I told him I don't need gifts or present to feel valued anymore, because I value myself now. But I do need to feel loved, to be shown. We talked about before we got married and him wanting to leave and me begging him not to because I love him and felt a failure. I said I have always wondered since then whether he only stayed because I begged and it was the easiest option. He told me he stayed because he believed in me and that he believed things would get better and they did. I can finally put that doubt to rest after 3 years of it being in the back of my mind.

Reflection: The problem with that was, people are not always honest, or as brave as I was to broach the subject. I didn't know it then either.

Notes:

01.12.15
My mind has been pretty calm today, until this evening when somebody broke down in tears, gut wrenching tears on television because they had lost their daughter. I suddenly felt that gut wrenching feeling and had the scene not changed, I would have broken down. What flashed through my mind was all the significant times in my life that things have been ruined by what happened to me, that I can never get back. Feeling safe, that first kiss, enjoying romance, first sexual encounter, getting married, my babies being born. I felt low on Monday evening.

Reflection: A sad evening but a noticeable connection with my own emotions.

Notes:

02.12.15
I looked after myself, stayed home, warm, meditated and my mind became calm. Feeling a bit sad, but not overwhelmed. Despite how I felt yesterday, I did sleep really well, for the first time in whenever.

Reflection: Finally I could tick the sleep box.

Notes:

03.12.15
I slept really well last night. I am meeting my Manager today and having a long meditation beforehand. I feel calm.
Meeting went really well. She has confidence in me and I felt very positive afterwards. A good day.

Reflection: What more could I do. I was on the up.

Notes:

04.12.15

Saw Jayne for counselling today. Talked about lack of self-worth, self-esteem and not being listened to. Or when listened to I have received hostile response. I was okay when I was in my appointment, but very shaky afterwards and when I explained to Alan I was in tears. Felt very low for the rest of the day. Why was I ignored, why when I asked for help were backs turned on me? What did I do wrong? My healing mind tells me it isn't me, but my irrational mind is asking why am I so worthless, why don't my feelings matter? Why, why, why have I never mattered enough?

Reflection: I was questioning now. A great tool to enhance understanding. I was trying to analyse why those experiences happened. I was beginning to pick it apart.

Notes:

05.12.15
My mind is working hard to disprove my belief that I am so worthless. Was it that path I took because I was sexually abused, a kind of learned helplessness? Did I feel I had no self-worth to fight for? I don't know. I read about somebody who had become suicidal due to his own personal circumstances and he was awoken to the fact that even though he used to teach about looking after people with suicidal ideation, it could happen to anyone.
Before I broke down and confessed to Jayne, I didn't know which way I was going to go. Within this article he talked about a website called recovery letters. I started reading the letters and it was very comforting to know I am not alone with how I feel. Simple daily tasks becoming a chore. Getting up and ready so difficult. Wanting to sleep to block things out. Even now I am hard on myself, I get frustrated for feeling like this, but I need to be so kind to myself. My mind is ill and just like a physical illness I need to take care of myself. My mind is not my enemy, it wants to be calm and peaceful. It is troubled and I need to take care of it. Those letters really helped to remind me.

Reflection: I was beginning to develop a real energy for understanding. I was beginning to seek solutions. A very positive step away from self-harm and suicidal thoughts, but they themselves needed to be dealt with.

Notes:

06.12.15

Feeling a bit out of sorts. Trying to work out why those things happened to me. Rationally I know it wasn't my fault, but why have I not been listened to? Is it because I was already so vulnerable so my response to situations resulted in me being victimised? I don't know, there was so much. Is everybody really that cruel? My eldest Son came to meditation with me tonight. That was so thoughtful of him. I enjoyed it because he was with me. What a special, beautiful little boy.

Reflection: He really got into it and I began to realise what I mean to my children.

Notes:

07.12.15
I have felt tearful all day. Everything is such an effort. I wrapped presents, I feel so down. I can't put my finger on it, but I have failed, struggled alone and I am tired. What is it about me that causes people to resent me? Alan got alcohol tonight. Big mistake! Charlie got upset about not being able to help with the Elf on the Shelf, I explained it was a mistake because it meant him being awake late. He was in tears. Alan let him help and said only if he goes to bed early. Everything I do causes a problem. Alans friends have organised a gathering for 27th December. That has made me feel very stressed as I know Amy from work. How am I going to face somebody who has no idea why I am off work? Everything feels such a mess. I just want to cry, I just want to sleep. I have messed everything up my whole life. I have been walking a very fragile line and now I don't feel safe anymore. I feel so afraid.

Reflection: I was all mixed up, trying too hard to find answers and yet I was only really beginning to recover myself. I was trying to run before I could walk and getting really frustrated with myself.

Notes:

08.12.15
Today wasn't a good day. I felt very down, almost paralysed to the spot. Feelings of worthlessness very strong and feeling like I keep making the same mistakes over and over again. I feel used, manipulated and my feelings ignored. I wrote down negative aspects of my life and positive to see if I could see what I am doing wrong. But I can't and the feelings of neglect, rejection, being ignored, worthless still keep happening and I hate the feeling because they all correlate to past sexual abuse and neglect feelings, so I associate with those memories and it makes me feel so hurt inside. I text Jayne and I talked to Alan tonight.

Reflection: I didn't know it, but I was grieving and I needed to allow it. I was constantly trying to get to the next stage because I hated the way I was feeling.

Notes:

09.12.15
Feeling generally subdued today. No major thoughts, just very low.

Reflection: Just a part of grief.

Notes:

10.12.15
Associated feelings of being raped all around me. Being manipulated by Charlie wanting to help with the Elf. Crying when he was told he couldn't then getting his own way because Alan gave in to him. Being praised for being a good Mum. Alan buying lager, me telling him I didn't want any, then being persuaded. When I got upset he agreed I had told him not to. I was manipulated and not listened to and all those emotions and flashbacks are with me now. I feel paralysed because I don't know how to stop the association, but also to stop being manipulated and to be listened to. Nobody listened to me until I was suicidal. Why won't anybody listen?

Reflection: Alan didn't listen because he was being emotionally abusive and controlling and trying in a very subtle way to keep me a victim, but I was too vulnerable at that time and I couldn't see it. I knew I didn't like it, but I didn't know what to do to stop it until much later.

Notes:

11.12.15
Saw Jayne today and talked about the difficult week. Done nothing but think about why people behave the way they did and still do towards me and I think I know. I was told I was strong, so I behaved strong, I suppressed all emotions, I didn't communicate when I didn't like something and I didn't stand up for myself. None of that was my fault, but a learned behaviour. A behaviour I can change, again it's about taking responsibility for myself. I want to talk to Jayne about what it was like with my ex-husband just like I did with that man. It worked to talk about him, to explain the depth of emotion and why I have these learned behaviours. That's going to be a tough one, but a necessary one. I don't feel better particularly, but I do feel focused and ready for the next bit. I feel things are building and coming to a head again, just like before. It has to come out.

Reflection: I was really focused at that point. I had some renewed energy.

Notes:

12.12.15
I feel like I have a virus, I ache all over, I feel fluey. I couldn't think about anything I felt so rough. I caught up with Carol today, I enjoyed that. Went to bed early.

Reflection: Says it all really.

Notes:

13.12.15

I must have slept for about 11 hours last night. I don't feel so unwell and I feel happier inside. I have been doing a lot of meditation yesterday and today. I text a very good friend of mine Cheryl tonight and I told her why I have been off work. A sure sign I am recovering, as I wasn't concerned or anxious about a negative response. Funnily enough I wasn't concerned about meeting Carol yesterday. I am beginning to feel an inner calm. A more together feeling of happiness, rather than the euphoric high I had experienced the last couple of weeks. Maybe it's because I am going to talk to Jayne about the other major part of the abuse with my ex-husband. I don't like it, but the thought of it doesn't make me feel suicidal, although when Alan gave me alcohol the other night and I had associated feelings, it did give me flashes of self-harm thoughts. That's why I want to get rid of the associated feelings.

Reflection: I don't remember being so focused, or understanding the next steps, but amongst all my vulnerability I appeared to know what I needed to do next.

Notes:

14.12.15
Wedding Anniversary today, cinema and lunch in the pub. I went to bed alone. Alan stayed up painting until 05.00am

Reflection: I still couldn't see the cracks and I'm not talking about the decorating.

Notes:

15.12.15
Last night I wrote a summary of my life with my ex-husband. I described how I was raped, humiliated, destroyed physically and emotionally. My plan was to read it out, then it would release the power, just like it happened when I talked in detail about being sexually abused when I was 10 years old. Except what happened was I started to feel sick and panicky before my appointment. When I spoke to Jayne I got a tickle in my throat so bad I couldn't stop coughing. I told Jayne I wanted to read it out, but I couldn't. I told her she should read it. She told me her priority was my safety. She said we could talk around it to chip away at it until I felt safe enough to read it out loud. She asked me if I had ever attempted suicide. I explained I had planned it, I said that my friend Melvyn came to see me from work. I told him I was going to drink a bottle of vodka, then before I collapsed I would swallow a load of pills washed down with bleach. I also gave Melvyn my suicide note. He talked to me and told me it wouldn't work, he disputed my ability to carry it through being so drunk. He then said *"Don't die, I don't want you to die"*. It took me totally by surprise.
I didn't look at is as death. I had been sexually abused, neglected, humiliated, ignored, degraded to the point where I felt absolutely worthless. I didn't matter, my feelings were never considered, I was pointless, my existence was pointless, so I just wanted to go. I was 27 years old, I was tired and I'd had enough. I really did have nothing to live for. Every day was a living hell and I didn't want to live any more. Melvyn was the first person to EVER tell me I was needed. He didn't want me to die. GOD somebody actually wanted me to be around – to live. I was shocked. Shocked enough to make me look up. He told me he would come back the next day to see me. I couldn't believe it I was wanted, somebody actually cared enough to actually want me to live. He has absolutely no idea how significant that day was. He saved my life. He made me look forward, when I had completely given up.
Later today I felt very disappointed, I thought I was going to get it all out, ready to move forward. However, Jayne said it's big and is going to take time. I am so exhausted by this. It is so hard, like trying to solve a puzzle constantly. It's frustrating at times, demoralising, agonising and endless. And always, always up hill. Today it felt like starting again, all over again. It's so maddening.

Reflection: My impatience added to my stress. An added stress I didn't need. The tight throat though, the tickly throat. It fascinates me the power of the body and the lengths my body was going to, to keep me silent. Jayne did read out what I had written, she asked me how I felt afterwards, but I said I felt no different because I hadn't read it out. I needed to do it and I would another day.

Notes:

16.12.15

My mind has tumbled into turmoil. Everything feels wrong. I have shifted to an emotional being and now I don't know how to come to terms with what happened to me with my ex-husband. That longing to be loved, being destroyed physically and emotionally by him. I want to be loved and cared for without prostituting myself to do so. I am in a dark place again. I am right back in that marriage. I am looking for a way forward. What I'm writing doesn't make sense, but that's how I'm feeling. Lost, confused, frightened. I want to live a life free from association with that time. But what he did to me was so horrific, I feel it is grained into my mind. I am continuing to look after myself, I am continuing to eat healthily, but it feels alien and strange and scary. But I want to feel strong and proud and confident. So going back to the start of this, that is why I feel in turmoil. Everything that is happening is suddenly giving me an association with something that happened to me when I was married. I am experiencing the emotional response from that time. He raped me, he humiliated me. He physically abused me and it all resulted in destroying me, so much so I wanted to leave this place because I felt I didn't belong. And when things go wrong for me now those feelings come back.

How does anybody ever move forward from that? How do I recover from being destroyed? Everything I do is a front. Everything I do is hard. I put me back together again, but I didn't repair the damage. I couldn't and I have never been able to. I feel so lonely, so hollow, everything is so fragile. I am recovering, but it's only skin deep. I need help, but I don't want anybody to be disappointed in me.

Reflection: It felt like I had gone back to the beginning again, but in reality I hadn't I was just tackling another experience of sexual abuse. All those emotions I understand now are absolutely normal in any unchartered waters. I was still being so hard on myself and still considering what others thought of me. So much pressure, as if there wasn't enough already.

Notes:

17.12.15
In London with my family to see the Theatre Production of Elf. Okay what normally happens when we have arrangements is I think about how long it will take, how I am going to feel and when, how and where everything is going to take place. When I am in an activity I am on the outside looking in.
Today we came to London and I just became engrossed in the experience. It was only when the interval arrived that I realised I was just going along with what was happening and doing none of the above. I would usually wonder how many people I am around have been sexually abused, how many people are pretending to be happy, but feeling like me. Like I am on the outside watching what is happening. This thought was only fleeting and I felt so happy it has gone.

Reflection: It was such a relief to not plan everything out in my head first. To just experience events as they unfolded. This was brand new to me and I loved it. I felt so free and so light in my head. To be free of negative thoughts. I couldn't remember a time it had happened before.

Notes:

18.12.15
Feeling exactly the same as yesterday. A good day, a good feeling. Except the sensation of my weight gaining body.

Reflection: I was determined I was going to eat normally and healthily. No restrictions, just immerse myself in the normal day to day of eating as the rest of my family did. But I have always been able to feel my body when I start to gain weight. How it feels when I sit down, or how my clothes feel. I wanted to ignore it, I wanted to be healthy, but the changes I felt made me feel very uncomfortable and I couldn't ignore them.

Notes:

19.12.15

A quiet day of reflection. Then I reflected on my last appointment with Jayne, because the images don't bring up the same emotion. What expressed it for me was the range of emotions I went through to try to cope with being raped. I said I didn't like it, I said "no", I cried, I binged to hurt myself more than he could, I drank alcohol, and I laughed at him. I had no emotion left to cope with the terror. He destroyed my mind.

Reflection: It would be a bit difficult to reflect on a reflection, so I will leave that to you, the reader.

Notes:

20.12.15
Thinking about my vulnerability and realising, low self-confidence, low self-esteem. My mind was destroyed, I was invisible in every aspect. My circumstances changed, but I didn't repair the damage. How do I repair the damage and learn to grow up? My body feels like it is growing. I want to stop worrying about it, but I can't whilst it's still growing.

Reflection: What I meant by this was I decided after my ex-husband I would not have a relationship of any sort with a man ever again for the rest of my life. I was protecting myself from further abuse, further torture and torment. And I did do that from 1996 when I separated from my husband, until 2005 when I met Alan. However, what I didn't do was learn from those experiences. Come to terms with them, so all I did literally was avoid the situation. When I met Alan I still had the same mind set. I still felt like an abused child. I was still vulnerable with low self-confidence and low self-esteem. This resulted in the same patterns of behaviour. Avoidance I learned does not solve any problem. Dealing with it head on is the only way to break the cycle.

Gaining weight felt horrible and it still does when I feel it. But I eat healthily now and I go to the Gym, so I am comfortable with my body. We work in harmony with each other my mind and body. At that time though, I still didn't feel in harmony, or even in control of anything and I worried horribly about the changes I could feel.

Notes:

21.12.15

This evening has been so frightening. I told Alan I was worried about money. He talked about cancelling the holiday, when I said it might have to be cancelled he said *"You're not serious, I've paid £1000 already"*. He doesn't care about me at all. I am invisible once again. I can't bear to look at him. He raised it again later because he could see I was upset. He told me I was being over sensitive, anxious about counselling tomorrow and it's my fault I interpreted what he said that upset me. I am in bed using all my strength to not tell myself I am a bad person, that this is all my fault. I am trying to tell myself I deserve to recover, I deserve to be healthy and well. He hasn't come to bed, so that tells me he believes he is right to throw everything back in my face. I can't live with that any more. I want to change the way I respond to people. I am trying so hard not to feel bad about myself. I need to go to sleep.

Reflection: I was becoming increasingly aware of my feelings and that they were valid. I didn't internalise what happened that day in the same way I had previously. I was holding on to my self-belief. I knew the answers and I was getting stronger in my convictions all the time. This was a big change to self-loathing. It was becoming more about his behaviour and less about the impact mine was having on him.

Notes:

22.12.15

Saw Jayne today, told her about last night. This is where the links came together. When my Sister died I was neglected by my Mum and Dad. They didn't listen to me when I said I was scared in the house on my own, or when I asked my mum not to go out.

I was sexually abused when I was 10 years old because I went looking for love elsewhere. I believed he did it because he didn't like me, I was rejected.

My ex-husband raped me. I was looking for love and he hurt me. I said "No", I cried, I laughed at him, I drank copious amounts of alcohol to blot out what he was doing, I became anorexic to at least have something to control. I said to Jayne that I had bought Alan a hot air balloon trip he really wanted. He humiliated me and threw it back in my face.

I saved up to take us all to Disney Land Paris for my 40th Birthday. Everybody moaned, Alan said he never wanted to go anyway. I did it to please everyone so I would get a reward. It was thrown back in my face.

I felt so bad about myself. What a mug, how stupid am I. How worthless are my feelings to be trodden all over like that. Alan told me I was selfish when I told him I couldn't stay up all day before a night shift so he could play cricket.

When Sam, my elsdest was young and Charlie was a baby I was pregnant with Elizabeth. Sam was being particularly challenging. I said to Alan I recognised he didn't love Sam as much as Charlie and he said *"No, I don't, I don't love Sam at all"*. I felt so vulnerable, my heart ripped in two. I was rejected, my feelings were destroyed, once again I felt so bad about myself.

Then finally 5 months ago when all this began. I was suicidal and Alan turned his back on me. He said he didn't want to know. But at the time I was too ill to understand. I told Alan I wasn't going to live with his callous, cruel behaviour any more. I now have to protect myself and my children. I deserve to be loved, cherished and looked after and I will not be silenced, ignored, or destroyed EVER again.

Alan listened, took it and said he would never do anything to hurt me again and he said he now understands the consequences of his actions as he had no idea how much he had hurt me before.

I talked to Jayne about London and she said I am now beginning to live in the present. To live mindfully. I told her how liberating that was. I asked her how to build my self-esteem and she said by continuing to do what I am doing. I said when she spoke about fight, flight and freeze with the men who had abused me, it had all made sense. I stopped blaming myself and suddenly realised why what happened, happened and it wasn't my fault. I said I need her to say something like that about my ex-husband. She asked me to try and view it the same way. It wasn't my fault what he did. I was looking for love and he abused me. My self-esteem and self-worth were so low I couldn't do anything about it. I told her I need to work on processing that.

A very emotionally charged session. I have opened up to Alan, now it is up to him because I will take care of myself now for me and my children.

Reflection: I can see from this entry that my strength is really growing. Jayne was incredible in supporting me and helping me to see situations from my perspective. Not hers, not anybody else's, but mine and how I could make sense of them.

Notes:

23.12.15
Woke after a good sleep feeling calm, self-assured and again living in the moment. I made snowflakes with Elizabeth this morning. I didn't realise I knew what to so. She listened and then we made them together. I was fully absorbed in what we were doing. NEVER have I done that. I have always looked for a way out. Being absorbed in play meant I couldn't be alert to everything else. I loved what we did this morning. It's so new and so liberating, incredible, wonderful, fantastic and exiting. We visited Alans family and I was relaxed, just totally part of what was happening. I have always felt on edge because I was conscious of Alans feelings, always putting other people's feelings before my own. But no, I was just me, living in the moment. Tonight I threw all the complaint paperwork away from Lady Jane Grey Primary School, and it didn't bother me. Although I didn't tear it up. Because it hasn't disappeared. If he truly is a bad person, I believe he will be uncovered. God what at 24hours. No wonder I feel shattered. It's not until writing this I realise just how much.

Reflection: I had made a complaint against my Son's Primary school because he had been inappropriately touched by another boy and when he reported it he was intimidated by the teacher and told to his face that he wasn't believed. I reported the incident to the police, Ofsted, The school Governors, everybody I could think of and there was no consequence for either the teacher or the head teacher. I was so angry, another teacher had ignored my Son's distress, told him they didn't believe him. I was terrified that my Son was going to be as damaged as I was and I needed him to be heard. It brought all those feelings back of not being listened to. Being ignored and that teacher Brenda Smith telling me "*These things happen*". I was more traumatised than my Son. All of those feelings, emotions, flashbacks of being sexually abused and ignored where tied up in that school complaint. Getting rid of the paperwork was me accepting that what happened to my Son wasn't the same as what happened to me. He was supported by me and protected. I was supported by nobody and completely unprotected. My Son was fine and getting rid of the paperwork meant I had separated his experience from mine.

Notes:

24-26.12.15 Been swept along by Christmas. Living in the moment and just enjoying the experience.

On Christmas Eve I messaged Alans Mum, I thanked her for a lovely afternoon yesterday. I told her I have been off work for the past 5 months dealing with historic sexual abuse spanning 16 years. I told her that is why I have appeared, cool, aloof, or distant. I realised the kids were shy of her because they hardly know her and if she wanted to then I would like to see her regularly. She sent me a lovely message back saying I had never come across and cold or aloof and she wished she could give me a hug and that they are there if I need it. I felt a massive weight on my shoulders just lift off. A secret had been unleashed. I no longer have to maintain that wall of silence or be alert or protective of the kids. It is a massively liberating feeling. To not be on guard. I loved it. We saw Daryl and his family on Christmas Eve evening and I felt so relaxed.

Christmas Day I could bask in the joy I witnessed seeing my beautiful children full of excitement and happiness.

Boxing Day we went to see Alans Mum and her partner. We had a lovely relaxed afternoon. I ate well and enjoyed a slice of profiteer roll cake. When we got home without thinking, I went upstairs to have a bit of quiet time to myself.

Reflection: I lived that afternoon for myself. I told his Mum of my experiences because I wanted to be me. I no longer wanted to put up a front, a mask of control.

Notes:

27.12.15

Went to town with Alan and Elizabeth. He wanted a suit, Elizabeth wanted a ruck sack for school. I didn't enjoy being in town at all. The boys stayed with my Mum and Dad. I just wanted to get home. I didn't want to be out, but didn't put too much meaning into it. It was hot and crowded. Who would want to be out? I am worrying about food. We went to my Mums, had a drink, collected the boys and came home. I am writing this on 30.12.15, I remember nothing else about the rest of the day.

Reflection: I used to get episodes, that I called black episodes. It would relate to a period of time during the day, or night where I would have no recollection of events. I don't mean not remembering, I mean no recollection, as if the event didn't even happen. I would be very distraught when I would get these episodes because it reminded me every time of when I was at Jack and Emilys and I woke up and Jack was getting out of my bed. I have no recollection of what he did. I have no memory, other than him getting out of my bed and whispering he had to get back before everyone woke up. Every time I had a black episode it took me back there.

I didn't know what these episodes were for a long time. Later when I did understand them, I realised they happened when I was so consumed with flashbacks and memories that I completely disconnected from the real world. Physically I was present, but emotionally and psychologically I was somewhere else. A bit like when you drive to work and when you arrive you have no recollection of the journey. But in that case you know you have travelled from A to B. In my case I had no recollection of anything. It was all blank until I was present again.

I recognise it when it happens now, although it happens a lot less frequently than it did. I recognise when I am distracted, so I don't panic if I don't recall a sequence of events, or a film. I recognise also that when this is happening I am becoming overwhelmed. I just need to trust those around me who I love to bring me back and ask me if I am okay.

Notes:

28.12.15
Still anxious about food, but wishing I wasn't. I can't remember this day.

Reflection: A black episode because I was overwhelmed by changes to my body and what I was eating.

Notes:

29.12.15

Alan went to work. I was a little anxious about that to begin with because I had found it so difficult during the summer holidays and October half term, but I was okay. It was a relaxed day, I played with the kids and I was beginning to get tired about 4pm, so when Alan text to say he was on the train home, I told him we would pick him up. I just needed some head space. But I was pleased I was okay and enjoyed the day.

Reflection: A new experience for me. I wanted to be in the car, so I could be alone with my thoughts. A healthier and more positive approach.

Notes:

30.12.15

I saw Jayne today, it has felt so long since I saw her. I talked about the week, Alans Mum and how good that feels, talking to Alan and how I was able to stick with how I was feeling and accepting how he was feeling without believing I had to change my behaviour to comfort or accommodate him. I talked about how good that felt, to stay with me and my thoughts. I talked about my rise in anxiety levels because of this recurring dream I have where I ask for help and nobody listens to me. I remember how those feelings affected me when I went off sick and I am afraid they might return.

I talked about the Safeguarding Consultant I spoke to a year last September when I felt overwhelmed by what Charlie was going through and how it was making me more sensitive to my caseload. She acknowledged I was struggling and agreed to meet with me weekly until I felt on top of things. Not only did she never do that, but she now completely avoids me and does not acknowledge my presence when she walks in the office when I am there.

I understand now that depression and anxiety develop because of a feeling of loss of control and inability to vent. I understand that so much that I don't want it to happen again and that is what is making me anxious.

Jayne supported me and agreed this is something we can work on. I left feeling anxious, but reassured. Then tonight something went wrong and I spiralled into despair. Alan had the box my 'phone was in on Sunday when we went to town as I needed a new Sim. He told me tonight that he had given me the box back, but I knew he hadn't or I would have put it away. Eventually, I found my earphones and charger in my drawer. I have no recollection of this or anything that happened the rest of that Sunday. I feel so upset, angry with myself. I didn't know what it was before, but I have been told it is due to the sustained trauma and the affect it has had on my brain.

That's what distresses me so much. That's why I like things to be put away in the right place. When I look back this has happened since I was sexually abused, but the first time I reflected on it was when I was living with a friend following my previous marriage breakdown. We were going on holiday together and flying from Birmingham airport. I told her I had never been to that airport and she told me I had taken her there and picked her up after she had been to a work conference several weeks before. I had no recollection of EVER doing that and I still don't.

This isn't about memory loss and being reminded, what's so distressing is having absolutely no recollection. And there just being a black hole, even when prompted. And I don't know if that will ever go away, because every time it happens it's a reminder of what happened. The trauma following what happened. The constant vigilance, fear, total state of anxiety.

Reflection: These black episodes were happening more and more around this time and they were really frightening me. I learned over time that grounding myself in the present helped to alleviate them. By slowing everything down in my mind, I could begin to recognise that I was becoming overwhelmed and either allow the emotion to unfold and accept I would be 'spaced out' for a while, or to gradually bring myself back to the present and not allow flashbacks, or memories overwhelm me.

Notes:

31.12.15
Tonight we went to the Village party. Parents knew each other, kids knew each other. There was music, food, drink and games for the kids. Sam was talking to a friend and ended up dancing, Charlie also had a laugh with friends and Elizabeth had a great time with her friends. I socialised and had a great laugh. How truly wonderful to live in the moment and enjoy what's going on myself. No longer feeling on the outside. A colleague from work messaged me last night and I responded, but also acknowledged that a few weeks ago I wouldn't have been able to do that because I felt so unwell. And that made me feel a little subdued.

Reflection: I felt like I was recovering, I was beginning to be more present and more myself. I felt no stress or tension, I enjoyed myself for being there.

Notes:

01.01.16
Woke feeling okay, but tired. Kept myself warm and nourished, then went for a run when I felt up to it. Looking after myself also feels truly amazing. Towards the end of the day I again felt subdued, looking back at how I have been.
Charlie and Elizabeth went to bed upset because of a disagreement with each other and Alan. I spoke up about how it made me feel and came to bed. I didn't feel angry or upset, but I think everybody is just a bit tired and emotional as even Alan is crying now. I don't like the subdued feeling thought, it frightens me a bit, because I am recovering now.

Reflection: Whenever I experience positive emotions I would cling to them so hard because they were new and refreshing and they made me feel alive. They made me feel like myself, myself that I was learning all about. However, when I felt low I would become anxious, because that is all I have ever known and I was afraid the low mood would consume any positive emotion and I would spiral back to where I had come from. A world of terror and torment, misery and pain. What I didn't know was that eventually all those emotions could live in harmony with each other. I would have good days and low days, but one no longer dominates the other.

Notes:

02.01.16
Today I think my mind is quiet. Went to Alans Mums and had a lovely afternoon. I love this freedom being in the moment. Still have this heavy feeling in my heart. It's like I can see, but objectively how bad things have been. I read about typical behaviours of survivors of childhood sexual abuse. Low self-esteem due to lack of self-worth, alcohol abuse to escape trauma, eating disorders due to fear of body, suicide attempts and self-harm, wanting to go to sleep to escape feelings and self-harm due to self-loathing. All of which I have been through and I feel sad.

Reflection: Those reminders were hard to wear, but I kept reading them because I wanted to see how far I had come. How well I was recovering, but I also wasn't ready to let any of them go. I still needed to read how hurt I had been. Those statements validated how I had been feeling and at that time I needed them to keep doing that.

Notes:

03.01.16
Felt very tearful today. Went to meditation, but it was closed. I really needed the comfort and support. I am afraid that my mood is going down. I messaged Jayne and Melvyn asking if it is normal to feel sad, even though I am feeling better. Melvyn replied that it was absolutely normal and healthy. I feel a little reassured. I talked to Alan, showed him the text messages and he gave me a lovely hug, reassured me it was part of everything and that things are good. I went to bed feeling a little better. I feel sad for everything I have been through. How did I do it and how am I still here?

Reflection: The fear was very apparent in relation to my low mood. Not only did I look to others for reassurance that it was okay to feel low and that I wasn't spiralling, but I would also ask how long it would last, because I desperately needed to know it wouldn't. I had been low for as long as I could remember, these new happier emotions were a refreshing experience and I didn't want to experience anything else.

Notes:

04.01.16
I have a feeling of dread. One emotion I appear to struggle with is sadness. Feeling sad scares me because I am frightened it won't go away. I have lived with sadness, but never expressed it. It somehow feels isolating. I feel so sad. Like I want to visit a grave where I can sit and be sad and nobody will question why. I am sad for my loss, my struggle and for all the bad things that have happened to me. I just feel grief stricken. There is no other way to describe it. But I have felt this way inside for so long. I feel better so I don't want to be sad, but I don't want to suppress it either. I shall just ride it out. That's the best thing to do.

Reflection: Once again I knew the answers. The difference with this sadness to the sadness I had always felt was, this sadness was coming from insight and understanding and healing. The sadness I had always experienced had come from hopelessness and despair. I just wasn't able to see it at that time.

Notes:

05.01.16
Today I saw Jayne. I talked a lot about my lack of memory on Sunday 27.12.15. About how it happens with books and films. How it happened with my Safeguarding exam. I revised 2 questions, but each time I revised one of the questions the other would completely disappear. It's as though my mind will not convert it to memory. It goes no deeper than reading the words on the page. I talked about when I went on holiday with a friend and we flew from Birmingham airport and I commented that I had never been. My friend pointed out that I had given her a lift to that same airport just a few weeks before and I had picked her up. I had no memory recall and didn't when we went. It was a black hole.
On 27.12.15 I went to town with Alan and Elizabeth. They boys went to my mums. Alan bought a suit, I got a sim card for my 'phone and Elizabeth got a rucksack for school. We went to my mums, had a drink and came home. I remember us all getting out of the car to go in to the house then I remember nothing about the rest of the day. I didn't realise until several days later when I was looking for my 'phone charger and earphones. Alan said he gave the box to me, but I had no recollection of it. I found it eventually, but that's when I realised I had no recollection of that afternoon. Alan tried to prompt me by saying I came upstairs whilst he tried his suit on. And as if a light switched on I remember seeing him in it and commenting that the trousers looked a bit snug on his bum and then it's like the light switches off and it all goes black. I was so angry and upset. Why can't I make my brain work?
Jayne explained that when one trauma happens It's like a jar of water with sludge in. Nothing can get above the gunk and the water on top sometimes can't get through it. I have had a lot of trauma so there is a shitload of gunk to wade through all the time. I also talked about feeling so sad about what I have coped with and it scaring me, but she helped me to understand. I am learning to express emotions. Over the past few months there has been terror, major anxiety, fear, self-loathing, depression, happiness, elation, euphoria. Jayne reassured me that sadness is just another emotion. I can't expect to be able to express all other emotion without sadness. Of course it makes perfect sense, but I panicked because sadness has been with me all of my life. Experience it, allow it and it will pass. I need to stop looking for goals and timescales and learn to live in the moment. I also talked about not getting attached to things because everything is taken away from me. My Sister, my innocence, my body, my mind, my baby. Every time something is taken away, another barrier goes up. It was a very emotional session and I am exhausted and my eyes are dry from crying. I feel a bit silly about the sadness thing. How obvious is that. Not suppressing emotion means not suppressing any emotion.
Lesson Learned!

Reflection: I learned a lot during that session. Sometimes this would happen, I would bring a lot to a session, but with the simplest of explanations they would fall into place. Often it was the most obvious of explanations. I would get frustrated even with this, but Jayne explained to me that when I have had no frame of reference, then I had nothing to bounce a problem off. There reason there was a blank sometimes was because the learning and understanding had never been there in the first place.

Notes:

06.01.16
I met Alans Mum for coffee today. I felt nervous before hand, we have never really spoken before. I saw a police officer walking through the shopping centre and thought I could just stop him and tell him I wanted to talk about something. It's still on my mind.
When we met it was so easy, she had her own story to tell which is not my place to disclose. We spoke non-stop for 3 ½ hours, only leaving because I had to get back. I started to feel less alone, less isolated. She has been through so much. She messaged me tonight and I felt really sad for her. I cried for myself, her and all the others who have gone through and are going through what I have experienced.

Reflection: Some people go through life as I had been. Cool, distant and aloof for fear that showing any emotion would amount to loss of control and falling apart. Some people behave in a similar way because they believe that showing emotion amounts to weakness, vulnerability and less credibility. For me though, talking about my experiences and expressing my vulnerabilities has the opposite affect for the majority of people I come across on a day to day basis. Discussing life experiences and vulnerability I have found give me more credibility. People appear to perceive me as strong and resilient. It even at times, as with Alans Mum leads to disclosure. A number of people have disclosed experience to me after I have talked openly about mine. It has sometimes made people feel better, sometimes people have gained understanding and insight into their own behaviour and for a few it has touched a raw nerve for them and they have avoided me, or at least distanced themselves from me. They are the people I feel sad for. But that is their journey, not mine.

Notes:

07.01.16

I am so tired today, Alan is away in Leeds and Elizabeth slept with me last night, or rather she didn't sleep, being full of a cold. I decided to go back to bed after I had dropped the kids at school and called in on my Mum and Dad. I wrangled with my conscience. I couldn't do that if I was at work, but I'm not, so I will. I slept for about an hour, induced by meditation. They are always the best sleeps. If I struggle to get to sleep recently, I meditate and it always works and I have lovely dreams. When I woke up I felt so calm. I only slept for an hour, but then I got a call from school to collect Sam who had slipped and fainted.

Carol messaged me the other night saying she had been an emotional wreck. I felt sad for her, she had been treated so badly and I thought what a bastard to do that to her. Then I thought about Alans Mum and thought what a bastard to hurt her. Then I thought about me. What a bastard my ex-husband was to me.

It wasn't Carol s or Alans Mums fault, those people who hurt them are very damaged people. My husband didn't rape me because I was damaged, he did it because he was damaged. I have understood for a short while now that none of this was my fault, but I understand so much more now that it didn't happen to me because I was damaged. It happened because he was damaged. To think Carol and Alans mum feel the same because the people they were with were sick individuals. I feel ready to let go of what my ex-husband did to me because not only did everything happen that wasn't my fault, it didn't happen because I was vulnerable, it happened because it was their fault and they are damaged.

That is a truly amazing enlightening moment. The 7th January has always been an important day, since 2002.

Reflection: I love it when I read about enlightening moments like that and it reminds me of how much I now understand. I wish everybody who has been hurt could get to this point. That's the purpose of publishing this book.

Notes:

08.01.16

I dreamt last night Jayne was asking me about my memory. Why do I get so upset? Why do I get angry with myself? I kept telling her it was because I don't remember and she kept pressing me, but why do you get so upset? Why does it make you so angry and I cried *"because I don't remember what he did"*. After I had been sexually abused when I was 10 years old, I stopped going to the house. But a short while later my mum bumped into Emily and they got talking and she told my Mum to bring me over.

I went back to and I started staying over again. It was lovely to be included again, be part of a family. I was aware of him standing on the landing looking at me, but I closed my eyes and when I opened them again he had gone. But one night I woke up. He was in bed with me. He got out of bed and whispered he had to get back before anybody woke up. I have been tormenting myself trying to remember if anything happened, but I can't remember. It's blank, just like my memory is blank sometimes. And that's why it causes me so much pain. But this morning I realised, the reason I don't remember is because I was asleep. I will never know what happened, not because it is blank, but because I was asleep.

The pressure this has released is phenomenal. I have been so distraught when I have had a blank about an insignificant occurrence, but now I don't need to feel that impact because my mind hasn't betrayed me after all. I was asleep. I also talked to Jayne about how when Carol and Alans mum had talked about how they felt, I was focused on how totally sick and damaged those men had to have been to cause them so much pain. I talked about how I had a sad ache in my heart for both of them, but recognised the pain those men had inflicted upon them was nothing to do with them.

This has helped me to re-dress the balance and I asked to read out what I had written about my ex-husband, describing how he raped me throughout our marriage and the profound affect that had on me. I started off vocalising the pain, telling him to stop, saying *"No"*, crying, then doing nothing, but controlling food to gain some control. Abusing alcohol to block the pain and remove me from the reality. Suicide attempt. I laughed at him, I humiliated him, I threw everything at him, but it never stopped. He destroyed me physically and mentally. But he did all of those things because he is damaged. So damaged by his incestuous upbringing and his controlling mother.

He didn't rape me because I had been raped before, or sexually abused as a kid. I was vulnerable and he needed a vulnerable person to control. It was not me. He didn't rape me because I had been raped. I told Jayne I was able to read it because I was letting him go. I wasn't my fault, any of it. I understand damaged people do damage to other people. It wasn't me. I am beginning to see this from a mature adult perspective. The freedom this has given me is enormous. A breakthrough moment that I didn't want to end today. I wanted to stay with those feelings, that realisation, I didn't want to return to the hustle and bustle of the day.

Today has been a profoundly liberating day. A day I never believed I would see. Thirty six years of a belief and it is being re-written and put into perspective. I truly cannot believe it. I could read my story about my husband with sadness. I am no longer afraid of sadness. It is just as much a part of me as joy, excitement, fear and anger. I am becoming whole. I am becoming brand new. I am healing, I am recovering and I never believed I would.

Reflection: Another incredible insight and a massive step forward for my recovery.

Notes:

09.01.16

I am so tired. I was so tired last night, but I couldn't sleep. My mind was doing that re-wiring thing. Everything falling into place. Physically drained, but mentally manic. I went for a run this morning, but I felt so tired, my body was heavy and my eyes wanted to close. I got back and tried to fall asleep, but I couldn't, I just lay with my eyes closed. I was frustrated because I couldn't meditate.

Alan is so distant from me now. We went to Daryls tonight and he sat as far away from me as he could. Daryl told his new partner we had had a row, but I reassured him we hadn't. I am so alone, Alan is so cold. I'm not sure how long we will stay together.

Daryl played 80's music, it reminded me of when I used to go clubbing and the rude connections I made to each song, but my friends were oblivious to it. It makes me feel so sad. I am so alone. With Alan.

Reflection: I think one of the saddest places anyone can be is lonely when they are with somebody. I had been sad and alone and lonely all my life and even then it was happening again. I didn't see Alan as a current abuse relationship though, I was starting to see him as another mistake I had made as a consequence of my past experiences.

Notes:

10.01.16
Still incredibly tired, I am seeing Occupational Health Consultant tomorrow. I am keen to go back to work, equally anxious about seeing everybody, being able to do my job now I am different, but also my fatigue is caused by my constantly working hard to process new ways of looking at things. When I go back to work, when will I be able to look after my mind? I struggled on Friday because I wasn't on my own and we had a busy weekend. My meditation skills are weak, but I don't want to lose sight of myself ever again. I tried to explain this to Alan. I enjoy meditating as I go to sleep, plus it gives me very lucid dreams. I am sure that must help, at least a little bit.

Reflection: I loved and still do love the lucid dreams meditation brings during sleep. I referred to my skills as weak, but I was in reality using it really well and it worked the majority of the time. It still works the majority of the time. Like any physical exercise which requires ongoing practice, exercise for the mind is no different. At times I can be very physically tired and have no energy to exercise, it doesn't make me weak. At times I couldn't and can't meditate. That doesn't make me weak either. It makes me human and makes me feel like I want to care for myself in another way, such as resting, or reading, or having a soak in the bath. I have learned that caring for myself comes in whatever form it needs to, to leave me feeling I am caring for myself.
I was anxious about going back to work though. My main anxiety was around people not listening to me. I was afraid that when I went back to work I would have to be 'normal' again, but what if I needed help and nobody listened? I did not want to get to the stage where I became suicidal again. I never wanted to get to that stage again, but I didn't know what I needed to do to make sure people listened when I needed them to and that scared me.

Notes:

11.01.16
Saw Occupational Health Consultant. I discussed what happened on 20th November and last Friday. I told her I was feeling calm and we discussed a therapeutic return to work, beginning next week. I am excited and apprehensive at the same time. I thought about my feelings when I left work of nobody caring, nobody listening. I don't want to feel that when I go back. It was the first meditation class tonight with Norpel. Being able to focus solely on what's happening in the minute is the medicine I need. I need that constant reminder to focus on now, on me and how I am feeling.

Reflection: Living in the moment really was and is the best medicine for me now. I no longer need that constant reminder to be present in the moment, I just do it. Life is so less stressful now I can do that. Anxiety about nobody caring was understandable, given only 6 months earlier I was planning to end my life. But the other part of that was that I still didn't care enough about myself to not need people to care or listen. I was becoming whole, but I was still living in 2 minds.

Notes:

12.01.16

Today I spent peacefully on my own. I meditated, exercised and read "The Monk who sold his Ferrari". I felt so calm and peaceful. Tonight I felt isolated from Alan. He spends the evening on his work laptop. I want to talk.

I am meeting Martyn on Thursday. Six months ago during one of his last lectures, I had decided I was going to sit on the window ledge because nobody was listening to my nightmare and I would, I believed, be better off no longer here. Better for my family, my kids, everyone. I believed I had let everybody down. The last time I was at work, that was how I felt.

I feel so sad for me now, but also I feel an association with how I felt and returning to work. It's difficult to explain because I don't feel that way now. But it's like when a person doesn't want to attend a certain hospital because the last time they were there a relative had died. I don't like this feeling, but I have it and I will talk to Jayne about it. I'm not sure how to get passed the feeling. I understand why I have it, but I think I'm afraid of being plunged back to that time and experiencing the same reminders when I get back to work.

Reflection: To explain that more in depth. The last time I was at work I was in a daze, I was on the outside looking in, I was suicidal. I was really frightened that returning to work would catapult me back to that time and I was anxious that those feelings would become real again and not just associations, or memories, or flashbacks.

Notes:

13.01.16

I don't want to write about this, but I am going to. Six months ago I was in complete despair and believed the only way out was suicide. No-one was listening, I was struggling, but nobody listened until I could cope no more and believed everyone would be better off without me.

Now I am due to return to one place that left me feeling that way. I have told close friends and family how I feel and they have been re-assuring, but I never, ever want to feel that way again.

I feel vulnerable and I am shaking just writing about it.

Reflection: Many people never do return to a place that caused them so much despair. You hear it often when people have traumatic experiences. I came to the conclusion though in my head that if I did feel the same I would resign from my job. I never told anybody. The most I could express was by saying I didn't want to return to the same job, the same building, the same people. But I did and I still do and gradually over time the association went as I continued to grow stronger and more grounded in myself.

Notes:

14.01.16

Today I woke with a slight heavy heart. Today I am going to meet with my tutor Martyn. Six months ago I was going to kill myself right there in his classroom. Well the window ledge to be precise. I had enrolled on a communication course. I was really looking forward to it. Looking forward to improving my communication skills and not being the most articulate of people, I was totally relaxed and ready to embrace the learning.

The course began with a 2 day workshop. We had actors playing the role of our client and we were asked to choose a difficult conversation that we may encounter during our day to day work. I chose a scenario from one of many similar scenarios where a teenager had been sexually abused by a relative. I briefed my teacher and the actor on the background of the story and our role play began.

The actor then got into role and a disclosure was made, I responded in the manner I was used to, by hearing and not listening to what I was being told and discussing how this person may be best supported by various professional agencies. However, this not being the purpose of the role play, Martyn interjected by saying "*hold on, this person has just disclosed something to you, you need to ask her more about it*". That was it, it suddenly dawned on me exactly what the purpose of the role play was and indeed the purpose of the course.

Inside I began to tremble and a voice inside me was saying "*No I don't, I don't want to know. I don't want to know anything, because nobody has ever asked me, nobody has ever heard my story*". But it was too late, my guard was down, I never dreamt for one minute I would be listening and asking questions to the actor (my client) whilst they shared their horrific accounts of sexual abuse.

Their horrific accounts were my horrific accounts and I couldn't bear it, but it was too late. Savage emotions were beginning to surface and suppressed and deeply suppressed memories were beginning to vie for my attention. Images, smells, voices, sensations were beginning to creep over me, beginning to invade my mind. Then flashbacks, panic attacks began within days.

Another candidate who was observing my role play on that day said she saw in me the minute the penny dropped and I realised the level of communication I was to be practicing and expected to engage in. Little did she know the sudden awful realisation I had experienced and what could possibly be to follow. The rest of the course was torture. We had a speaker attend one day who was delivering a session on various mental health challenges faced by various people, this included a discussion about suicide and suicide attempts. I was shaking so badly inside.

I asked to see Martyn following that session. I was holding it together so tightly, I could only say I was struggling. Struggling to avoid vicarious trauma? Martyn listened, supported me and advised me to speak with my manager. I was screaming inside, I was tortured, frightened by the overwhelming emotions I was experiencing, but I couldn't say any more. I left, keeping myself together.

I spoke with my manager about support, but was faced with a negative response.

As part of my assessment I had to undertake an OSCE. A video recorded interview with an actor playing the role of a client. The scenario was based around sexual abuse, alcohol abuse and suicide attempts. That interview was one of the longest 20 minutes of my life. Eliciting information I didn't want to hear, whilst a voice I my head was screaming "*STOP, STOP, STOP*". I was frozen in error and all I could hear coming back from the actor was my experience. She was me sitting there, me telling me exactly what had happened to me and how I was feeling. I can't articulate how destroying that felt.

Following my OSCE I returned to work and sought out a trusted colleague. I could barely articulate how I felt, but she looked at me and asked me if I was going to do anything stupid. I just stared at her and whispered "*I don't know*". She contacted Martyn and he called me to meet him the next day. The first thing he said was he'd had a call from and he understood I had thoughts of self-harm. I was so stunned. Stunned that somebody had cared enough, listened and contacted Martyn, but also stunned that he had listened, cared enough to contact me. Not only that, he listened to me then too.

He was calm and unhurried in his manner and I started to unravel right then. He spoke quietly and slowly and he didn't make me feel panicked. I began to talk about what happened. Everything just seemed to slow right down. He didn't panic me when he asked me to seek help from my GP and also consider accessing counselling. He was so none threatening, he gave me space, he was patient, calm and quiet. Despite everything that was going on in my head and my body, he created this very calm, quiet space. He listened to me. I told him how very bad I felt and that I was going to sit on the window ledge if nobody listened. He told me he was listening. He saved my life.

I had nothing left and could see no way out, but he listened and that slowed everything down. During my next lesson, I sat away from the window. The temptation to go through it was overwhelming. I spoke with him again that day. Gave him a graphic written account of the sexual abuse I had experienced. I expected to feel better, but I felt worse, and worse came, as illustrated in this journal.

I accessed my GP who put me on anti-depressants. I accessed work counsellor. I was having panic attacks. I went on annual leave to Majorca a week later with family and friends. I returned to work and lasted 2 days, I had totally lost my focus. I went off sick on 24th July and began this journal.

I have met Martyn a couple of times whilst I have been off, but today I met him because I wanted to say thank you and goodbye. Of course I told him about events leading up to today and reminded him of the impact he had had on me. I was finished, I had given up and I was ready to die, to do everyone a favour, but he listened, he gave me time, he made me feel safe and by doing that he stopped me from killing myself. I can never express my gratitude or begin to know how to articulate what that meant to me then and means to me now. I was so unwell, so totally vulnerable.

Martyn is a hugely significant person in my life and I will never forget what he did that day and on the days following when we spoke. I also felt an element of guilt. Guilt for putting him through that. And now I am here looking at it from a healthier perspective. How could I put anyone though that? To have to hear what I said. But he did it and that makes him a lovely special person.

I said goodbye to Martyn today, but I will ever say goodbye to the life he gave me. I felt more at peace following our conversation today and just talking to him gave me more confidence as I look forward. A truly remarkable man.

Reflection: It makes me feel emotional reading that entry. Martyn was one of those people who I have described in this journal. He was none judgemental, he was calm and unhurried and he listened and listened and listened and that was all I had ever wanted. Counsellors reading this need to understand that there is a place, always a place for listening. Listening can do more healing at the right time than any practical action, or objective response. I'm not suggesting if somebody is in immediate danger then a counsellor should listen whilst they articulate their demise. I'm saying there is a difference between physical action and emotional torment. I needed somebody, anybody to listen to how I was feeling. The action could come later, but I just wanted somebody to listen to me and he did. He was the first person to ever do that and I will never forget him.
Survivor guilt is also very common and I have read a lot about it and I understand it and I no longer feel that guilt. I have come to terms with what I said to Martyn and what I was going to do. I don't have any reason to feel guilty about wanting to end my life. I had been shouting and screaming and never been listened to for 36 years. I was completely justified in my feelings and once I was listened to and validated and supported I began to heal. There is nothing to feel guilty about in that.

Notes:

15.01.16
Spoke to Jayne at length about my anxiety about returning to work and the perceived weakness if you ask for help. Then driving home I thought I am a damn good midwife, never given anyone any cause for concern and always given my absolute best to everything in relation to my career and if I ask for help, I defy anyone who questions my ability to cope. How does Jayne do that? How does she plant the seed that makes me see things from an alternative perspective? I don't need to be anxious about it, it's not my weakness, it's their failure if I ask for help and I'm not supported.
Tonight I saw Carol. We had a takeaway together. We caught up with what's been happening and then we had a laugh. Carol has been a terrific friend to me right from the beginning and she heard my story as it all began to unravel. A truly amazing friend and I will never forget the support she gave me. Talking, texting, supporting, listening. Talking me through urges to self-harm. She was there. She really was there. A truly amazing friend. I will never forget the time and emotional energy she gave to me. Really kept me going and dragged me out of despair on many, many occasions. I feel sad to remember, but also grateful and thankful that she did. She means a lot to me, that time will always be there and I love her for that.

Reflection: A reflective piece in it's own right I think. I will leave it there for your thoughts.

Notes:

16.01.16
Today my mind has been quiet. I went for a run today. I love the solitude. It's so new, so unique. I have always hated being on my own, not because of loneliness, but because of what I didn't want to think about. I would have the television on, every radio in every room would be on. Now I marvel at the peace and quiet. I crave peace and quiet. I love peace and quiet, it is so new, so novel. It's incredible. I just love it.
When I run I do have music playing, but that's so I am cocooned in the with the music. I can enjoy my environment if I want to, but more often than not I am in a trance, just completely zoned out. I love it so much. I did take some time out today though to think about my memory. Norpel at meditation talks about training our mind to be calm and peaceful, because if you let it, it will think random thoughts constantly and it's an effort to make it stop. In relation to memory, I have been told and I understand that when you have experienced abuse, you process things very quickly and dismiss what you don't need. This makes sense because I don't remember a lot.
Today I tried to concentrate on something I was doing, really focus. But inside I was thinking I can't be bothered to do this it's too hard. I deliberately tried to do this and when I realised I didn't want to I remembered what Norpel had said about the mind. It needs training. Just like skim reading, I skim process. I have always done this because of the constant background noise of abuse that occupied my mind. It is just like a radio in the background. Now that radio of abuse including memories, thoughts and emotions has been turned right down and is increasingly switched off for longer and longer periods of time. I now have the ability to focus and concentrate, but I find instead of being distracted by abuse, my mind just simply wanders off. I wander off into any old thought. I hope this makes sense. So what I have to do now is train a wayward, roaming mind to concentrate and that's my next aim. My mind hasn't been focused and now because it hasn't been focused for so long, it doesn't want to. But I will train it, now it is no longer distracted, or hyper alert. I have always been hyper alert to everything going on around me. Had to be to stay safe, to maintain the guard of protection. Now I don't, I need to learn to focus. I really hope this makes sense.

Reflection: I'd had 36 years of abuse there in my mind, invading every aspect of my life. Simmering away in the background, just enough to distract me from enjoying life, or immersing myself in any life experience. Now that abuse had been dimmed, turned down, my mind suddenly had this free reign and it wanted to wander like a baby let out of it's pram. It wanted to think and wander and ponder anything it felt like. It was untamed. It probably sounds bizarre if you have never experienced it, but I really did have to train my mind to concentrate on tasks. Simple tasks, any tasks, because it had always dealt with things on a superficial level. This is why I never learned anything at school. I heard the words going in, but I didn't process them, or think about anything long enough to gain any understanding. The words just came in and then they left again because the abuse was playing over and over and over in my mind. Now the abuse had started to leave my mind alone, it just wanted to roam wherever it wanted. It really was very tiring. I had to learn to concentrate. I had to train my mind to focus. Not because the abuse was invading it, but because it had never had the opportunity to focus on anything. Once I was able to start focusing, I started to learn, I started to remember things. It was brilliant, but so very tiring too.

Notes:

17.01.16
Alans relatives came round today, a good, but hectic day. I tried hard to focus and I kept finding myself drifting away. I hadn't realised quite how disconnected I have always been. Also when we woke up this morning it had snowed overnight and we all played in the garden. Normally I would have stayed inside making an excuse why I couldn't join in. It's so lovely living in the moment, but also time goes much slower and I have been sitting here wondering why I am so tired. And now I know.

Reflection: I think I have just explained that in the previous entry.

Notes:

18.01.16
I have contacted my manager to let her know I am able to come back to work this week on therapeutic hours. To my initial astonishment she messaged me back to say she had no time to meet with me until next week. Astonishment soon lent itself to that familiar feeling of worthlessness. I feel completely devalued as a member of staff and completely worthless. I didn't allow the feeling to dominate my day. Following completion of household chores, I exercised, then meditated. I took a nap, then read for a while. I did feel calm until my parents arrived bickering and both turning to me for support. I felt the irritation growing inside me, then I left to go to my meditation class and felt calm at the end of the day.

Reflection: I was beginning to fend off negative distractions. Yes they were affecting me, but I could see they were affecting me instead of just being absorbed by them and I took steps to make myself feel better.

Notes:

19.01.16
I saw Jayne today. I told her what had occurred regarding the text exchange between myself and my manager. Described the worthlessness I feel inside, but recognised it is up to me to make change happen. It gives me a focus, but not a happy feeling about returning to work. I talked about my Mum and Dad yesterday and whilst I accept she is the way she is and I accept the way he is, I can't cope with the way she speaks to my Dad. She is cruel, cold and heartless, provocative and rude. Through conversation with Jayne I understand that the emotions I feel are because I am outnumbered. Both of them are incredibly selfish and have vied for my attention since I was small and those feelings are raw. Neither can see beyond the end of their nose. I feel angry that work has hijacked my last two appointments, but through conversation I understand the connection of returning to an environment of being worthless, ignored and not valued are all the same emotions related to being sexually abused. I have to find out how to resolve this. It may mean leaving midwifery altogether. There is uncertainty there, but through meditation I am continuing to practice living in the moment. I feel uneasy today. Horrible emotions returning.

Reflection: My Mother is narcissistic, my Dad has since passed away. My Dad had Alzheimer's and his vulnerability was used against him by my Mother. She would speak to him like he was nothing. Like he was worthless and not fit to be valued. I was outnumbered then and it took a long while, but I have learned to not respond to her narcissistic behaviour and she has responded to that by disconnecting herself from me and my children. I feel sad for my Dad who lived all his life with her being treated like I had been treated. Not knowing any love, warmth or compassion from her. Feeling scared and alone. I am lucky that I have broken that cycle. On occasion it makes me feel sad that I have been rejected by a Mother that should have loved me, abused because I was neglected and destroyed because she had no capacity to be there for me when I needed it most. Sad because she has never liked, never mind loved me and that was apparent throughout my whole life. But I accept that she is what she is because of who she is and not because of who I am. It's just so very sad and has led to a terribly damaged life for me and her.

Notes:

20.01.16
A quiet day today. Trying to focus on what I was doing. To be mindful. I had a good meditation, but cannot fend off the creeping anxiety of returning to work. I have to find a way forward. That at least gives me focus.

Reflection: Really there wasn't anything I needed to do expect continue to get stronger. Work would be the same as it had been before I went off sick. Nothing had changed, except me and that's how I would get through it.

Notes:

21.01.16

I met with my Supervisor today. She was supportive in terms of my absence, but had no insight or understanding of the need for support, but overall a positive meeting. I saw Carol in the office, I felt very nervous, but a positive first step. I was looking forward to a meditation and relaxed early night, but my Dad arrived at dinner time and stayed until 9pm. He has argued with my Mum and needed to sound off many times. That's his Alzheimer's. I am looking forward to my meditation course tomorrow.

Reflection: I had enrolled on a Mediation teaching course. I wanted to be a qualified meditation teacher so I could hold classes and help people to benefit from the positive experiences I was getting from meditation. Sadly that never happened, but it was great in terms of being able to really look into my own mind and helped my healing greatly, so it was beneficial in more ways than I had expected.

Notes:

22.01.16
I enjoyed my course today. I met Kim Lowrey and Mary Pearson the Co-founder of the British School of Meditation. We looked at Benefits of Meditation and it re-affirmed my feeling about changing my whole way of life. I have been striving to achieve more and more in terms of job status, academic achievement and both are because my Mum is so disappointed in me. I don't have that expectation to live up to any more. I have realised that I am enough and that's what makes me happy and fulfilled. I need to do it, I want to change my life.

Reflection: The determination to live a better life was a great step forward for me in terms of my recovery. It meant the bumps in the road along the way didn't take me back to those darkest of days. I had found something to aim for, for myself, not anybody else.

Notes:

23.01.16
A truly amazing thing happened today. I did a silent meditation on my course and my mind was completely still. No external thoughts or distractions, except the thought that kept popping into my head. *"I can't believe I'm not thinking about anything"*. I felt so elated, empowered and euphoric. My mind has not been calm and peaceful for the last 36 years and today for just 10 minutes it was completely still. Indescribable.
Alan was agitated when I arrived home. We all did a square breathing meditation and everybody felt tired afterwards. Yesterday we did a teddy meditation which the kids liked. Today has been a lovely, tiring day. Thank you.

Reflection: The more I became calm and present, focused and together. The more agitated Alan became. I spoke to Norpel about it, I couldn't understand why being a more balanced, articulate person could irritate somebody so much. Norpel expressed the opinion that some people don't like change. I challenged him and asked how that could be, when that change was for the better. He didn't reply, but just gave me a knowing look. I had no idea what that meant at the time.

Notes:

24.01.16
Last day on my meditation course. Very enjoyable, but lots to do. I have to rely on my memory and that concerns me greatly, but I have thoroughly enjoyed my course and I have been present. So please let it kick in. I think I have always relied on not forgetting something, rather than memory retrieval. Please memory help me out. Lovely meditations today.

Reflection: Well my memory served me well. I did remember what we had been taught and I did pass the course. Committing something to memory is completely different to not forgetting something. To explain: You try not to forget to put the bins out. You don't need to commit it to memory if somebody asks you to do it. Committing something to memory can be revising for a test and then being able to recall relevant information that has been revised when it's required. I had been living on trying not to forget. Holding information right at the forefront of my mind, because I was incapable of committing anything to memory because it was full of abuse. My meditation course provided the first opportunity to test out my newly refurbished mind and it worked and I was so excited and so proud of myself.

Notes:

25.01.16
I met with my Manager today. She has concerns about my ability to do my job because she is concerned that the compassion I feel will drag me down. I know It's not the job that will drag me down, but the way I am treated a work. Feeling sadness and compassion is healthy, but is viewed as weakness. My Manager said she wouldn't be able to do my job because she would lose her cool. The client group just wind her up. How is her attitude any healthier than mine? Am I missing the point somewhere? I went to meditation class tonight and the focus is always love and compassion. I will never lose my compassion. This is why my head remains mixed up. This is where the clash is in my head. My true genuine feelings and the way I am being told I should feel again. I am not weak, I am stronger than ever and I will not have my personality challenged again, but it leaves an uncomfortable feeling when once again your feelings, or should I say my feelings are being challenged. It's horrible and I feel trapped.

Reflection: I hadn't developed that strong self-belief at that point. I have bucket loads of compassion for my client group. I can really empathise with their experiences now and feel sad for them. The difference is, it no longer makes me feel sad about my own experiences. I no longer attach their feelings and emotions to my own because I own all of my experiences now and I will talk about them whenever I want to. Some people do judge me at work, they think I am weak, but since that entry and it did take a long time, I have developed all the self-belief that I need. I am strong, resilient and self-assured. I don't need to be aloof, cold or arrogant. I don't have a chip on my shoulder and I don't need to pretend I am something that I am not. I am calm and gentle and caring and incredibly strong, because that's who I really am.

Notes:

26.01.16
I received an e-mail today from Dr David Hamilton. It was explaining vulnerability and when it can be used to say or do something that leaves somebody feeling exposed, is actually a declaration of self-love. That give me a bit more courage and when scary things feel a bit less scary, then opportunities can expand.
I can make a difference, I believe I can. I should stop feeling uncertain when challenged and stick up for myself. It's a good day, plus I did an amazing twenty minute silent meditation this morning and I loved it.

Reflection: Positive affirmations really helped me to secure my self-belief and confidence in my own abilities. I was beginning to surround myself with like minded people. Dr David Hamilton is a published author of many books about the mind and body and how they are connected and how meditation and mindfulness benefits us in terms of our wellbeing. I enjoy reading his books.

Notes:

27.01.16
Spent three hours in work today because I am beginning my return. I felt so relaxed because I had done a thirty minute medication all the way to work. I feel more confident in myself, experienced no anxiety. I felt calm and composed. One day at a time.

Reflection: Practice, practice and more practice and I was doing it. I was believing in myself in terms of what I needed to do to look after myself getting back to work. Reflecting back, I can see I had more confidence than I believed at that time.

Notes:

28.01.16
I felt subdued after work today. Feels like my Manager has lost credibility in me. I don't have to prove myself to anyone, yet I feel I do so she doesn't think I am going to go off sick with work stress.

Reflection: This was just one of the challenges I faced going back to work. Other people doubting me and my ability. From a personal perspective it was very demoralising and I felt judged negatively. From my Manager's perspective, she knew I went off sick 6 months ago with suicidal thoughts, she knew I had a demanding and Professionally stressful job. What Manager wouldn't have reservations about that person returning to work in the same environment? A Manager who had no understanding of what I had been through and no confidence in her own ability, never mind mine. Had I known that then I wouldn't have felt subdued, but I didn't know myself how I would feel, so I could hardly blame her.

Notes:

29.01.16

I saw Jayne today and told her about my Manager and my Supervisors attitude towards me. My Manager saying "*Can you see a time when you won't need counselling?*" I told her I feel trapped, but I am making an effort to change that, by looking for another job. I recognise it's not me that's at fault for being caring and compassionate, but I'm being referred to as weak for voicing it. My ability to do my job is being called into question. Jayne acknowledged how hard I am working and said I was strong not to be crushed by what my Manager had said. She has no idea how hard it is, how vulnerable I feel and how easy it would be to doubt myself, but positive affirmations, Jayne and meditation are holding me together. We talked about my memory. I said I think instead of committing things to memory I realise what I do is just try to hold something in my head.

For instance if she asked me to bring say £2.50 next week, I would recite it over and over in my head so I don't forget. Jayne explained to me that when someone suffers a trauma it stays in the front of the brain going round and round, so when other information comes in that goes round and round too, or just isn't taken in. That's why I couldn't remember my two exam questions for Safeguarding. I read notes for one question, got it in my head, but when I revised the notes for the second question, I forgot everything about the first. Now it makes sense. It was because I wasn't committing it to memory. I was keeping it at the front of my mind. And I can't remember what it's called, but she said she will bring me a diagram to show me next week.

As the day went on I felt very sad. I feel very tearful now, because once again it affirms what happened to me and secondly all those years and memories lost. The kids when they were babies, the things I did with them. I know I took them of lots of days out, I was always going with my mum or Joelle. I just can't remember where or what we did. All lost. If I could have got help sooner, if someone had helped me I could have had all those memories. I feel so, so sad☹ Jayne said meditation will help, but she will also help me with strategies to learn. Today it hit me, I have been through so much and I'm still trying hard. I'm so sad.

Reflection: One of the questions I asked Jayne was now that I am able to commit things to memory and the abuse is no longer constantly playing on a loop in my mind, would I regain some of that lost memory. Jayne couldn't answer me what I wanted to hear. Sadly, it hasn't. When I think back to that period in the '90's and my children as babies and our experiences together all I see is black. A blank screen. I have lost all of that time and I feel devastated about that. All I can do and all I am doing now if focusing on every second of my life. I can remember things now. I can remember everything I feel I should be able to remember as part of a normal memory. But before that time, it's just a blank screen. A time erased, gone for ever and that is the saddest thing to have to write.

Notes:

30.01.16

The urge to self-harm today began with a fleeting thought. I dismissed it and went for a run. It improved my mood, but I felt low again. The urge to self-harm got stronger as the day went on. I started to feel a bit scared. The urge to self-harm is not anger at myself or frustration, but to show people how hard this is to overcome, to come to terms with, returning to an environment that challenges how I feel, which is basically compassion and empathy. Something I have always been challenged on; that is expressing how I feel and being ignored, or told I'm wrong to feel that way. To self-harm, to have a scar, would show everyone just how painful that is.

I meditated today and it felt all wrong, but I persevered. My mind was full of negative power and emotion, but later a thought popped into my head. What would be the reaction if I did self-harm? Proof that I couldn't cope. That I am still vulnerable, I am still unwell. So whilst the thought scares me and is in my head, that's just where it is. The correct response is for me to be able to accept for myself just how hard it is. Stay focused on caring for and looking after myself. I know it's hard, I know it's painful. I can cope with my job, my role. What I can't cope with is being told how I feel is wrong. I will keep meditating to keep me strong. But I am so frightened. So, so frightened. A moments weakness! I have to stay focused to respond, not react and that is so hard, so hard. I am so scared. I feel so lonely.

Reflection: The urge to self-harm remained with me for a very long time. When I was feeling emotional pain, I really wanted to cut to get that scar. I wanted the scar so that when people saw it, even if they didn't say anything I believed they would recognise that I had experienced terrible emotional pain. When I saw it I would be able to see that I had experienced terrible emotional pain. And if I was at a low point I could look at it and it would validate my emotions. At the time of writing the journal I didn't self harm for fear that people would have a very negative response towards me and injure me further by taking negative action against me in terms of my job and my life in general. I would feel out of control as people would take matters into their own hands and I didn't want that to happen, I was gaining control for the first time ever. It took a long time for me to view self harm as a negative reminder of emotional pain that I no longer felt, or thought about and although I was recovering really well, I couldn't see a time when I no longer felt such emotional pain and turmoil.

Notes:

31.01.16
I slept so well last night. I feel lighter this morning. I'm glad I didn't message Jayne in my panic. I went for a run in the rain, it was great to clear my head, although I had the image of him in bed with me. But in relation to my memory, I'm sure it isn't a black hole. I'm sure I just woke up and he left the bed. I was asleep and I have to accept that I will never know. I took Elizabeth, Charlie and her friend to play crazy golf this afternoon and I thought of nothing else but what we were doing and I didn't realise until we had finished that I had been totally focused on the game. It felt great. I had a lovely contemplation meditation this afternoon. I thought of the word 'calm' and all the connotations it brought up in my mind. I then was able to focus on making my mind still. It was so lovely I didn't want it to end. I feel so calm. I always want meditation to work.

Reflection: Well take it from me it does. It works every time, even when it doesn't. Think about that one.

Notes:

01.02.16
Feeling very emotional today, concerned about my mental wellbeing fluctuating from thoughts of control and empowerment, to thoughts that I am not strong enough and feeling a little spontaneous. How quickly and easily it would be to self-harm. Went to meditation class and spoke with Norpel. Discussed care and compassion being viewed as a weakness. He tried to reassure me that it is okay to have that professional balance as well as feeling compassionate. I understand, but it's hard. Thirty six years of suppressed emotion and six months of released emotion. I don't want to have to suppress it again. Equally I don't want to be told that what I feel is wrong. I've had that all my abused life. And it's that that triggers the self-harm thoughts. Look how painful those words are to an already damaged mind and self-esteem. I'm so frightened, I don't want to slip backwards.

Reflection: I was still slipping back into the idea that I needed to behave in a particular way in order to accommodate others. I was able to articulate that I didn't want to do that, but I didn't have the courage to state that I wouldn't do that. Instead I was fearful that I would and slip backwards. I still hadn't grasped that I am the owner of my own destiny. I was getting there slowly, but the pain it caused. Partial insight is hard to manage.

Notes:

02.02.16
My calm and peaceful mind has been taken over by conflicting thoughts of self-harm. A scar to show how painful it is to be told your distress is wrong. Or a scar to show I am still not strong. Distress at the reality that abuse has caused this short term memory problem. Distress at those lost pleasant experiences that were never committed to memory. I wrote a letter to my ex-husband, I text my cousin. I feel like I gave the memory back to them, but the man. He who started the damage, it still feels open ended and I don't know what to do. I need to be satisfied if only in my own head that I have given the memory back to him. I hate that it is causing me so much distress. I want my calm and peaceful mind back, but I recognise I can't push these feelings away. I have to look at them and work them out. The self-harm thoughts are lessening as I continue to believe in myself. The memory loss is turning to anger and that in turn is wanting to drive me to give it back to him. Then I really feel I will be able to close the chapter. I really want to be calm and peaceful again. I want to put this in its pace and move forward.

Reflection: As difficult as those emotions were I was taking more control. I was about to embark on a new wave of self-belief. It's strange, I didn't consciously set out to do it, it kind of came as the next natural step. The subconscious mind, the soul, whatever you like to call it is incredible. It knows when to take over. The organismic self I have since learned.

Notes:

03.02.16

Today I felt apprehensive driving to work, so I completed a squared breathing meditation. I was very calm when I arrived at work. I stayed for 2 hours and came home. It went well. My mind feels like a ping pong ball. I'm glad I felt calm and well, then I'm thinking just how hard this all is. Working all the time to be calm and peaceful, accepting my emotions and trying to rationalise negative thoughts. Then feeling so tired and wanting to scream *"I was just a child, I was raped and this is so hard to work through!"* Then being rational again, this is just happening because I'm returning to work, things are changing, but stick at it, it will get better. It's just so hard. This is so, so hard.

Reflection: Everything was so hard. Adjusting to working life and adjusting to an ever developing mind. It was all very tiring and yes hard because I was working hard. My mind had been given a direction and whilst I consciously didn't know how to connect it, it was making connections all the time. It felt like every morning I woke up something inside me had changed, or developed, or connected. I felt like I was just the passenger.

Notes:

04.02.16
Meditated on the way to work, calmed my busy mind, but I felt subdued all day. I just want to talk about how hard it is to carry on, to release the pressure. I scratched my arm today on a match. Just a scratch. I need to release the pressure.

Reflection: I have no recollection of doing this. An indicator that I was becoming overwhelmed, but I had nobody to explain it to who could watch over me.

Notes:

05.02.16

I cried a lot today. I saw Jayne and talked about the strong urge I get to self harm, to have a physical scar that shows how hard it is to be rational when my mind wants to be irrational. Also the scar will show how much it hurts to not be listened to. We talked about addiction and old habits. Is it either or both? Self harm is all I have ever had to fall back on when things have got hard. Breaking the habit is tiring. Feeling spontaneous is common. Jayne helped me by getting me to visualise the blue cushion on the settee (my favourite colour). When I am calm I can reason with my negative emotions, it's when I'm not calm that I feel spontaneous. She got me to close my eyes and visualise the cushion. I did it and it worked. She said that can be my stop sign when I feel spontaneous. To close my eyes and visualise the cushion. I hope it works.

We talked about how I have felt bad for getting angry these past weeks, talking about the failures of people at work who don't understand what I am going through. Jayne reminded me when I said It's not their fault, that it's actually not my fault either. People are so scared of mental illness. I talked about my image of Jack Kilbourne in bed with me. I said I kept thinking about it, needing to re-assure myself that I was asleep. I also talked about the possibility of talking to the police. I wrote a letter to my ex-husband letting him know I had realised he was raping me. I sent a text message to my cousin letting him know I had never forgotten him sexually abusing me, but Jack Kilbourne has had no reminder. It's left open and I don't know what to do.

Alan is worried about repercussions, not me. I feel so alone and very tired of always trying to work stuff out. So tired. Jayne told me I am working my arse off to recover, but people keep letting me down. It just feels good to have her support, I couldn't do this on my own. I re-connected with a friend today who I wasn't very good to. I am going to visit her and her husband to discuss my options about going to the police.

I have huge guilt and shame about the people I have humiliated myself in front of and behaved badly towards. I am trying to forgive myself, but I was so horrible at times. I would say or do the wrong thing and portray myself in a bad light, either because I was scared, or because I was trying to look hard. I think my friend may forgive me in time, I hope she will. I feel so bad about everyone I have upset. I cried the whole time I was messaging her. Walking round shops, in the toilets, outside, it just didn't stop. I am so, so sorry. So sorry for everything I have done wrong. I am so sorry, please, I have learnt my lesson. I am so tired, I don't know if I can hang on much longer. I am desperate to stop feeling pain. I'm not strong.

Reflection: I was in fact incredibly strong. I was about to do the strongest thing I had ever done. I was about to report Jack Kilbourne to the police. That took incredible strength, but it was all coming from within. It was like my inner self was driving me and I was being swept along with it. If I hadn't been strong I wouldn't have done it. If I hadn't been strong I would never have messaged my friend and asked for her forgiveness. I had been a cold, callous person for a long time. It was all about self preservation and control, but of course nobody knew that. I wanted to explain everything to my friend and risk her not forgiving me. That took strength.

Her husband was a police officer and I wanted to be able to talk through the process and potential consequences of me reporting Jack, before I decided whether to embark on any action. I didn't tell Alan I was going because he didn't want me to report it. He wanted me to forget it.

Notes:

06.02.16

My life has been difficult for me today. I feel exhausted from what feels like constantly rationalising or cancelling out negative thought or emotion. Self harm and the technique Jayne gave me. Flashbacks of what Jack did because I feel I need something to close him off.

I wrote the letter to my ex-husband describing in graphic detail what I'd realised he'd done to me. I text my cousin reminding him that I'd never forgotten and I have been able to let both of them go. I was raped when I was 13 years old and violently raped when I was 16 years old, both times by strangers and as horrendous and terrifying as they both were, I can even let them go because I see them as a consequence of what had already happened. So low self esteem, no self worth, due to feelings of being ignored, or belittled, or not valued. Those attacks are closed off by damaged feelings. But Jack, I have talked about him, what he did and my feelings around that, but have not been able to close him off. In my mind my feelings were heard and validated by my ex-husband and my cousin. Particularly because I described back to my husband that I now understood that for years he was raping me. I sent the letter to him, his parents and his brothers and heard nothing at all. That validated it for me.

Then my cousin, I text and described to him that I had never forgotten how he sexually abused me. His denial and cutting contact with me was also enough to validate it for me and let it go. That's why I need to be able to do it with Jack. The torment is there and I just want it to stop. I've experienced life without it for a few short weeks and now it's back.

I'm not suicidal, I don't think I will ever be that low again, that desperate, because I will never allow anyone to not listen to me again. Even if they don't agree, I will make my feelings and my presence felt. But I do so desperately want the pain to go away, to stop hurting, to stop feeling like his abused victim. I need to give it back to him and the sooner the better because I just need it to stop! I am so tired, I've been tired all day. I am totally drained, totally exhausted. And I feel so lonely.

Reflection: I was becoming driven with this need to give back to Jack what he had done to me. To let him know that I now knew what he had done to me was all his fault. Of course I was tired, I was exhausted, I was working really hard and I had no support other than Jayne. No support in the outside world. That hour a week in that room was my only space to be free to explore everything. One solitary hour.

Notes:

07.02.16

Had nightmares last night and generally upset. Feel flat today, went for a run, but can't get the thoughts of what might be able to happen to help me out of my head. So both positive and negative. However, I did a visualisation meditation and my daughter came and laid her head on my knee. So filled with love and visualising all the things that are causing me so much heartache being taken away by a hot air balloon, actually cleared my head for most of the rest of the day.

Then my clothes felt tighter and I was given cake by my husband's mum. Of course that made me feel agitated and anxious. I have been anorexic in the form of controlling food since I was about 20 years old. That's 26 years controlling food. I guess that's not going to relinquish easily after just a couple of months of no longer controlling what I eat against the calories I burn. But it is just another emotional difficulty. I am fed up of being mentally ill. I want to feel okay. I want to feel normal emotional reactions to daily life and it's challenges. I just need the penny to drop. Everything to click into place. I know it's happening, but I am so exhausted. So tired of trying all the time. So tired.

Reflection: This was like the longest assessment of my life. If you are taking an exam you have a couple of hours where you are expected to focus on a topic and put all that energy into expressing all the knowledge around that subject. I had up to that point, had 7 months of working out how to repair my mind. Well firstly how I could destroy my mind, that took a lot of time and energy, then conflict around whether to destroy my mind once and for all. That also took a lot of time and energy and then trying to work out how to repair my mind, with all sorts of external factors being thrown into the mix. So big hug to me for feeling tired all the time. It makes me feel tired reflecting on it.

Notes:

08.02.16
Thoughts all over the place, developing such a strong feeling that I need to report Jack, both to give it back to him so he no longer holds the power of torment over me, but also because of the guilt which comes in waves about not reporting it and possibly other children just like me being at risk.

Reflection: There it is, that driving force, that determination again.

Notes:

09.02.16

I hardly slept last night, going over and over in my head what might be the negative consequences of reporting what he did. I concluded at 03.34am this morning that I am sick and tired of being scared. I don't want to be and don't need to be scared any more. I made my decision and I called the police this evening. I rang the Police and was told to call the Police Constabulary where the offence happened. I did that, they took some details and told me to contact my local police station to make a statement. So I called them and they said that's not how it works, they told me to call somewhere else. In the end the guy at my local Police force rang the appropriate Police Force and they are going to fax through the details and I have been told I will be contacted in the next couple of days to arrange to meet me to take a statement.

The point of writing about the left hand not knowing how the right hand works is that it alleviated my anxiety about talking to the police. It humanised them and brought them back down to my level. Even though I have only made the initial contact, I already feel lighter. If they come back to me saying there is not enough evidence to pursue the case, then at least I will feel as though I have given it back to him. He will no longer hold his power over me in my mind, because he will know that I know what he did was wrong. If it does go further, well maybe it will make a difference and save another child from being sexually abused. Either way I will no longer hold any guilt. I will have exposed him and freed myself.

This is a major step forward for me.

Reflection: It was about to be a huge step forward.

Notes:

10.02.16
I have an appointment with the Police to make a statement on Saturday evening. It has already made me feel liberated. There have been flashbacks of anxiety, but mostly I feel ready to do this. I was pre-occupied thinking about it, but I did a ten minute breathing meditation and everything calmed down. Even though I understand how meditation works, it still astonishes me that it works for me.

Reflection: The excitement was growing inside, I was beginning to feel powerful again.

Notes:

11.02.16
Spent a few hours at work today, I can feel my confidence growing. Still a few flashes of anxiety about Saturday, but mostly enjoying feeling more confident.

Reflection: Taking control of a situation if a great way to alleviate fear. Even if the situation itself causes fear. It's the control that makes it easier.

Notes:

12.02.16
I saw Jayne today. Talked about work. The CQC criticised the Trust I work for, for inadequate provision of Supervision. Also another colleague revealed that she is accessing regular supervision via a different route. Why are my opinions, my voice, not heard? I talked about the need for this not only when I returned to work, but also 6 months ago and it was viewed as a weakness. There is conflict in our office between 2 staff members and it is not being dealt with and I am picking it up.
Jayne therefore helped me to recognise that this might in fact not be about me at all, but about somebody else's inability to deal with difficult emotive matters. I have always de-faulted to me being in the wrong if somebody questions, or discredits my opinion and I had never before considered that it might have to do with the other persons weaknesses. Now I have recognised this, I will try harder to believe in myself.
We also talked about me giving a statement to the police and the possible outcomes. Such as no further action due to lack of evidence, right through to the possibility of it leading to a court hearing. I talked about my reasons for pursuing this, to be free of him. To stop him having this hold over me, the guilt of never coming forward and the possibility that he has abused others. Whilst I know I did nothing wrong – now. I always live with the philosophy that I am the one in the wrong when someone questions me about anything I do. Making a statement is giving it back to him. Letting him know I was never in the wrong – he was. I can live by believing in myself. Whatever I do for the good of myself and others can never by wrong. EVER. And starting by giving what he did back to him, I can start to live by that. After thirty six years.

Reflection: I knew then what I needed to do to get Jack out of my head, out of my body. This was the right path for me. It might not be what everybody needs to do. The important thing I believe, is finding what is right to get the poison, the nightmare, whatever it is removed. For me it was reporting it to the Police, because that was giving it back to Jack. Giving the responsibility for sexually abusing me back. Giving it to the Police was me recognising that I knew it was wrong. I didn't need it to go any further. Giving it back meant I no longer carried that burden.

Notes:

13.02.16

Trying so hard not to think about my appointment with the Police this evening. Flashes of anxiety when this happened. I do recognise that avoiding feelings is not the right thing to do, but today, I really, really had to do it or I would have been a complete nervous wreck. I spent 5 ½ hours at the Police Station. I was calm, I was okay. The Officer taking my statement was excellent. He obtained the facts as if he was taking down a recipe and method.

For example:

Police Officer *"When you were sitting opposite him and he had his legs open did you notice if he had an erect penis?"*

Me *"No!"*

Then next question, no hesitation. It's the first time I have spoken about what happened without becoming emotional. He was very supportive, he made me feel safe to talk. I arrived at 7.50pm this evening and I left at 1.20am. As I was driving home I began to shake. By the time I arrived home I was shaking like a leaf. I have made my statement, I can't do any more. I accept whatever the outcome. But I have done it. I am no longer controlled by him, I no longer feel like a bad person, guilty or ashamed. He did this to me. I was vulnerable, trapped, even more so having to wait for him to come home for me to be abused by him. But no more. His secret no longer has any hold over me, no power, even if there is no evidence to proceed.

I know now after thirty six years and he knows exactly what he did to me. I now know it was wrong and he will know I know what he did was wrong. The reason though I hope it does proceed is because I never want any little soul to suffer at his hands like I had to. He destroyed my life. He destroyed my childhood, my innocence, my adolescence, my 20's, 30's and 40's to date. He destroyed my self-esteem, my confidence, my self-worth. God the damage he has done is immeasurable. I can't allow myself to feel guilty about not reporting this earlier, because I can't take time back and because nobody until Jayne was able to help me understand what he did was wrong. Now as soon as I understood and felt strong enough I have done it. What makes me feel sad is now I recognise it's wrong, I don't care for me if it goes no further. I am beginning to re-build my life and I have given it back to him: But if it does go no further, nobody can protect any other children, babies, or child relatives in his care. I am surviving – just, because I have had inner strength from somewhere to keep going. Despite suicidal thoughts and attempt. I can't bear to think another child could be destroyed, not cope and maybe not make it.

Suicide is such an easy way to stop pain and torment. I never want a child to have to endure the torment of sexual abuse at his hands. God it is so painful, soul destroying, life destroying. I have never believed in God, but if there is one for other people, then please put this degenerate, deviant, maniac, pervert, psychopath away for those people. I am not about revenge – I am no longer a victim, but a survivor, so for fucks sake if there was EVER any justice, please, please, please, whoever you are, if I deserved the pain for whatever reason, I have learned my lesson, but for God's sake don't put anybody else through this, please whoever the fuck put him on this planet, babies do not deserve to have their soul destroyed at his hands.

Reflection: It was quite cathartic talking to the Police Officer. I expected to be taken into a comfortable room, with comfortable chairs and soft lighting with cushions and a dear sweet lady would come in and gently extract an experience from 36 years previously. What I got was a big burly police officer who took me into a back room behind reception. I sat on an uncomfortable desk chair and it was cold. He was very matter of fact. He wasn't embarrassed, he was calm, patient and thorough. After I had made the statement he made me a drink and told me I had done well to come forward. He walked me to my car and wished me all the best.
I was shaking when I got home. I was wide awake, I couldn't believe what I had just achieved. I felt pure elation. I got home, Alan was tired, he poured me a glass of wine and went to bed. Summed it all up really, but not he or anybody else was going to take away from me what I believed I had just achieved. I was just so lonely that I wasn't able to share that with anybody at that time.

Notes:

14.02.16
Numb today, feeling a little spaced out. Not thinking too much about last night except, I wonder when they will call me.
Reflection: Disbelief too I think about what I had done. I was so much stronger than I had ever given myself credit for. I'd done it. He was gone, it was back to him.

Notes:

15.02.16

Feeling a bit high today, almost invincible. A sense of elation that I've done it, but a little disbelief as no outcome yet, so the full extent of what I have done has not hit me. Waiting for a 'phone call. Thoughts have entered my mind such as they can't find him so are not pursuing it. I don't know what to expect, but I want to know so I can move forward, deal with whatever. I suppose I feel a bit in limbo. It feels a bit unreal too. I disclosed everything, yet the world has kept turning, noting has changed. I want to put this away, I just need to be patient. I am coping okay.
I've been told I've been very brave, but it doesn't feel brave. I can talk about it now without my world falling apart. I needed to give it back to him. To let him know, I know what he did was wrong. I'm waiting to hear that he has been given that back. As for how things go after that, I don't know how to deal with it. I guess that is my nagging concern. But as of tonight, I am okay.

Reflection: This was the first time I had experienced anything like this. So: You give something back, you feel justice has been done, you feel elated. But then very quickly you come back down. Because in reality nothing has changed. Everybody is going about their day in exactly the same way. Nobody other than myself and the Police Office knew what I had done. Elation soon turned to despondency and despair and it's really important that victims, survivors, or whatever word you choose to use are aware of that. You feel like when justice is done it will somehow change everything, change you, the world, the universe. When in fact the 'hit' you get from doing something so brave and courageous, crashes very quickly when reality strikes and in the real world nothing has changed inside you and you have still been abused, anorexic, tormented, lost and suicidal. Yes I had given it back, but I had only given the responsibility back, I hadn't given the consequences it had had on me back. They were still there living within me. That was a really hard lesson to learn and it took a few more times for this to happen, before I learned that I still had the responsibility of my trauma to live with. That was such a hard blow, every time.

Notes:

16.02.16

No longer feeling high today. Not heard from the Police and a nagging doubt creeps in. What if my statement wasn't sent, what if nobody has read it? What if they can't find him and decide not to bother? So suddenly the impact of what I have done is beginning to hit me. Thirty six years of carrying this monster, fear, guilt, shame, self-loathing and I think I can shake it off finally when I give it back to him. I am becoming more and more anxious to hear they have given it back to him. So he will know that I know what he did was wrong. I feel very low because I have heard nothing and beginning to dread I will hear nothing.

So I looked up anti-climax and it would seem what I am feeling is normal. People who experience massive highs, huge achievements, naturally experience an anti-climax. The higher the hit, the harder the drop. The advice I read is not to ignore it or fight it, but to recognise it, acknowledge it and understand it. Then focus on what that milestone was.

I calmly spoke about being sexually abused thirty six years ago. Thirty six years I have carried guilt, blame, shame, embarrassment, self-loathing. Thirty six years a monster has scared me, affected me, ruined how my life could have been. That is enormous, huge beyond comprehension. That is no small achievement, realisation, enlightenment. Seven months ago I was suicidal because I believed the monster within had destroyed me, after thirty six years of tormenting me, the monster had won. Now, not only have I broken the monster down. I have almost thrown his poison back in his face. Almost destroyed him. That's why I need to know. That's why I need to get rid of almost. His stale breath is hanging on, I need to kill it off. That's why I need to hear. Please, please let me stay strong enough to see it through. I DID IT!!! I REALLY DID IT!!! I just need it to be finished. Please, PLEASE.

Reflection: Already I am moving the goal posts. Firstly all I believed I needed was to give it back, but as I came down from that high, I needed another hit to get me back up there. So then I needed to hear back and I needed to know that some action had been taken. For any counsellor who is looking after somebody for the first time, don't believe that the only thing a survivor needs is to somehow give back the responsibility to the perpetrator by whatever means. I truly believed that that was all I needed to happen, but I didn't. I was still looking to be exorcised of all the abuse I had experienced and the impact it had had on my life. It wasn't a conscious thought, it just developed. Any survivor reading this needs to be aware of that. The abuse, the impact on your life, that will never go away. You will come to terms with it, you will be able to lead a fulfilling life, but it will always have happened. Deciding to confront a perpetrator will only ever possibly achieve consequences for their actions. Possibly! But it will never take away what happened and I made the mistake when I reported Jack of believing somehow it would cleanse me of everything.

Notes:

17.02.16

I heard from the Police today. The investigation will start now. I feel excited again. Not because of him, but because it has reminded me that I am doing the right thing and I am actually being listened to. I spoke to someone at work about not knowing where his daughter is. They said maybe she committed suicide because of what he did to her. When I remarked how insensitive I thought that was, given what I've just experienced these last 7 months, the response was *"Yes, but you're over that now"*. I felt very upset. I've lived with his ghost for the past thirty six years and on more than one occasion it has almost killed me. Just because I am learning to put my abusers in their place, doesn't mean I'm not still coming to terms with the impact all this has had on my life. I am moving forward, I am re-building my life, but God it has taken it's toll. I am not 'over it now'.

What he did was life destroying and I don't know where I found the strength to carry on sometimes. I will never be *'over it'*. But it will start to become a memory, a chapter in my life I have held on to for so long. But I can feel that very soon I am going to let it go. Let it drift into a memory, no longer a part of my present. I am ready to let it go, I just need him to let go of *'little me'*. He will do that when adult me lets him know I know what he did was wrong. He destroyed my childhood, all those years of crying alone in bed, desperate for someone to hear, but nobody ever did. All those years not sleeping, all those years trembling which turned me into an anxious adult, always thinking I was in the wrong.

All those years of living on the outside of everything, existing, not feeling, not living. Watching and feeling different to everyone else. Isolated and so terribly sad and lonely. Just a child. A part of me died inside when he sexually abused me. Gone forever, the wonder of just living, seeing everything through fresh excited young eyes. Replaced with fear and dread and a very dark space inside. A dark, dirty space that made me feel just horrible and completely lost, wondering what would happen next. How bad am I going to feel, how much worse is this going to get and when will it stop?

When I cried at night I thought nobody would ever hear my tears, never hear how much I was hurting, never see how lonely and scared I felt all the time. Thirty six years later and they have. I am 10 years old inside, I am all of the above, but I am being listened to. I am an adult, but 10 year old me is getting comfort from being cared for and loved. And when he knows I know what he did was wrong, the little me I can see inside will finally be able to rest. To allow the rest of me to grow up. She will be able to stop tugging me, *"What about me? Don't forget me"*.

I will never forget me, I will always love and care for me. Then she can live with me as and adult. Loved and cared for , listened to and comforted. He will never hold that power over me again. I can become whole. I need to stay calm and trust all of me. Love me and put me first. Then I can be a good mum, wife, friend. I will be whole. I will do it. I just need him to let go of me and he will very soon now, he will.

I cried tonight because everything just seems too hard. But it is hard and nothing will ever be this hard again. I felt better after I cried. It will be okay.

Reflection: I see this entry as a little bit of self-soothing. A bit of self-re-assurance. I needed to because what I didn't know what life was about to become a whole lot more challenging.

Notes:

18.02.16

I was calm today. I am also very, very tired. I got home from work at 2.30pm, lay on the bed and slept until 5.30pm. I am exhausted. I know why and I am taking care of myself. Still thinking about Jack, about what is happening and will they be able to find my friends to corroborate what I am saying. I don't want to think about it until next Wednesday, but I can't help it.

The image in my mind has changed from him sexually abusing me, to him being questioned about me. I don't have any more to write today, because I just feel in limbo. Not happy, anxious or scared, just waiting. Yes – limbo.

Reflection: The problem with waiting is it gives the mind time to think about all the possible outcomes. It gives the mind time to decide if it actually wants more. Reporting a perpetrator is the easy part. Understanding that it is a lengthy, challenging process isn't what anybody tells you. I really believed after I reported Jack that it would all be done and dusted within a few weeks. I thought the Police would interview Jack, he would deny it, the Police would state not enough evidence and the case would be closed. To anybody thinking about reporting a crime be prepared for the strength you will need to see the process though to the end. It is absolutely worth it, but it does require all of your strength and determination.

Notes:

19.02.16

I saw Jayne today. We talked about Sarah-Jayne. I hope she didn't commit suicide. I have had waves of guilt throughout my life. I thought if I reported him I could stop it happening to someone else. But I felt so bad about myself, so guilty and ashamed of taking myself to that family, that I thought if I did report it I would be told it was my fault. But now, now I know it wasn't my fault. Everything could be innocent with Sarah-Jayne, but of course I don't know yet. If something has happened to other people, I don't know what it will do to me. I hadn't thought about it too much until now.

I dreamt about snakes last night. Even after I woke and went back to sleep I dreamt about snakes, so I googled it's relevance and it all applied to what's going on now. I don't want to dream about snakes again. I hope nothing has happened to Sarah-Jayne. But equally if something has, or has happened to someone else, it gives strength to what I am saying. Validates it somehow. This is so mixed up in my head. I just want her to be okay. Because nobody understands the damage it does, only those who have been damaged.

At best it kills, because that means no more pain, at worst it is never disclosed and the torment sees out a painful life. Then there is me. Half a life of torment and disclosure, then half a life of ???? I just need her to be okay. If she believes in God, then please, please, let it have looked after her. I am so sorry for everything I did wrong, please, please, don't let my weakness have killed, or worst still destroyed her. Please no!

Reflection: I thought about Sarah-Jayne a lot as I was growing up. I particularly thought about her when I knew she would be 10 years old. I had lots of episodes of guilt around that time, but as well as holding on to all the responsibility, I believed it was too late to report it. I angst about Sarah-Jayne on and off for many years.

Notes:

20.02.16
Shattered today, did not have a restful nights sleep. Busy day due to family commitments, but half an ear out for the 'phone and wondering what is going on. So tired, just feel like I need to sleep. No other thoughts except I hope she is okay and everything else today just feels like such a huge effort. I am shattered. My mum and Dad argued, both giving me their sob story. It doesn't usually affect me anymore, but today I felt I have enough to cope with and I just watched them both and thought this is what you have always done, but never a thought for me. And look what happened to me. And now I am going through it, they have no interest or inclination. They are blind to everything except their own misery and just today it made me feel sad.

Reflection: Neglect, I would say is probably the worst form of abuse. Neglect does all the damage it did to me and then I had to live with the consequences of that damage. Watching them argue only intensified my feelings of being neglected.

Notes:

21.02.16
My meditation class teaches us to observe out thoughts. So I deliberately didn't try to block out my thoughts of Sarah-Jayne. I have decided in my head that she has died at his hands. Through drug overdose, or suicide and I was almost in tears to-day. So I observed that thought for a while. I don't know why she has not been found yet and the reason could be perfectly innocent. I will hopefully find out on Wednesday when I get my update call. I didn't get angry or upset with myself for having these thoughts. I had these thoughts because I was projecting how I have felt about what Jack did to me, on to Sarah-Jayne. So in reality I still feel very hurt, sad and upset with Jack sexually abusing me. I think about how bad I have felt and how desperately I have wished to die over the years just to end the pain. Just to make it stop.
Jack ruined me, inside and out. He destroyed me and almost killed me and nobody can see that. I have to tell people if they are going to see how injured I have been. But you don't tell people things like that. Not like a physical injury. I guess when someone commits suicide through the trauma of being sexually abused, it makes me want to say – *"that's how hard it is. That's how sexual abuse destroys someone. It is harder to stay alive and live a nightmare over and over again, than it is to just give up. Suicide is so easy".*
I desperately don't want anything bad to have happened to Sarah-Jayne, but equally I want people to see how unbearably hard it is to live a life when you have been completely destroyed as a child. My Dad came round again today full of anger, bitterness and self-pity. Then my Mum rang me later full of anger, bitterness and self-pity. I am not a child now, but I was then, and this was them then. Full of self. I never stood a chance.
Some days the only thing that is not hard is to breathe. Today has been one of those days. I long for the day that life is no longer hard. Please, please, whatever I did wrong, I am so sorry. I am so, so sorry. I just want to live again. I want to stop hanging on. Please give me some peace, I am so sorry.

Reflection: It took me a long while to realise who it was I was saying sorry to. I will leave it for you to work out, I talk about it later in my book.
That sentence ending "suicide is easy". I really believed that at that time and logically. When everything was hard, overwhelming and the answers just weren't there, it was my belief that suicide was the easy way out. If you have a headache, you take a pill. If you have an infection you take antibiotics. If you are emotionally tormented, my understanding was get rid of the emotion. The only way to do that was to get rid of me. No me, no feelings. But that was because I didn't understand that I could get rid of the torment. If you have a headache you don't have your head cut off, you get rid of the pain in your head. Etc etc. What I hadn't worked out was I needed to get rid of the emotional torment and still live and live a better life without pain. I feel devastated when I hear that somebody has committed suicide because they, like me back then, had no idea that with work, and a lot of it, the emotional torment, the emotional pain will go. A full life can be lived. Going back to the headache, you know the headache will go. Adverts for painkillers tell us this, shops full of medications for every physical ailment are in full view. But where is the advert for over-

coming emotional torment, trauma and despair. We hear about suicide, mental health issues. We don't see adverts for Counselling organisations, we don't hear testimonies from people who have overcome adversity. We don't see an advert of a before and after with a little story in the middle with a person skipping off into the sunset. What we do see and hear is the damage that trauma and abuse does to people. Of course it does, but where is the 'pill' that helps us to overcome it. Mental health is still something to be scared of, not talked about, pitied and judged. It's about time we started seeing some adverts for positive mental health. It's about time people started talking about it as much as they moan about their physical ailments. People will do that for hours, but if you tell somebody you're depressed, you risk alienation from friends, family and work colleagues. It's wrong and with this book I intend it to change.

Notes:

22.02.16
A quiet mind today, more focused at work, but very tired.

Reflection: Says everything really.

Notes:

23.02.16
I heard from the Police today. Jack is being interviewed on Friday evening. A witness has been found and I am told he is very worried. I had to talk to my mum to let her know she would be contacted to make a statement. To say she was cold about it is an understatement. She is so unfeeling. I need to find photographs of when Jack and Emily took me to London with Sarah-Jayne. I saw the photo's before they moved, but I look through a load tonight and they weren't there. She said she had probably thrown them all out when she moved. She showed no compassion, no caring, no understanding. She didn't care, just like she didn't care when I was 10 years old and she didn't care when I told her what had happened when I was about twenty three years old.
She is and has always been so completely and absolutely wrapped up in herself. I meditate to understand why she behaves the way she does, I do understand, but I don't like her. I don't like her at all. I feel and have always felt totally rejected by her. She doesn't love me, or anybody. I have a Mum that has never accepted me or loved me and I am damaged because of that. She really is horrible and I have never had that unconditional love or approval. Now I understand why I have always felt so alone.
My Sister loved me and I loved her, when she died I lost the other half of me. I am empty. I am sad. I have no solid ground. I am alone, I feel so very alone. I have dealt with me all of my life. I'm not a child any more, but I never got to know how feeling safe and secure felt. Not after my Sister died. I used to talk to her, ask her why she left me. I used to look towards the school doors in assembly and expect my mum to be stood there with my Sister. But she never came. I held on to that hope for so long and then I met Jack, Emily and Sarah-Jayne and I belonged all over again. I was accepted and loved like a true member of the family. I loved it so much, why did he have to take that away from me? Why did he have to hurt me? What did I do so wrong? I am so sorry, for everything. I am so sorry.

Reflection: I remember the time I went to London with Jack and Emily very clearly. I remember Emily asking me if I wanted to come and I was so excited. I took Emily to meet my Mum and my Mum agreed that I could go. I didn't realise though what Jack had planned to do to me and before I went to London with them Jack sexually abused me. I was so frightened and I didn't want to go, but I had been so excited up to that point that I couldn't think of a reason to say I no longer wanted to go. We stayed with some relatives of Jacks, I didn't know who they were. I slept in the same room as a teenage girl. She was really friendly, Emily and Jack slept up in a loft space, with open slat stairs that came down into the bedroom. I was frightened, but thought I would be safe with this other person in the room. I can't remember what we spoke about, but I do remember thinking I wanted to ask her if Jack has ever touched her. I didn't because I was frightened she would tell somebody and I would get into trouble.

Notes:

24.02.16
I wasn't expecting a call today, but a DC investigating my case rang me. Jack has been in to give a voluntary interview. He still denies knowing me, but Emily remembers me now. Jack is a supply teacher in a primary school, but he has been suspended pending investigation. When the Detective told me that I felt sick and guilty all in one go. Sick for what he might have done to kids and guilty because I haven't said anything before now. She told me he was angry that he will never work with kids again. I said "*Good!*" She said he was also angry that he had been searched for on Facebook and was going to close his account down. She told me Sarah-Jayne is estranged from the family when she had a baby two years ago. Jack was very angry because he was made to listen to my statement.
Now the Police are going to try to contact Sarah-Jayne and she is going to speak to Sharon to see if she remembers. My emotions are all over the place. I feel powerful and elated. Angry that he says he doesn't remember me, yet I have never forgotten him, or what he did to me. He destroyed my childhood, how dare he not remember me. I feel I need to sit down quietly and work through it. It is all happening so fast. He's held this power over me all these years. I have been hiding, afraid.
He remembers me alright!! You don't have your fingers in a ten year olds knickers and not remember it. He's a teacher, he's not stupid. I don't know if I will find the photographs, I don't know if Sharon or Sarah-Jayne will disclose anything. I am still searching for an answer and I'm not sure what it is.
What do I want? I want my childhood back. I want all those years he robbed from me. My youth, my adult life, my mind. I want my young innocent mind back. I want my life all over again. I want to be able to grow up when I am ready. I will never get that back.
Jack you stole it all from me. You destroyed me and I want it all back. I want my innocent childhood back. That's what I want. I really want it all back and I can't have it. You destroyed everything, my innocence, my right to be safe, to just be me. You stole it all. My sleep, my peace, my mind. You stole everything from me. Ripped my soul apart when you sexually assaulted me.
You killed me!!! I want it all back. Don't you understand. You have lived your life, but you destroyed mine. I have had no life. I have existed, gone through the motions and when the pain got too bad I tried to kill myself. You ripped my heart out when you stuck your fingers in my knickers. You completely destroyed me and I just want it back. I just want my childhood back. I hate you, you bastard, I HATE YOU!!

Reflection: Sharon was my best friend when we were 10 years old. We would play together with her brother and his friend who we called Piggy, for reasons I have long forgotten. Anyway after Jack sexually abused me I confided in Sharon. Sharon stopped being my friend when I spent so much time with Jack and Emily, but after Jack sexually abused me I re-connected with her. Her Nan and Grandad used to live in the same flats as Jack and Emily, but they lived on the ground floor and they had a lovely garden. Sharons Nan had a heart condition and we used to walk to bingo with her. Anyway, this particular day I confided in Sharon. I told her what Jack had done to me, how he had started off tickling me and then put his fingers in my knickers. Sharon then shared with me that a neighbour had done something similar to her when she was in his house alone, only Sharon told me that he put 'milk' down there. (Referring to where her knickers were). I remember clearly asking Sharon where he got the milk from and how did he carry it from the fridge to put it down there. She kept telling me she didn't know. I remember feeling confused. I remember asking her if she wanted to go round again, but she told me she didn't. I was so curious about that milk for a long time.

Notes:

25.02.16

Today I was proud of myself for the first time ever. I dealt with a conflict at work between two people and it was successful. I used the skills I learned on my communication course and also what I have learned these past six months. I went to my Mums tonight and Alan found a bag full of photo's and in one pack there was a photo of me, Jack, Emily, Sarah-Jayne and Jacks Dad. Jack lied about not remembering me. I know it and the police know it. I felt so sick and light headed when I saw the photo. I have felt sick all evening.

The emotions, the fear I felt after Jack Sexually abuse me came back in a rush, a big wave. I thought I was going to cry, faint, I don't know. I feel very sick inside. His behaviour to me, all this guilt and seeing him in that photo, past and present emotion flooding together. Fear from my past and true real validation from me now. Validation that makes me feel sick!

I have lived with Jack in my head for thirty six years. Now what he did to me is being reflected on the outside, because of his statement. He has lied. It validates just how awful it was what he did to me. He wasn't playing, he was sexually abusing me, no mistake, no mis-interpretation. But because it's now being reflected back to me though what's happening now. What he said, it's still a shock.

Just like when someone knows somebody is going to die. You know it's going to happen, you imagine what it's going to be like, you are watching that person die. But when they do die, you find that you are shocked! I knew what Jack was doing to me, I just didn't trust my feelings because he was so calm when he'd done it. Now it's here in the present, really happening and that's just what I am – shocked! My feelings then and now were absolutely right. He destroyed me. He violated me, he ruined me and I was just a child. I just wanted to be loved. He didn't have to hurt me. He left me broken.

Reflection: Seeing those photographs had the same impact those people I have described earlier did. Being told I had been terribly abused, shocked me to hear the words said. The photograph made Jack really real all over again. It was proof, it was real proof that he had sexually abused me and that's what made me feel sick. It was literally being pushed in my face again.

Notes:

26.02.16
I saw Jayne today. Told her about the events of the week and how I am feeling. The investigating officer called me tonight. Emily denies I ever stayed over, she said my mum always took me to their house and collected me. She is colluding with Jack. My old friend Sharon doesn't remember me disclosing anything. I expected it, but I feel sad at the same time. Alan helped me tonight by scanning the photo's of when they took me to London. I don't think it will do any good. Without evidence they have nothing.
I was very disappointed that the Police didn't ask Sharon about Jack and Emily. The reason we fell out was because I was there all the time. I know this is all going to come to nothing, it was too long ago, but I need to get that sniggering face out of my head.
Emily even asked if I was getting confused with Jacks Dad. How desperate is that!! My God!! If the police don't find enough evidence, I will make sure by staying the right side of the laws, that he is never going to 'forget' what he did to me. Not only that, but I will make sure that everybody knows. He is a disgusting, filthy paedophile. He knows it, Emily obviously knows it because she is now lying for him. I can't abide liars, so I will nail him. He will be sorry he EVER stuck his filthy fingers anywhere near my knickers.
That Bastard is going to pay and I will do anything in my power to make sure he does!!

Reflection: My Mum had no idea where Jack and Emily lived. She never went to their flat. I saw Emilys lie as further validation that Jack had sexually abused me. It made me angry that she could live with a man who she knew had sexually abused me. Her own husband. What I wasn't able to see was the torment she would now be going through, because she knew she was lying for him. She knew exactly what Jack had done to me the minute she needed to lie. I just couldn't see it at that time. Using Jacks Dad, I could see that was desperate, I just couldn't see that she would be horrified by what she knew Jack had done to me. Using a dead person, somebody who couldn't even answer for themselves in order to protect her paedophile husband. Was Emily also a paedophile?

Notes:

27.02.16

I was reading about the patterns of abusers and how they think, yesterday and it obviously sunk in overnight. I understand why Jack is behaving the way he is. It's because it's his coping mechanism. Jack denying all knowledge of me, not wanting to hear my statement is all text book typical. Emmily colluding with him is also textbook typical. That helps me to understand.

What makes me feel totally worthless is my Mum. How can she not remember me going away with them and staying with them? She was so wrapped up in her own life, I could have danced naked on the table as long as it meant she didn't have to deal with it, or I didn't get in the way of her drinking. I feel so worthless to her. I grew up feeling worthless, because I was.

Alan doesn't understand why I haven't cut her out of my life. It's because I am better than her and I am not her. She made me feel so worthless, invisible, shit. She totally neglected me, how shit am I!

Then everybody after that totally demolished me. My cousin, the man in the park, the boy when I was 16, my ex-husband. I should have committed suicide years ago. Nobody would have cared or even noticed. What have I done? What did I do? I am so sorry for whatever it was. I don't feel suicidal now, but I still feel worthless and I don't want to any more. I want to build my self-esteem. How do I do that? My past is reminding me constantly how worthless I am. I want to let it go. I am not worthless. Why did everybody do that to me? I hate myself and I shouldn't. I didn't do anything wrong, but my mere presence made people work really hard to show me just how worthless I really am.

Reflection: My Mum was and still is a negligent parent. I could see that then and I can see it now. What I couldn't hold on to was that she was negligent because of her failings and no mine. I was abused because of their weaknesses, not mine. The only part I played in any of it was being vulnerable. Being vulnerable made me a target. My past wasn't reminding me how worthless I was, my past was reminding how awfully I was treated by those who abused me. But lack of self worth and self esteem, fostered that belief and that's what I really needed to be working on. I was trying to solve the wrong problem.

Notes:

28.02.16

Kept wondering if the Police were going to call me today. They didn't, but the intensity of emotion I was feeling yesterday has gone. I enjoyed being engrossed with my children today. I can't keep giving Jack thinking time, but I can't get him out of my head. He's been in it for thirty six years. Now I want him to go. And as bad as it sounds, I think as long as my Mum is around, he will be here in my head, because every time I see her, she reminds me of why I was driven to him.

Reflection: Coming to terms with why Jack did what he did to me means that he isn't in my head because my Mum is still around. They are 2 very different people and they abused me for very different reasons. She doesn't remind me of Jack, she reminds me of a very damaged person, who inflicted her pain onto me.

Notes:

29.02.16

Felt calm again today, I don't hate myself, I just hate what has happened to me. I want a life back that I can't have. I have to accept that and learn to let it go. For some reason though it is not ready to go. He sits on my shoulder hovering over me sniggering. The image in the living room is with me daily. I just want him to go. He's been with me for thirty six years, why won't he go? I understand why he is behaving this way, I understand why Emily is behaving the way she is, it stops me from feeling hurt. It stops it destroying my mind, both their response is text book. So what is it going to take to make the image no longer threatening? Maybe I am trying too hard to make it go. I have to trust it will go. The other images have gone. Patiently I will wait – for now!

Reflection: I needed time to process what was happening. Jack sniggered at me when I told him to stop. I had that image of the arrogant, confident man. Maybe he wasn't scared because Emily knew what he was doing to me and she allowed it to happen. I hadn't processed that Jack and Emily had been made explicitly aware through my statement of what Jack had done to me and that would be having a huge impact on their lives. He definitely wasn't sniggering now.

Notes:

01.03.16
Started off feeling calm and positive today. Prepared to accept what will be will be. I can't influence any outcome. But this evening feeling very angry and tearful. Angry at my Mum for neglecting me, resulting in me seeking love elsewhere. Angry at Jack for sexually abusing me when I had found the love I needed. Angry at Jack and Emily now for lying and so angry at my Mum, because her current cruel, negligent behaviour towards my Dad just mirrors her behaviour towards me as a child.
The behaviour that lead me to Jack, the behaviour that caused me such low self-worth, low self-esteem and self-hatred. I am angry that whilst I am feeling more rational and able to function, at times it is a very difficult battle. Everything feels too hard and I just want it to stop. I can sense and end to this, even though I don't know what that end is going to be. I can predict it, it feels so close now, but it just needs to happen. All I know is that when it does I will be able to let Jack go, or he will let me go. It's coming and it's coming very soon. I just need the strength to hold no, because I am tired and sometimes I think I am going to go mad. I feel like my brain is going to lose all sense of rational thought and that scares me.

Reflection: There is nothing more exhausting than having questions constantly going round and round in my head. Anger is a particularly draining emotion, but when I couldn't figure out myself how to stop feeling so terrible about myself, I would occasionally throw it back at them and blame them. It gave me a focus, but it was like a hard tennis ball constantly batting back and to in my head, from why do I feel so bad about myself, to why did you have to make me feel so bad about myself? It was absolutely exhausting because I couldn't find the answers. I was looking in the wrong place still.

Notes:

02.03.16

Today began quite calm. Later I spoke with my friend who saw I was struggling in July last year and said to me "You're not thinking of doing anything silly are you?" I stared at her for some time, barely able to make my lips move. "I don't know" was all I could force out of my mouth. She contacted Martyn and all this began.

Today she told me that when she was twenty eight years old, her brother committed suicide. He was thirty two. I felt so sad for her and so very bad for putting her through my experience. I wanted to cry, but didn't want to make it even more about me. I felt and still feel so ashamed. I felt suicidal because I didn't know how to cope with the pain. I wanted it to stop. I still want it to stop. I want it to go away, but listening to her today I realised, nobody recovers from suicide.

As much as my pain feels like it's destroying me, it fluctuates and I desperately hope it will go away so I can feel free. But to have committed suicide at that time, I believed everybody would be better off without me. But my god! The lives it destroys forever! I hope I can hold on to that feeling I had today, because I am so deeply sorry for making her experience that time.

I am truly sorry.

Reflection: I really couldn't articulate it any better in order to describe the impact suicide has on those left behind. This isn't to make anybody who has suicidal thoughts feel guilty, but it's to perhaps get people to think, before things get so bad. Reach out to family and friends. You will soon know, as I did how they feel about you. Those who can't be there for you are not worth your time. But those who can would much rather listen to your shit, than listen to your eulogy.

Notes:

03.03.16

Today I have such a heavy sadness. I worked in clinic today and felt so disconnected. Conversations and gossip felt so trivial. The longer I was there, the sadder I felt. I cried all the way home, I feel I don't belong to anything. I e-mailed the investigating officer, no update, but the teacher not only doesn't remember being told, she doesn't remember me. I can't describe how insignificant and worthless I feel right now. Of course people don't remember insignificant things, but it wasn't insignificant to me. My Mum and Dad had already drilled it home how worthless I was. I loved going to see Sarah-Jayne. Jack ruined all that, now he denies me, but I know he is lying. Nobody would even notice if I wasn't here at all. Today I wish I wasn't.

Reflection: It was so difficult to be back at work, get back into the mentality of work when all this was going on around me and inside me. It was like I was still 2 separate people and that was incredibly hard.

Notes:

04.03.16

A very emotional day. I saw Jayne today and talked about the whole week. My Mum not remembering me sleeping out, her neglecting my Dad. Trying to cope with the insignificance of being sexually abused by everyone else. My friend talking about her Brother committing suicide. It all got too much today and I couldn't stop crying, or shaking. Today my mind is so overwhelmed. I felt supported with Jayne. I felt so lonely the rest of the day and this evening. This is hell. I just want to feel okay. After all this disclosure I thought things were becoming easier to come to terms with. Suddenly it all feels very current again. Very overwhelming. I am so tired. When will it end? I hope by the time I reach the end of this book.
Please let it end. Whatever I did before I am so sorry. Please.

Reflection: I likened my recovery to renovating a house. In order to renovate a house you have to strip it back to the bare bricks. It gets messy, you can find things you didn't know where there and for a while you are clearing up endless mess and nothing appears to be improving. This was exactly how I felt at that time. I felt like I was clearing up a lot of mess. Dealing with a lot of stuff, even stuff I hadn't realised was there. But I still wasn't feeling better. But as with any house renovation, perseverance and determination will see results. The problem was I couldn't leave the mess behind and go home. I was living in the mess. I had to live with the renovations going on in my head.

Notes:

05.03.16

I feel numb today, overloaded with the events of previous days. Then I had a 'phone call from the Investigating Officer. She told me she had spoken with Sarah-Jayne and no disclosure had been made. She told me she had spoken with Kim. Kim initially denied any disclosure, but when the Officer returned to her office Kim had left her a message saying she remembered a disclosure. She is going to see Kim to take a statement on Friday next week.

Sharon is niggling away at my thoughts. Sharon met Emily and Sarah-Jayne, she took Sarah-Jayne for a walk with me a couple of times, but wasn't interested. Sharon told me her neighbour had put 'milk' on her 'down there', I asked where he got it from, she said she didn't know, it was just there. Sharon told me this after I had told her that Jack had been touching me down there. It was our secret.

I can understand the teacher not remembering me, but me and Sharon shared a secret, that's what I can't understand. She told me about the neighbour because I told her about Jack. I am going to e-mail the Police again tomorrow. She also has tried to contact my mum. She left a message yesterday. I rang my mum and told her – disinterested is the only word I can describe. When I told her the Police want her to make a statement her only response was "*Oh! Bloody hell*". How inconvenient am I! But I don't care. Kim remembers. Somebody thinks I am important enough to be remembered. I am not reeling high, or low. I am just patiently waiting to see how this will unfold.

Today I am okay – Today.

Reflection: One of the hardest things was to hear back that people did not remember my disclosure. I would never forget a disclosure like that. I didn't understand. The Investigating officer told me that maybe Sharon was not in a place to deal with what happened to her, so she had to deny it. She asked me if I would have honestly been able to support her if I hadn't been ready to disclose. I couldn't answer that, because it hadn't happened and all I could think of was that I would. I would say I remembered. But then when I think back to the communication course and Martyn saying I needed to ask further about a client's disclosure and in my mind I was adamant I didn't want to. Maybe that was/is the same for Sharon. To acknowledge my disclosure would have meant she would have to acknowledge her own. I still hope that one day Sharon will be able to do that.

As for Brenda Smith, the maths teacher from Comprehensive School. Why would she remember me? As far as the was concerned "*These things happen*". Why would you remember something that you didn't think was abnormal anyway? Perhaps it had happened to her and she was told it was 'normal'. I don't know, but at that time and at times now it doesn't help. She doesn't know that she contributed to my mental decline, but she should.

Notes:

06.03.16
Very, very emotionally drained. My mind flipping back and too between flashes of belief at my complete worthlessness and insignificance and my mind trying to rationalise my complete insignificance not being about me. But if it isn't about me, it's about them, then why did so many people treat me with such insignificance. No thought, without caring or compassion.
My mind is so, so tired.

Reflection: It was coming. I was starting to have thoughts that it was the perpetrators responsibility for abusing me, but I couldn't quite make the connection and quickly internalised it. The sorting and figuring out I was doing was going on all the time.

Notes:

07.03.16

Very flat today and very, very bored and unmotivated at work. Everything just seems so trivial to me. I know it's me, I just feel so disconnected. Had a really negative experience at my meditation class tonight. Love and kindness, the focus being our Mother. I tried hard, I really did, but I just can't see it. My muscles became so tight that my back and left arm was so tense, the pain was awful. I felt so irritated afterwards. Insignificant, worthless me. How do I develop a sense of self-worth until I understand why I was so insignificant and worthless to so many people when I was a child. I am so sorry if I was so bad that people just backed away from me. But why?

Reflection: And I had flipped back to self-blame again. This went on for a long time, like those irritating lights that flicker on and off. I would have flashes of insight, but then they would go again. I remember that meditation class vividly. I can say it wouldn't end well even now if I had to listen to it again. It was all about what our Mother had done for us. That was like saying, look at what's happened to you, it's all about your Mother. Nope, I didn't need reminding.

Notes:

08.03.16
Numb. Not much else to say. My mind has temporarily bailed out. Extremely tired.

Reflection: I still don't know whether that was a good thing or a bad thing. Good in the sense that I had some temporary relief, but bad in the sense that it literally just closed down and I thought and felt pretty much nothing at all. Interesting to hear what the experts say on that.

Notes:

09.03.16
Had a nightmare last night about Jack trying to find me. Disturbed me in as much as it woke me up early, but I felt okay and felt calm all day. It feels as though Jack is so far away. My heavy feeling has gone. I felt numb again today. My weight is really bothering me though and I wish it didn't because that makes me feel tense. I want to feel okay with my body, but haven't since I was ten years old. I guess it will take time. I really believe something is going to happen soon, I've got that feeling. And when it does it will lead to a big change in my life. It's coming, I can almost feel it. Before I get to the end of this book.

Reflection: When I had an image of Jack, it was no longer the sniggering face magnified in front of mine. It was an image of a long straight road and Jack was standing a long way down the road looking at me. Not sniggering, not laughing. Just looking at me as if he was waiting for something to happen.

Notes:

10.03.16
Had a nightmare last night about a petrol bomb pushed through the letter box. Still didn't feel scared, just annoyed that I woke up. Felt calm today, some thoughts about Kims statement tomorrow. But it really is out of my hands. Jack feels so far away, almost invisible at the moment.

Reflection: It's a shame I didn't articulate at the time, the time when Jacks face was no longer sniggering. Perhaps it was the day before this day when he seemed far away. It was lovely not to have that face in mine any longer and he no longer felt like a threat. He looked so small in the distance.

Notes:

11.03.16

I saw Jayne today, talked about Jack being a tiny figure at the end of the road. I know Kim is going to be making a statement today. I think I feel calm because somebody is validating my experience. It somehow justifies everything that has happened since. I had another nightmare about Jack trying to get to me, but he couldn't. It doesn't scare me, it just wakes me up, then I am frustrated because I can't get back to sleep. I keep expecting a call to say Jack has killed himself.
The Police didn't call tonight, my anxiety levels shot up at 9pm tonight. I felt something was happening.

Reflection: At that time it really didn't matter to me how much Kim remembered, just knowing somebody remembered made me feel important. Important enough for Kim to go to the trouble to make a statement. I really did think Jack was going to kill himself. I felt the way the Police described his behaviour, he would deny me my voice again and end it all.

Notes:

12.03.16

Another nightmare. This time Jack set fire to the house with him and Emily in it. Anxiety levels really high about 0835am, again a huge sense of foreboding, like something bad is happening somewhere. It spoiled my day. I have decided not to call the Police for an update. I want to hold on to the reassuring belief that Kim has validated my experience.

Jack is beginning to fade out at the end of this road. His image is so small and he keeps almost disappearing, like he's going, but trying to hang on. I'm not going to let him spoil one more day of my life. I knew I was always grasping at straws reporting him so long after it happened. I am positively resigned I have done all I can. He is disappearing, I just need the nightmares to stop. I'm nearly at the end of the book. Something is going to happen.

Reflection: Perhaps that's why I was having nightmares. Jaco had dominated my days and nights. He no longer dominated my days, so he was trying to get to me through my subconscious. Only now it didn't scare me, it irritated me. He no longer held on to the power he'd always had over me. He was recoiling, because I had outed him. If I'd realised that at the time I would have been so much happier, but I couldn't see it.

Notes:

13.03.16
No nightmare last night. Hurray!! Maybe because part two of my meditation course yesterday and I was relaxed, calm and very tired. Fleeting thoughts of the Police calling, but otherwise no thoughts. Today was an okay day. Jack is no longer at the end of the road. It's now just a road, with baron land either side, like route 66. I don't know what that means. I don't care. He is beginning to leave me alone, or is it I'm beginning to leave him alone. The image of the living room has changed, to me sitting in it, him next to me, but it's beginning to feel like it was a long time ago. In a different life almost.

Reflection: This illustrates just how incredible the right counselling can be. Jack was leaving me, or I was leaving Jack. It really doesn't matter which, but he was going and the flashbacks were becoming really distant memories, they no longer held any power. My mind was letting go and he was drifting into space. Bliss.

Notes:

14.03.16
Awake most of the night because Elizabeth was up and down, so shattered today. No real thoughts about anything.

Reflection: Brilliant!

Notes:

15.03.16

Had a good sleep last night. And a calm day today. I had a missed call on my 'phone and a message and thought it was the Police, but it wasn't. That was my only thought in relation to Jack. I feel calm at work, I am able to concentrate on information I am receiving, in meetings and I am even asking questions and putting my opinion forwards. I did get annoyed because I have requested a car park permit for my safety and the person I am requesting it from is being difficult. I have no patience any more with people who are deliberately obstructive. Particularly when it come to my own safety.

I did e-mail the police into all my correspondence, just in case anything should happen. I will not compromise my safety for anybody. EVER AGAIN!

Reflection: How incredible that as soon as the trauma is released to drift away, new information is able to be retained. I felt like I had an opening in my mind that could now receive information, like a space had been cleared. I remember clearly that day asking questions and expressing my opinions. I remember smiling to myself because the questions were out of my mouth before I realised and I was there thinking where did that come from? It still happens now 3 years later and I still smile and wonder in the same way.

Notes:

16.03.16
I had a couple of calls, but not from the Police. It's there at the back of my mind and I don't want it to be. She has not got back to me about Kims statement and she has not tried to contact my Mum as she said she would. I want to know what has happened, because I'm sure something must have. I just don't know.

Reflection: My lack of understanding of the investigation process led to a lot of frustration. Investigations are incredibly long and I didn't know that then. Having that information at the start would have really benefited me in terms of my recovery. I am quite a literal person anyway, I didn't know it then, but it really helps if I have an idea. It doesn't matter if it's going to be three hours or three months, as long as I have an idea in my head.

Notes:

17.03.16
I e-mailed the Investigating Officer today. She had had to cancel Kims appointment last Friday due to another incident, but was going to see her at 4.30pm today. She then e-mailed me to say that appointment had to be cancelled too. I felt so disappointed. Now I feel sad inside. I just need a turning point, this has been a large part of my life. Jack has disappeared and there is only open road. But I can't go down it until the road is clear. It won't be clear until I get my outcome. Whichever way it goes, because Jack is no longer sniggering at me, he's not laughing at all. But like me, he is waiting to see which direction his life is going to go in. But he will never snigger at me again, because for the past few weeks he has only been able to think about me.
I feel tired and lonely. It's my path that only Jack and I have trodden and we are both waiting. Nobody can feel that, but me. I need to move on now. I want to move on and leave Jack and the nightmares. I need this to end really soon, so I can be free. I don't want to die anymore, I want to live. A life without Jack. Please let it be soon and I promise to make the most of every single day. I am so sorry for what I have done, I promise to be a better person. I promise - please let him go. Please.

Reflection: I had Jack where I wanted him now. Gone, but I needed to close the door in my mind. He had disappeared, but the door was still open. I didn't know where he had gone and I needed to know. Waiting was torture. I still didn't know who I was apologising to.

Notes:

18.03.16
I saw Jayne today and told her I am beginning to feel better. Since last Friday I have begun unconsciously to stop responding to people's behaviour and have begun to start voicing my opinions and feelings. For example, I spoke up in my meditation class, because I don't agree with obtaining other people's health details just to attend a meditation class. I spoke up at work regarding a safeguarding referral form I feel needs changing in layout and space for answers.
My Mum was being completely self-obsessed and cruel to my Dad, she was verbally attacking me. I stayed calm, announcing I wasn't sitting round to hear any more and I left. This has been going on all week, it wasn't a conscious decision, it just seems to have started happening. I talked about Jack and how I still react to him. I wait and wait to hear, wait for the next step. I am still waiting to see if he is going to dominate my life or not. I want him to go, I really do, but he holds this influence over me. Please make it stop! Please. I am so sorry.

Reflection: I was developing a real sense of myself at this stage, but I didn't realise it because it was a conscious decision. It was happening naturally because Jack had gone out of my head. I'm still apologising, but who to?

Notes:

19.03.16

I had a nightmare last night about Jack. I don't really remember what it was about, but he was in it and I wasn't happy. I keep getting this flash of emotion, but I don't know what it is. When something emotional happens on television I get it, but I don't explore it through fear. Next time it happens I will, because it triggers something inside me, but I don't look at it. I noticed it again tonight.

When somebody is sad about something sentimental I get a trigger response, but it quickly passes. Before I disclosed all this back in July last year, whenever something happened to me, say I got ill and it brought me some attention, I always got this urge to say – *"Help me, I can't do this, I need to tell you something"*. It's that kind of feeling about an emotion I have not yet explored. It's coming though, because it keeps happening.

Reflection: Okay, so what was happening was when I felt a flash of emotion, I felt like it was going to overwhelm me and I was going to fall apart. Just like the example I gave in this entry. When something sad happened I felt and overwhelming sadness, not for them but for every single sad thing that had happened to me. When I was unwell and feeling vulnerable, I felt vulnerable about every single thing that had happened to me. I was anxious because the emotions I was feeling towards external situations were new, but they were very powerful within me and I was worried that if I cried over a sad television drama, I might just fall apart. I needed to learn to release my own emotions and also learn to regulate my emotions at other times. I felt like I was no longer 10 years old in my mind, but reaching adolescence. My mind had been stuck at 10 years old, but suddenly it was moving on and I wasn't sure what to expect.

Notes:

20.03.16
I didn't feel very calm last night. An important part of my recovery I feel is to deal with my needle phobia. I spoke to Jayne about it on Friday and I feel well enough to talk about it now. I had to come to terms with what Jack has done to me before I could look at it. I have to take blood as part of my job. Since I have been back at work I have not had to take blood, but when I thought I had had to I wasn't sure if my spike in anxiety was associated with the association of anxiety, or the needle phobia itself. So I thought about it last night and it is the needle phobia.
The tourniquet represents being held down, trapped, gripped forcefully.
The needle going in is the sexual abuse, rape.
The twisting and turning and pain is rape and the removal, sudden and sharp is rape.
The smile, the patronising chat is Jack, being laughed at and humiliated by my Cousin and ex-husband, being discarded by those who raped me.
It's not the image so much as the emotion, the feeling afterwards. The bruised feeling, the ache after being raped. I don't want to feel like this. If I have to take blood those feelings come back, if I have to take blood from somebody who is anxious about it, it is almost unbearable for me. I want to stop because I want the flashbacks to stop, but also because I know I am taking blood, or having blood taken. I am not being raped. But it takes me back there every time.

Reflection: Being able to describe my needle phobia was really important to me. It was like an abuse that I had kept inside. Now I no longer held on to it in my mind I could begin to deal with it more rationally.

Notes:

21.03.2016
Today was okay. Only fleeting thoughts of Jack, but generally okay.

Reflection: I'm wasn't counting the good days, I was just glad they had begun to creep in.

Notes:

22.03.16

Feeling a bit down today. The Investigating Officer called my Mum who gave an account over the 'phone. But she relayed it back to me just like she was recounting a memory of an old acquaintance. She couldn't understand why I hadn't told her. She is and has always been so cold and disconnected, I feel like a piece of meat. Not a human being who has been emotionally destroyed and put back together again. That is the thing that has been flashing through my mind. I have had no compassionate back bone. Of course I am getting help now, but it's structured, formal, matter of fact. I miss and will always miss being unconditionally loved. I don't mean my kids. I mean somebody who is there for me unconditionally. My Sister was, we were equal. I can't help it and I wish I could, but I just miss her so much. She would have been there for me whatever. And I for her. That's where I feel my emptiness. Knowing there really is no-one there. I am just a piece of meat. Today I feel worthless and so very, very sad.

Reflection: It's sad to read this, because how I felt was completely justified. Growing up without unconditional love is beyond destroying. Being abused as a consequence of that and neglect felt so unbearable. I believe I was right to feel worthless, but just to her and my abusers, because to them I was. However, I wasn't a worthless person and I think I was beginning to see that because I felt sad and not self-loathing.

Notes:

23.03.16
Everything feels wrong. I feel so out of sorts. I e-mailed the Police a list of people I disclosed Jacks sexual abuse to. These people from my past, the most humiliating times of my life. Judging me, talking about me, I feel like a piece of meat. A friend cancelled an appointment to make a statement today. These are my emotions, my devastating past they are going to be talking about, all now on display. I feel exposed, and objectified when I should be grateful they are going to speak for me. I felt paralysed today, almost unable to move. It's like my life stops all over again. It is physically hard to move. I don't know what causes it. I am still held back by Jack. He still has a hold over me. I feel really down, like I don't own myself. Because after ten, I never did again.

Reflection: I had to recount events to the Investigating Officer. Events that I had only just begun to get my head round. There was thoroughness in her questioning, but there was no compassion, sympathy or emotional understanding. She had a job to do and she was doing it. But it didn't stop me feeling like I was just an object and I had always felt like an object. It was very difficult to understand that this process would only ever treat me as a set of facts and evidence. It didn't nothing to help me connect with myself as a person, a real person with feelings. Feelings that had always been ignored. It was a strange experience the whole investigation. I had to distance myself from emotion, when what I was trying to do the most was the entire opposite.

Notes:

24.03.16

Everything is wrong today. I am overwhelmed and every movement is such an effort. My needle phobia and association with rape. My any association with rape. I am tired of being reminded all the time. Today it all feels too much. My Mum, my Auntie, my past. Everyone treating me like a piece of meat. A novelty, someone to blame, humiliate, I can't cope today.

Even my family now. Alan is cruel, he uses my vulnerability to hurt me, just because I can't take information and remember it quickly. I try to stick up for myself, but he says it's a waste of time, no good reason to help me or wait for me to understand.

I am trying so hard to believe in me, trust me and be kind to me, but it's so fragile. God I'm pathetic, why can't I be stronger? I wish it would all go away. I can't take much more, I am trying so hard to recover, so hard. Why do people have to be so cruel? Why have I never been important enough for anybody just to care? Why am I so bad? Whatever I have done I am so sorry. So sorry, please stop hurting me, I can't do this anymore.

Reflection: If only I could see who I was apologising to, I wouldn't have berated myself. I was being emotionally abused by Alan now, he was driving the nail into the coffin, but all I had at that time was confusion. I felt bad because I couldn't go at the speed he wanted me to. I could see he was being cruel, but instead of being angry at him, or seeing him for what he really was, I became angry with myself. I believed if I didn't annoy him, then he wouldn't need to be cruel. How sad that a person can destroy another person like that for their own gain.

Notes:

25.03.16
Today it is so hard to write. Today is the darkest of days. Today I am completely consumed. Physical association of rape and sexual abuse have consumed my body. I can feel, am feeling the sensations of being trapped, raped and sexually abused. This is unbearable and I don't know how I can get through today. I am on the outside looking in. I am distracted, disconnected and completely removed from everything around me. I can't shake off the sensation and I can't live with it.

Reflection: Days like these hit me really hard, especially when I had days in between that were better, sometimes even good at that stage. I felt like the abuse knew it was going to be overcome, but every now and again it would surge to fight back and when it did it absolutely floored me.

Notes:

26.03.16
Exhausted today. Very tired, then the Police called. My Auntie said I was abused by a teacher. God, how completely de-humanising. My Auntie who called me her fourth daughter, even though her fourth daughter died. The person I was closest to, who I confided in, who blabbed to my Uncles about Jack. Values me so much, she has no fucking idea who sexually assaulted me.
Kim remembered and Jane remembered what Jason did. He really did fuck me up. I couldn't feel any more worthless to my family. I can't describe how insignificant I feel. My life has been worth nothing. How do I recover from that? Because all my belief that I am worthless is completely valid when it comes to my family. If they have validated anything, it's my total worthlessness. I meant nothing to them and I mean nothing now. None of what I have felt has been exaggerated. They have confirmed what I always believed and felt.
I am a worthless waste of space, I really am. I have always felt it and they have confirmed it. My sexual abuse and worthlessness are all as real as I felt they were. Jane telling the Police about Jason shocked me, but also validates how fucked up it made me. I was friends with Jane when I was about seventeen years old until I was about twenty six. I used to talk to Jane when I was drunk, because I couldn't cope with how I felt. Jason fucked me up as much as Jack. The rapist in the park, the rapist when I was sixteen and my ex-husband. I am so fucked up. I have to let this out and I don't know how to live with it. I can't go on.

Reflection: This was another blow. My Auntie and I were very close when I was growing up. I spent a lot of time with her and I talked to her about things I couldn't talk to my Mum about, which was pretty much anything. Anyway, my Auntie drank very heavily, she always did and so did I at that time. I would talk about anything and everything. One drunken night I told her about Jack and being anorexic. I told her not to tell anybody. Sometime later at my Cousin's 18th birthday, she blabbed and told my Uncles. They got really angry, demanding to know who it was and threatening to beat him up. So I told them. I told them his name was Jack Kilbourne and I believed he lived in Liverpool. That was the last it was ever mentioned again. I didn't know if Jack was a teacher when I was 10 years old. I didn't know what he did. I never thought about it. But to be so disregarded by another member of my family, by all members of my family was another massive blow.

Notes:

27.03.16

Nightmares again last night. I remembered I had told my Manager in my first job about the abuse. He was a social worker, so I e-mailed the Investigating Officer the information and I was astonished when she e-mailed me back to say Jane had 'phoned this morning, been in and made a statement. Now they are bringing Jack in on Wednesday to show him the photograph with me, him, his dad, Emily and Sarah-Jayne. I am exhausted, so much emotion racing round my body, consuming me. I have lost this week of my life. A truly awful week, I just cannot describe. I just wish it would stop.

Reflection: I would have given anything for a hug at that time. I was so tired of shouldering everything.

Notes:

28.03.16

I had a disturbed sleep, but I'm trying to pull myself out of this hole, so I suggest we visit relatives and then take the kids to the circus. They loved it and I enjoyed it too. It really did lift me, even though I didn't want to go because of my depression. My melancholy mood kicked in later, but I could smile for a while and hold on to the positive feeling. I'm proud of myself for doing something despite every sinew in my body wanting me to just curl up and cry.

Reflection: I remember that night and I remember getting comfort from watching my children enjoy the show. When I was with my children I always felt safe and comforted. They were living an innocent life and I wanted to be part of that with them. I thought if I forced myself to do normal things then I would start to feel what I considered to be normal. But with everything going on around me and inside me, that was a pretty impossible expectation. Part of the problem at that time was my expectations of myself were always so high. They are not any more. I now expect me to be me and if that's on a good day or a bad it's absolutely fine. Feeling low, or vulnerable or upset provides enough pressure without adding to that by self-admonishment.

Notes:

29.03.16
Constantly sleeping and waking throughout the night. I spoke to Carol today, explained why my emotions and self-esteem are in my boots. Who even needs me? Who thinks I'm important, valuable and worthy? And if the answer is nobody does, then how do I cultivate any self-worth? How?

Reflection: I still couldn't see the answer lay right within me.

Notes:

30.03.16
Telephone call from the Police. Jack has been shown the photographs and he denies knowing/remembering me. It is now being referred to the Crown Prosecution Service. I have been listened to.

Reflection: This was huge. Jack had lied, he had denied knowing me, denied taking me to London and there was a photograph of him, Emily, Me, his Dad and Sarah-Jayne stood right next to the Thames in front of Tower Bridge. Now everybody knew he was lying and he had been exposed as such.

Notes:

31.03.16
So tired, but relieved. I can stop obsessing over my 'phone. I don't expect to hear anything now for several weeks. I'm just riding a roller coaster of emotions. Just Stop!

Reflection: I knew now that the case was progressing, so it gave me more expectations. It really was a roller coaster, it could never have been anything else. I understand that now as the evidence grew.

Notes:

01.04.16

I saw Jayne today and I talked about low self-esteem. I'm not feeling sorry for myself anymore, I'm passed that, but my self-esteem is non-existent, I don't feel confident. Here's why.

My Mum and Dad neglected me, I went to Jack and Emily, he sexually abused me, the abuse went on, my thoughts, feelings, even voice ignored. Even as recent as Alan. My mum continues to validate this. How with this constant reinforcement can I even begin to develop, when I keep being reminded how insignificant, worthless, pointless I am. Jayne said we can work on it because it feels like I am banging my head against a brick wall trying to figure it out.

Then I saw Carol tonight and she explained it in a way I had never ever thought of. So, because I am vulnerable, I focus on things people say that relate to my self-esteem. For instance we talked about when I asked for Supervision at work last year. It was viewed as a weakness, inability to cope with my job. So I felt ignored, worthless and all the other things I label myself with that adds to my low self-esteem. Carol however reflected that back and said if it had been her that was asking and she'd had the same response, she wouldn't have internalised it, she would have thought that they were crap.

So my Mum and Dad being negligent is about them. My Mum is cruel to my dad. Jack sexually abused me because he is a pervert, not because he didn't like me and wanted me to stop visiting. Alan attacks my vulnerability because he is cruel and needs to do that out of some twisted need to come out on top, be more powerful. What an epiphany!

It doesn't suddenly make me feel confident, or have a better self-esteem, but it does make me understand that it doesn't KEEP happening to me. It's my Achilles heel and I need to start reminding myself that I am okay. Because I am a good, honest, loving, caring, person. People who treat me badly are damaged people who would treat anybody the same. It's not me. Wow! What a Wow! Moment!! I refused to pay Carol £35

Reflection: This was a significant turning point for me. Often the answer to a problem, or a question is to turn it around and look at it from a different view point. It's so simple, yet genius. I live by this philosophy today. It doesn't always work, but then that might be because I am looking at the wrong thing as the problem. But I have the ability to step back and evaluate that when I can't find the answer. I question myself, what is the real problem?

An example: Recently my Mother has disconnected from me. At first I was really angry. How dare she ignore me, how dare she ignore my kids, how dare she treat me like I have done something wrong. I was angry for a good few weeks and it wasn't looking like it was resolving anything. So instead as I was driving to work one day, I thought about it again. I was spending all my time being angry at her, that wasn't making me feel any better and I wasn't coming to any conclusion about it, so instead I concentrated just on the anger. Why was I angry? I was angry because I felt hurt. I felt hurt because she had rejected me again and that tapped into her rejecting me when I was seven years old after my Sister died and she told me nothing was special any more. So I began to cry. I cried for a few minutes, then I reminded myself that being rejected by her is in fact nothing new, I had been aware of it for many years. So I stopped crying, I was no longer angry and by the time I got to work I was thinking about something completely different.

Sometimes the thing that we think is the problem, isn't actually the problem at all. Stepping back and approaching a problem from a different angle is sometimes all you need to do. It certainly isn't going to make anything any worse and at best it provides some clearer insight.

Notes:

02.04.16

I slept so well last night. I am okay 😊. I am going to grow, step by step. I had an e-mail from the Police, my case has gone to the CPS. It will take up to five weeks to summons. I have to prepare for the fact I may have to go to Court. I have five weeks to work on my self-esteem and me. I am going to do it, because I do not want to stay down here a second longer than I have to.

Reflection: This was great in terms of progress, but I believed I would be going to Court very shortly after the outcome. The Police really need to provide information on the process during an investigation.

Notes:

03.04.16
I slept really well again last night. Day one of living life, being part of it, being active, deliberately pushing negative thoughts to one side. I will improve my life and I will improve my self-esteem.

Reflection: Renewed vigour.

Notes:

04.04.16
A busy day with the kids, no negative thoughts. A good night's sleep last night.

Reflection: Things were looking up because I had started to pin all my hope on that 5 week deadline.

Notes:

05.04.16
Another busy day doing activities with the kids. Laughing and having fun. Still conscious of what I am doing, thinking about it a bit. Not fully immersed, but periods of time go by when I am immersed with them. Sort of consciously making it happen, rather than spontaneous, but loving it all the same and time also appears to slow down. I am really enjoying this new experience.

Reflection: This was really liberating for me.

Notes:

06.04.16
A good day with the kids. Feeling good.

Reflection: Every day moving forward, every day hope building.

Notes:

07.04.16
I didn't sleep well last night, I don't really know why, but feeling very tired today. Being determined to stand up for myself is causing tension and I hate it, but there is nothing I can do. I have to continue to feel better about myself and that means not humiliating or compromising myself any more.

Reflection: This relates to my relationship with Alan. I was beginning to voice my opinions and he didn't like it. He was becoming more abusive and that was becoming very stressful for me.

Notes:

08.04.16
I saw Jayne today and talked about how to build my self-esteem. I talked about the conversation I had with Carol and how it's causing tension with Alan. So we talked about how we would approach it without confrontation. I talked to Alan about vulnerable aspects of my personality. This includes my lack of knowledge, issues with food and my memory and how he uses that to laugh at me and that I won't tolerate it any more. Alan acknowledged it all. We will see. But in order to get better, I have to feel better about myself. I am caring for myself physically, I am meditating, so I need to build my self-esteem. I have to do it, because I would never survive this again.

Reflection: It was very difficult to work on my self-esteem when Alan was chipping away at it. Interesting that the police investigation went naturally quiet, which gave me time to address issues closer to home.

Notes:

09.04.16
A good day. Had friends round this evening and I was a little apprehensive. It has been a long time. I was also a little worried that Alan would put me down, but he didn't. Maybe he has listened. I just want to be accepted for who I am on the day. Just one thing, I am feeling a little paranoid about being watched. Not because anything has happened, but because I don't believe nobody is going to try to find out anything about me in the next five weeks whilst I wait to hear from the CPS.

Reflection: I was beginning to feel anxious because I wasn't sure if I was safe. Alan had told me there might be repercussions reporting Jack for me and the kids. Several weeks of silence allowed that thought to grow in my mind and I was anxious that somebody that Jack knew might find me and attack me or the kids.
Not much domestic violence going on there either, feeling afraid and then grateful that Alan didn't humiliate me in front of friends. It was a very stressful time at home.

Notes:

10.04.16
A good relaxed day at home with family. Only fleeting thoughts about work tomorrow, but no anxiety. Daily meditation really helps.

Reflection: Speaks for itself. Feel free to comment.

Notes:

11.04.16
I felt a bit out of sorts today and I don't know why. Elizabeth was watching a programme about a girl who repeatedly self-harmed, then died. This took me back to last year just before I told my tutor Martyn I was suicidal. On the outside I appeared normal, inside I was hysterical. I was repeatedly climbing on the window ledge and jumping out of the window, or I was screaming hysterically in the office at work and running out into the middle of the road. I played this over and over in my head. Each time becoming more vivid, more determined, until it stopped being an 'if' but became a 'when'. I was ready to go. I was waiting for somebody to say something, it was like waiting for somebody to pull the trigger. Just one person to say how terrible it is to be sexually abused when I was on my course and waiting for my Manager to have a go at me at work for something I hadn't done well enough.
My adrenaline was racing, I felt I had so much energy, I just needed the trigger to release it and I was going. Out into the road, or out of the window. My mind was being flooded with flashbacks, images and feelings of sexual abuse. I was drowning in it, terrified. Everything was coming at once. I thought I was going mad. Everything was racing so fast. Like a speeded up movie, images, terrifying images racing in front of my eyes. I couldn't suppress it any longer, it flooded like vomit, spinning me round, completely consuming me. I was petrified.
Anyway, the programme, her repeated self-harm , each time reminded me of the pattern my mind was racing round. Images, petrified, overwhelmed, petrified, racing petrified. Jump - Die...... God that was such an awful time. Now knowing when the flooding was going to stop. More and more and more rushing out with such force. Martyn Geary saved my life. With everything rushing and racing and frantic, he was calm, he spoke slowly and quietly. He was like an anchor. My racing petrified mind could hear what he was saying. I felt safe when he was present. He didn't rush me, he didn't take control, or force me to do anything. He listened to me, he let me speak, he gave me some space and time. He calmed me, then he guided me so I took his advice. God how close I came.
If he had reacted, panicked, reported me, took away my control I would have died. When I spoke to Martyn I was over the edge. I couldn't see a way out. I was flooded with terror. It wouldn't have been his fault if I had died. I was ready for someone to pull the trigger. I was racing with adrenaline, I was ready to go.
Martyn if you ever read this. You are the reason I am alive today. Even thinking back to the knife edge I was on still terrifies me. You did the right thing, you saved my life. In my head I was jumping out of the window, I was jumping in front of a car. You spoke to me, you listened. You did it? Every sinew in my body was ready to go. I can never repay you for what you did. I don't know how to thank you enough except to say. *"With all my heart Martyn, thank you for saving my life"*.

Reflection: I intend to thank Martyn when I give him a copy of this book.

Notes:

12.04.16
Today I feel tired, emotional and just want to hug myself. I have been so frightened, so brave, so sad, so scared. So lonely so lost, so strong. Today I feel it. I feel like I have been through it, and then some. My mind and my body have battled and fought to live, not to die. To get well, to learn to grow. Today I just wanted to hug myself, comfort myself for being so brave, so strong whilst all the time feeling so clobbered.
Tomorrow will be a better day.

Reflection: It reads to me that that day was a good day. It was a day of self-reflection, self-care. I still saw sadness as a negative emotion. I see it now as a recognition of what I have experienced and how I have come to terms with it all, but still respect the impact it had.

Notes:

13.04.16
Today was a very busy day at work, so I was carried along with it. Then when I got home I just wanted peace and quiet, but there was none. Why do I want quiet? I feel I want to reflect. I had to deal with my needle phobia today and nobody knew. It was horrible. She had been sexually abused and she was almost hysterical. She consented, but couldn't hide her terror. She was venting, just like I do. I feel so sad for her, for me.
My manager was so matter of fact today talking about why I was off sick. Part of me was very relieved that Jack hasn't damaged my career development, but part of me wanted some compassion, acknowledgement. I still need that hug. It still feels like yesterday. I'm just growing. I want a hand to hold. Hugging myself isn't always enough.

Reflection: How strong was I on that day. I even answered my own question. I will always want that hand to hold, that hug. That's not trauma, that's just being human and we all want that loving interaction.

Notes:

14.04.16
I had to take blood today. She had been raped. She was almost hysterical, but consenting. She cried and buried her head in her carers arms. And there I was in that scenario again. I put the tourniquet on her, she flinched, that's me being touched. I put the needle in and she cried and I was being raped all over again. Afterwards she had smudges of blood on her arm, just like I always had between my legs after being raped. I couldn't wait to wash it off because it constantly reminded me of being raped again. She was okay after, talking about unrelated stuff, but I was recovering from the flashback of being raped. It happens every time.

Reflection: This was very traumatic for me, every time. Every time I had to take blood, I was being raped again. I needed to deal with it, but I had to be ready, I was still trying to avoid it.

Notes:

15.04.16
I saw Jayne today and talked to her about blood taking and my association. I talked to her about how I felt last year when I was suicidal. It was a very hard session. I felt really shaken afterwards and most of the day. I also had an e-mail from The police, this completely threw me as I wasn't expecting to hear from her until the CPS had made a decision, so I automatically thought something had happened. In fact she was just letting me know my case has been allocated to a prosecutor and I could have up to a four week wait. My emotions are all over the place again and I feel battered. It's been a hard week for me and I feel really low. The hard part is not being able to talk about it except to Jayne. I really didn't think I would get to the end of this book. I thought it would either be read after I died, or there would be some kind of resolution/outcome that released me from the grip.
I feel I am being held.

Reflection: Limbo. The worst place to be whatever the situation.

Notes:

16.04.16
Very tired today. Just very low. A day feeling stuck again. Stuck, banging my head against a wall. I can't seem to get over, or round. It destroys me every time.

Reflection: There was nothing else to do except go round in circles because I was completely focused on the CPS outcome.

Notes:

17.04.16
I can't believe my baby girl is eight years old today. All I can say today, she is safe, secure, happy and confident. She is doing more than okay and today I will take credit for that.

Reflection: Hurray, some self-recognition.

Notes:

18.04.16

Today was an emotionally quiet day, but I did feel real empathy for two young people in my care. I felt empathy without attaching it to me. I have always attached a sad feeling to me, to give me permission to feel sad about myself. But today I made no comparison. I felt empathy, sad for them, then I let it go. For me that's good. It's new, but good. One step at a time.

Reflection: This is when I knew I had come to terms with Jack. Before I made any disclosure, I would be very objective about disclosures. I would offer practical support and that was as deep as it would go. I had an invisible shield around me so that I could not absorb anything that anybody disclosed about abuse, because I knew what it would do. (What it did on the Communication course). Anyway, being able to feel empathy for what those young people had experienced meant I owned my own stuff and their stuff belonged to them. I owned it, I no longer hid from it, buried it or ignored it. Good for me!

Notes:

19.04.16
An emotionally quiet day.

Reflection: Another good day.

Notes:

20.04.16

Some days I get tired of trying. Today I am tired. Imagine having to practice speaking a different language every day and you have to practice just to get by, to able to survive, get the essentials because if you don't you will die.

Every day, every single day I am trying. I meditate to be calm and rational, I read, google, research to understand my deluded thoughts to make them rational. I strive to be the person I want to be, to build my self-esteem. Because the alternative is not compatible with life.

Today a friend asked me if I had any news. I told them I have to wait four weeks to hear and her reply was "*It's taking so long*!" I only started this bit on the 13th February, just two months ago. She has no traumatic emotional attachment to it and SHE thinks it is taking a long time. After the reality being thirty six years, her thinking two months is so long has suddenly made me feel very tired. So very tired.

I need some help to carry on. Today this all feels too hard.

Reflection: Another unhelpful comment. A better comment might have been to ask me how I was feeling, or to give me a hug, or buy me a coffee. Just in case anybody reading this is faced with the same situation. Support, don't put the responsibility back on the person, it is tiring enough carrying such an emotional heavy load, it really doesn't need any wait adding to it.

Notes:

21.04.16
Feeling drained and so very much in need of help.

Reflection: I needed that hug, that cup of coffee. I had nobody.

Notes:

22.04.16
Really struggling. I saw Jayne today and I think she is at a loss to know how to help me overcome the emotional feeling I get when something triggers a memory of sexual abuse. That what takes me straight back to when it happened every time. Thirty six years is going to take a little while longer. A lot worried.

Reflection: Like any grief it was going to take time, but I was impatient. Who wouldn't be?

Notes:

23.04.16

Today has been so difficult. Charlie is reading a book from school about the Yorkshire Ripper. In it was a sentence that said *"It is not unusual for women to be violently attacked"*. This book is aimed at eight year old kids and above. Why would I ever want my Son to think that is an ordinary occurrence and why would I want my eight year old daughter to ever read and believe this is what happens.

The last two weeks have been so difficult for me and now reading this I feel like I am going to blow. Everybody has been so calm and rational about the sexual abuse I went through. I have been and I'm still trying to be calm and rational. But this is why, it is because it's so normal that people don't see it as being out of the ordinary. This is fucking HELL on earth. Being trapped, held down, violated, raped, humiliated. It pushes a switch in your brain and you want to scream. I want to scream. I am so scared, so angry, I cannot be rational about it any longer and it terrifies me how vicious it is going to come out. I feel raped to my core, I feel sick, dizzy, ANGRY, so fucking ANGRY.

I spoke to Alan tonight about how I feel, I text Jayne. I am so scared. A lid has come off, as massive lid. Oh God, I'm scared.

Reflection: What I did with that fear was I e-mailed the head teacher my disgust at my Son being given the material to read. To have violence against women normalised. The head teacher in return apologised to me, spoke to the teacher who had deemed it acceptable to give my Son that book and withdrew the author from their school library. I was listened to.

Notes:

24.04.16
So, so tired today, and so very scared!

Reflection: I was scared because I thought I was going to 'blow'. I couldn't handle the thought that rape, sexual abuse, violence against women could be normalised when I had almost died trying to get through it. Absolutely justified. I think now, I would blow at somebody who normalised it, but I was afraid then that I would fall apart. I felt so fragile.

Notes:

25.04.16
So very, very tired. Everybody is carrying on as normal and I am being left behind.

Reflection: I just needed to process how I was feeling. I didn't need to keep up with anything.

Notes:

26.04.16
Two things happened today. I spoke to the phlebotomist at the hospital and I am going to work with her to try to address my phobia and negative association around taking blood. I saw a young person for the first time and could properly empathise and show compassion. When we parted company she gave me a hug. I didn't think about it again until tonight at meditation when we did a loving and cherishing meditation and she came straight back to my mind. And I suddenly realised I had been congruent. I was completely professional, but also compassionate and I got the balance without being conscious of it. It just happened . That was an incredible moment for me.
Thanks again Martyn for the Advanced Communication Course.

Reflection: If only I could have recognised the steps I was taking. I externalised any progress and internalised difficulties. I don't do that anymore.

Notes:

27.04.16
I am so tired, I feel angry with everyone and to top it off money has been taken from my salary without authorisation. So anger on top of anger. I haven't had an e-mail reply from school regarding the inappropriate book Charlie was reading. So I must meditate, my money will be returned and I will contact school for an explanation. Everything will be okay.

Reflection: And it was. As previously explained the e-mail was responded to, just not quickly enough for me and my racing mind.

Notes:

28.04.16
My mind feels like a stalled car.

Reflection: Thank goodness it did stop, or it might have blown. The mind needs rest as much as the body. I couldn't make it do it at that time, but it was clearly an automatic car.

Notes:

29.04.16
Come on mind!

Reflection: Nothing to say that hasn't already been said here.

Notes:

30.04.16
Alan threw everything he had at me today. Tried to destroy me with words. Ridiculed how I talk, what I say, how I behave. Had this happened last year I would have slashed my wrists. All I am doing is speaking up for myself now. I deserve to be heard. This journal is about my recovery, so I am writing this from that view point. I am hanging on to self-belief.

Reflection: This was exactly what my Mother did to me often when I was a child and it tapped right back into that. But I was beginning to see Alan for who he really was. I was really frightened of him, but determined not to show it.

Notes:

01.05.16
I can barely bring myself to talk, I am devastated by being ridiculed and mocked.

Reflection: Awful!

Notes:

02.05.16
Today has been another bad day. Everything feels wrong.

Reflection: My fragile sense of self was being attacked daily by Alan and I was really struggling to keep my focus.

Notes:

03.05.16
I am trying to save our marriage, but I have to be able to talk. He tried to tell me expressing emotion was wrong. I have now said I have to be me or we will not survive.

Reflection: I was hanging on with everything I had and it was so hard.

Notes:

04.05.16
I worked with a phlebotomist today. I explained to her briefly why I needed support. I learnt a lot in two hours. Not least that although she is very kind, she is focused, so she could empathise with anxious patients, but their anxiety did not become her focus. I began to realise that that is where I have been going wrong. I get hung up on the emotion and forget that taking blood is for a specific reason. It is not sexual abuse or rape.

Reflection: In my role as a midwife I am required to take blood. I had the advantage of being able to contact the phlebotomist at one of our hospitals to arrange to work with her for a morning. I was very, very nervous. Watching her take blood was very anxiety provoking for me, particularly those women who were anxious about having blood taken.

Notes:

05.05.16
I really did not expect to be writing in a second book (Journal). My intention has always been to write until I felt I had reached a point where I was ready to step back into life and begin living again for real. I believed that would happen before the end of my first journal. But it hasn't and I will continue until I am ready.
Right now everything feels wrong. EVERYTHING

Reflection: Change is difficult at the best of times, but my mind was changing, my attitude towards life was changing, my home circumstances were changing in that it was very tense, my attitude towards work was changing and I was coping with recovering and embarking on the police process. All of it was strange to me. Everything was changing and nothing felt familiar anymore. That's why it felt wrong. I didn't recognise me anymore.

Notes:

06.05.16
I spoke with Jayne today about everything feeling wrong. My work, my home life, my body. Then I realised it's not possible for EVERYTHING to be wrong, it's just I am changing, thinking and feeling differently about everything. So nothing fits at the moment. It feels very hard and I don't know what to do about it, but what I do know is things don't stay the same with me for very long.

Reflection: Again this was just something else that needed time.

Notes:

07.05.16
Today was a very busy day. Positives about eating properly – I have more energy. I feel better and I look better with clothes on. The negative is I don't like the look of my body naked. It has lots of chubby rolls now. It doesn't help that Alan never comes near me, so I feel more and more self-conscious. But I want to stay healthy, energetic and look better. I guess this is what's called a shit sandwich! Or a happy sandwich, depending on my mood. I do feel anxious though, slightly out of control.

Reflection: I was definitely enjoying having more energy and sleeping better. It wasn't until I started feeling better because I was eating well, that I realised how rubbish I had felt for so long not eating properly. I have always ate just enough to get rid of the feeling of hunger. Feeling full I always associated with binging. Eating just enough didn't make me feel uncomfortable, it just made me feel shit, tired and lacking in any energy. I need to find the balance.

Notes:

08.05.16
Busy day out, trying to feel involved, but it's there at the back of my mind.

Reflection: I couldn't stop thinking about the potential outcome from the CPS. The wonder was always there in the back of my mind.

Notes:

09.05.16
Thinking that the 'phone could ring any time.

Reflection: So distracted. I don't know now reflecting back how I managed to carry on at work and home. I was so very strong and so very tired.

Notes:

10.05.16
I called the police today, starting to feel down. I just need to know. The Officer wasn't there, but a colleague told me there is a slight delay.

Reflection: Great! Just when I believed the outcome was almost there I'm smacked with a delay. I could have burst I was so wound up.

Notes:

11.05.16
Saw phlebotomist today, my hands were clammy just watching, so she told me to have a go. I took blood and she told me my technique was terrible. That made me laugh. She taught me how to do it properly. It felt very cack handed, but I was delighted to learn my new skill. I took blood from several people using my new technique and I actually enjoyed it. Not least because my focus was on my technique. I can't wait to do it again.
GET ME!!!

Reflection: At least having a different focus gave me a break from association.

Notes:

12.05.16

Feeling very anxious this morning, distracted, images of Jack sexually abusing me very clear in my head today. I feel I could cry at any moment. I called the Investigating Officer this afternoon, she was very supportive. She said it could just be a few more days. We talked a bit about the process.

Tonight I told the kids off for being naughty. I my head I'm saying "*You will hear my voice.*" My Dad's CPN talked about giving him medication to stop him getting angry. He gets angry because my mum's cruel, negligent and nasty. He never gets angry with anyone else. I felt so sad to think they will gag him. Take away his voice. My head is banging back and too. If it does go to Court I get my voice heard, then I can move on. If it doesn't go to Court I don't get my voice heard. I'm gagged by people who don't know me. I feel so angry inside. People who have never met me are going to be making a decision whether my voice is heard or not. Then on the other hand if it doesn't go to Court, I don't have to go through it all and I can let go. My head is really banging and I had a memory black hole yesterday and now I know why it happened, it still makes me angry and upset.

Reflection: So that memory black hole was happening because I was so disconnected from reality and so preoccupied with the ongoing investigation and waiting for the CPS outcome. Feeling uncertain about which way the process was going to go was crippling for me and I was trying to second guess everything to prepare for the outcome.

Notes:

13.05.16

Today I felt anxious, light headed, nauseous and panicked. I am afraid I won't be able to remember stuff for a job interview. I saw Jayne and she suggested maybe I could call the police and ask them not to contact me until after Thursday (the day of my interview). All day I thought it was a good idea, but then this evening I thought no! This is part of me, I have to say calm and accept it in the moment. Deal with the emotions as it comes. I know I have to focus on my interview, but my memory black outs happen when I am panicked and anxious. I know what is coming, so I will patiently accept. If it upsets me I won't panic, I will be upset. It's okay, my reaction has always been to run from it, but I won't. Not anymore.

I forgot where I parked my car today, I knew when I got to work I had no idea where I parked it. So I knew before I needed to go back to it. I was panicked and my mind was everywhere, but I realised beforehand and I realised I was panicked. I just need to recognise when I am panicked and allow myself to slow down. Think about why I am panicked and take a breath. Look at where I am and what I am doing before doing anything else.

I feel much calmer. I am tired of avoiding emotions. I have to feel them. I do feel very low, very, very low.

Reflection: I felt overwhelmed. I was trying so hard to do the 'right' thing to control the situation, to prepare myself. I was actually putting myself under so much pressure. I felt so low because I was just trying too hard. It makes me feel tired just reading the entry for that day. At least I recognised one thing and that was when I was so disconnected, so distracted it really affected my memory. The answer was not to be distracted, to just allow things to play out, but I didn't know that then and I was still trying to anticipate every outcome so I could prepare myself to deal with it.

Notes:

14.05.16
Today I kept myself calm, very, very, calm. I used my subdued mood to help me focus. I read a lot and did remain focused. I allowed myself to think about Jack whilst I went for a run, that was all.

Reflection: Everything about my behaviour was so controlled. I used every emotion for a purpose. How exhausting.

Notes:

15.05.16
Today I remained focused and thought about Jack very little. I am tired and I know my mind is working hard for me. I am keeping myself calm and slow to allow feeling to arise calmly. I am actually doing it. I am controlling my thoughts. I forgot where my car was because my mind was scattered. If I stay slow and focused, that won't happen.
I CAN DO THIS!

Reflection: This is something I do unconsciously now, but then I needed to really concentrate in order to slow everything down. So yes I could do it and I still can. Occasionally I will be caught off guard and swept along with events, but as soon as I realise what's happening I am able to stop and reflect and slow back down.

Notes:

16.05.16

Today I felt restless all day and tonight I feel very, very irritated. I am ready and absorbing, but my body wants to feel the emotion it wants to feel. I really do want to get this job, but I have to be true to my own feelings. I am really finding this so difficult. I don't feel I can talk to anyone because I worry they are tired of hearing it. I feel very lonely.

Reflection: The job I was applying for was in Safeguarding. I was worried that I would forget everything that I had read and researched because that had always happened before in exams. The vicious cycle with that is, the more you worry and panic, the less you remember, or can recall anyway.

Notes:

17.05.16
I feel more and more concerned for my mental health. Part of me is looking forward to an optimistic, brighter future. The other half, well, I feel powerless by Jack. If this goes to Court I will be heard. If it doesn't I have images of be being on my own, deciding on my future. Of course I don't want to die, I have my children, but I feel so sad, so tearful, so disengaged. I don't want to let anybody down, I really don't, but if this goes wrong, I'm not as strong as everybody thinks I am.
When somebody really listens to me I can express that I feel so sad, so alone, so damaged. This isn't happening to me now, but it's the first time I am looking at it, so it feels like it is. I am so divided inside. Life is pulling me along, but I feel stuck.

Reflection: I felt I was at a real crossroads in my life. I could see a brighter future, but I was worried that a negative outcome, or experience might just tip me back over the edge. I was actually stronger than everybody gave me credit for, I was just so lonely and not able to confide in anybody how I was really feeling, because everybody had an opinion. I had to wait for my hour once a week to let everything out and it didn't feel like it was enough. Too much was happening in the real world to contain it I felt.

Notes:

18.05.16
Feeling very, very sad. If I go to Court, then that demonstrates to everyone how awful what Jack did makes me feel. If it doesn't go to Court then he gets away with it and I feel my life has been wasted. I feel so sad.

Reflection: I couldn't see that those who did know, the Police, the CPS, Jayne, those trusted few around me knew how awful what Jack had done made me feel. I felt after 36 years I had wasted a life and for it not to go to Court meant those wasted years would not be validated. It was a really sad time.

Notes:

19.05.16
I had to focus for an interview today. Every time I relaxed my concentration, Jack slipped into my mind and the possible outcome. So I was either concentrating hard for my interview, or concentrating hard to keep Jack out. Then I heard from the Investigating Officer. No news from the CPS and I won't hear now at least until next Wednesday. A new Detective called Dave is taking over. So much pressure. I tried hard all day to meditate and it did work. I am drained.

Reflection: I believed the interview went well. I went to the hospital chapel beforehand and meditated. It was funny really, I didn't think the meditation itself worked, but it did distract me. I was focusing on my breathing and I was deliberately breathing steadily and counting the breaths. However, my heart was thumping so hard with nerves, I could hear it in my ears. I became distracted by what I was feeling, thinking how can I be breathing so calmly and yet my heart be pounding so hard. It became an amusing distraction as I wondered what would win out. After 10 minutes the thumping heart beat in my ears won. I still don't understand how it could do that, but it fascinated me enough to distract me.

Notes:

20.05.16
Cock up with interviews, I have to wait two weeks. I have had enough of being controlled, manipulated and disregarded by people. If my feelings matter, they are going to be listened to. I am angry, trapped and feel claustrophobic. I hate it, I really hate it!

Reflection: The reason I had to wait two weeks was because one of the candidates was on holiday. I took the delay very personally and it was completely out of context. I was struggling with the wait.

Notes:

21.05.16
I had a nightmare last night about Alan leaving me. He'd had enough. I was upset and asking for him to help and he just walked away. It was horrible and I felt tired all day.

Reflection: On reflection I would see that as a premonition, but that was yet to come.

Notes:

22.05.16
I had another nightmare last night that my eldest Son was kidnapped along with eight other children. I found one of them, but nobody would help me find my Son. I felt very tired again all day today. I just have this constant horrible feeling inside. I just want to be free from worry and I feel so trapped at the moment. I can't shake it off. Bad thoughts keep flitting through my mind. I'm scared, but I need to keep my head above. I have no problem getting to sleep because I meditate, but I wake up through the night wide awake and struggle to get back off again.

Reflection: Well I can't analyse dreams, maybe you can. I can only put it down to my anxiety about the risk I may have put myself and my children at by reporting Jack to the police.

Notes:

23.05.16
Shattered, just so very, very, tired.

Reflection: Enough said.

Notes:

24.05.16
It's like my brain has switched off. I'm not stressed, angry, anything, just numb.

Reflection: That numb feeling again. The power of the mind never ceases to amaze me.

Notes:

25.05.16
Feel nothing.

Reflection: Perhaps this was when my mind was knitting more of itself together. Perhaps this was when it was carrying out it's own maintenance.

Notes:

26.05.16
Quiet day, although I'm sleeping and feel I'm sleeping well, I am waking shattered.

Reflection: The quality of sleep was obviously not good. How could it be when I felt everything was upside down and I was in limbo with my relationship and the police.

Notes:

27.05.16
Saw Jayne today, talked about growing as a person. I realised I have become too focused on Jack and the outcome. This is about me learning to be me.

Reflection: That was understandable. I don't think I was too focused, it was the extreme wait that caused the ongoing distraction. I was still learning about me. I was learning that being made to wait did my head in!

Notes:

28.05.16
Realised for the first time in a very long time, I have normal stuff to feel excited about. I am getting a new car, going to see David Hamilton and taking the kids to see a friend next week. Proper stuff to look forward to with energy and excitement I have never felt before. No dread.

Reflection: Dr David Hamilton was a Pharmaceutical Scientist. Whilst testing new drugs he became interested in the mind, body connection and now gives talks on the subject and has written many books about this theory. I found his work inspiring and could relate to it. I was privileged to attend one of his talks in Manchester along with the two people I completed my meditation teaching course with.

Notes:

29.05.16
Went to Manchester today with two friends. Today I actually did something I am completely interested in. David Hamilton talked about everything I have always believed in when I had always thought I was on the outside – didn't belong. Now I know I do. I didn't feel nervous about going and wasn't waiting for the day to end. I was totally absorbed and I loved it.

Reflection: It was great to feel like somebody, or should I say many, many people think and feel the same way as I do. I always thought I was different to everybody else and the only person that held the beliefs I held. Understanding that I wasn't alone was a great strength to me.

Notes:

30.05.16
Saw Alans family today. I felt sad because they were talking about historic family tree. I don't know why, but not ever having unconditional love is making me feel a bit sad at the moment. I just have this feeling that something is missing.

Reflection: I felt sad because I didn't have that family connection. I felt outcast. I didn't think, feel, or interact in the way that I thought other families did. I felt very alone and isolated.

Notes:

31.05.16
Quiet day at home, baked with Elizabeth. She said she enjoyed doing it with me. I love that my kids will always feel unconditional love, but I still have that empty feeling inside, I don't know where it has come from. I have started running regularly, only half an hour a day, just to keep fit, not to lose weight. Hopefully it will be okay.

Reflection: That feeling came from realising I had never had unconditional love. Those secure foundations had been lost when my Sister died. I was empty because there was nothing there where I believed the solid roots should be.

Notes:

01.06.16
Today was a good day, living in the moment really makes time go fast.

Reflection: I was having more good days. Bad days were broken up with some good days. That was really positive for my recovery, but I couldn't see it.

Notes:

02.06.16

I called the Police today. It's been seven weeks. The Investigating Officer is on holiday and away until next week. The person I spoke to said she has been waiting nine weeks. She said they are waiting too to sort cases out. And that's all I am – a case! Not thirty six years of being trapped in sexual abuse post-traumatic stress, finally finding the courage to speak out, to then be referred to as no more than a 'case'! How is anybody ever to feel any self-worth.

This destroys people, even kills people and always fucks people up, but to be referred to as a case is so dismissive, so belittling, negating every flashback, suicide attempt, self-harming behaviour. I have a voice now and I will be heard. Nobody will EVER dismiss what I am going through, or have been through EVER again. I just want to move forward, I just want to live again, but not until I am heard.

Reflection: I couldn't see that I was actually being heard. Yes, she referred to me as a case, but she took the time to explain. I was mistaking being heard with having an outcome. For me being heard had become all about the outcome and that wasn't a good way to be thinking. I was hinging everything on a positive outcome.

Notes:

03.06.16

Today has been an emotionally charged day. I began the day calm, talking to Jayne about beginning to find a balance. For example, yesterday, although the police were insensitive, I can see the balance. To them I am just a case, because that is their job. But they do their job because they care. Just like I do my job because I care, but I don't always remember who people are talking about until I see their detail.

It's a great balance to have that feeling. I asked my Manager when she will tell me about the job, she said Tuesday. Then at 4pm today I got a 'phone call from the Police. I had been allocated another Investigating Officer called Fern, she told me she is taking my case. She spoke to the CPS lawyer today, she has a case and a half to deal with, then she will be looking at mine. She said by Thursday next week. Oh my God! I am in a spin. Two outcomes next week. Then payroll didn't pay me what they owe me when they said they would, so my mood plummeted. But just at the end of the day Alan told me I could look for a dog for us to get when we come back off our holiday.

I don't know why, but I have fallen in love with the idea of a dog. A little life to love, that will love me back unconditionally. I have never had that. Of course my kids love me, but I can't put all my needs onto them like I can with a dog. I can love and protect a dog, but I can tell it anything and share anything and still get unconditional love. That gives me such an amazing deep feeling inside. Now that turned my day around.

Reflection: I was still waiting to hear if I had got the Safeguarding Job. Fern had taken over from another Officer who had been seconded elsewhere for a period of time. I didn't like the changes, but Fern sounded nice. She was much more human. Where the original Officer was very efficient and very professional, Fern had the human edge as well.

Notes:

04.06.16
Today I am very anxious. I have a swollen gland in my armpit. It has been tender for a few weeks, but since last week it has been getting more sore. I have been reading about visualisation today, mental health and viral illness. I am going to try to relax, but I will make a Doctor's appointment. Was I ever destined to be okay? Now all I want is to be okay, Why? I'm sure it will pass. Maybe it is a test.

Reflection: I'd had a pain in my right breast for several weeks and the lump in my armpit was very sore. I was convinced I had breast cancer. It was a bit of a wakeup call. I'd spent so long wanting to end my life, then I had started to see a light at the end of the tunnel and now this. I was quite frightened and it made me realise how much I wanted to get better.

Notes:

05.06.16
Feeling worried.

Reflection: Another wait, for another appointment with the GP. How much waiting can one person stand?

Notes:

06.06.16
I find out today that due to another HR cock-up, the interview won't be until tomorrow. I am angry at being messed about. My arm really hurts and payroll will not give me my money back.

Reflection: I'm surprised I didn't have a lump sticking out of my head, never mind my armpit. The tension was incredible. Everything appeared to be conspiring against me and I was more and more wound up.

Notes:

07.06.16
Today has been a bad day. I didn't get the job, then I find out the person who did doesn't even work in safeguarding. I work so hard, I believe I know my stuff, yet somebody who doesn't gets the job. My self-esteem has taken a big hit. What is the point of working hard when it's not recognised. I feel so angry and frustrated.

Reflection: I was angry and upset because I had completed a Safeguarding module at Masters level, I had worked in safeguarding for the previous four years and I had read a load of stuff around the subject. And I remembered it in my interview. The injustice I felt was really big. It hit my self-esteem hard because I doubted my ability. I had worked hard to prove myself to others, I still didn't have a sense of myself.

Notes:

08.06.16
Today I spoke with my manager who confirmed I didn't get the job based on my personality. That is really difficult to accept, so difficult to accept when I am supposed to be good enough as I am. I don't want to pretend, but I was told I lack passion. How can I not be angry with myself? I work so hard, but I am not good enough because I am calm for fucks sake. Why am I attacked for being me?

Reflection: I attacked myself in there too. It was sad that I was angry with myself and believed I was not good enough. I still couldn't see that other peoples' reactions to me are none of my business. I am proud that I am calm. I am also very glad now that I didn't get that job. But then I just wanted to be accepted. I just needed people to see how good I was. I still had no sense of myself.

Notes:

09.06.16
My mind feels like it's going to snap. I heard from the police today. The CPS want a statement off my Mum, Jayne, Quetzal and Martyn. All of which the original Officer could have got, now once Fern has the new information, my case goes back in the queue to be reviewed. I feel like a puppet being manipulated. After I spoke to her today I felt shaken, sick, and dizzy. I thought I was going to faint. I feel used, abused, exposed and humiliated. And after all that they could drop the case. I don't know what there is between feeling good and thoughts of self-harm and suicide. I either feel okay about myself, or I hate myself, there is nothing in the middle. I hate feeling this way. I hate it. I can't cope with it, I can't do this.

Reflection: It was very difficult to understand that I had made the statement, I wanted my voice heard, yet the Police wanted everybody else's opinion in order to validate what I was saying. I felt invisible, worthless and insignificant. That pendulum feeling either feeling good, or suicidal. They were poles apart and it was a dangerous time for me. I didn't have a sense of myself. I had no resilience. Whilst things were good, they were good. But if they weren't good they were life threatening. That makes a response very unpredictable, very spontaneous, very reactional. And I felt like that a lot and it did scare me.

Notes:

10.06.16
Saw Jayne today. Talked about feelings of self-harm. I am really struggling to cope with being controlled by other people. People who trap me by telling me I am not good enough. I lost my voice years ago, now I have it back I am still being told I am not good enough. How fucking loud do I have to shout? My anger scares me.

Reflection: There is the fear I spoke about in the previous entry. Any rejection of any kind and I internalised it immediately. My anger made me feel unpredictable. I would get flashes of slashing my wrists, or stepping in front of a bus. It was always a bus. Nobody was telling me I wasn't good enough, they were just gathering evidence to build up my case. To support what I had disclosed, but I couldn't see that. I saw that I was being talked about and my feelings were being ignored and only validated by other people because I had no sense of myself. I didn't have any confidence in myself.

Notes:

11.06.16
Read more about meditation and accepting myself. But if I do that then everybody still tells me I am not good enough, not worthy, then I will end my life because I will have accepted that I am not good enough. If I had told the truth when I was young, shouted and screamed from the roof tops, fought my corner, then even if I wasn't believed I would have kept screaming, repeating the same thing over and over again. Jack sexually assaulted me and now I have to rely on GP's, Counsellors and witnesses to support the disgusting horror of my experience. And if they don't, or it is watered down, then the horror, the nightmare, being pinned down and silenced will become nothing. Not even enough to make me worthy of being heard, being looked after and cared for, being accepted and listened to for being broken into a million different pieces by Jack.
I am a million different pieces and I am not strong. I AM NOT STRONG!

Reflection: I couldn't see that the police were trying to help me. I was really struggling and I had nobody outside of that counselling room to hold me up, to support me. I was broken, I did feel shattered and I was still looking for answers, so in fact I was incredibly strong. I was just alone in my battle to survive and when it got hard, I didn't want to survive. It all felt too much. It felt easier to give up, but I didn't.

Notes:

12.06.16
I heard from Fern today. She has spoken to Jayne and Martyn and now needs a statement off my Mum. She who drove me there in the first place and who is disinterested and dismissive. She who made me first believe I was worthless and now I have to rely on her to support me, but to do that will make her look bad. I feel so low.

Reflection: My Mother never wanted to give a statement. She told me that. She told me she couldn't remember much and I was disgusted with her. When I told friends what she had said they defended her and made out that it was too difficult for her to talk about. I felt like they were siding with her. They felt sorry for her for and she was the reason my life was destroyed. I felt sick, so very sick. She is an evil woman.

Notes:

13.06.16
Nobody would ever choose to feel this low. I don't choose low self-worth, low self-esteem. I wasn't born thinking "*Yeah, I'll have a shit life.*" I don't want to feel so low I can barely talk. I don't want to believe I am worthless. It just is who I am, I feel trapped and so desperately alone.
People think they have to try and solve it. Then they get frustrated because they tell me to feel grateful for what I have. I love my children with every breath in my body, but that doesn't change my self-worth. I feel worthless because I have been told I am, because physically and sexually I have been made to feel worthless, by being used for sexual gratification, irrespective of my cry of pain and emotionally I have been made to feel worthless when my thoughts, feelings and distress have been ignored to satisfy somebody else's needs.
I have been destroyed by all of this and it is only now that I am trying to repair this damage. So being told to be grateful that I have a new car, a job and arms and legs that work, sadly does not touch my self-worth. I don't want to look at how worthless I have been made to feel, but I have to so I can heal. I just don't know how to and challenges just knock me back.
Being sexually abused and raped destroys, violates your soul to the core and that is so hard to find and repair again. And I don't know how to do it. I just don't know and I feel such despair.

Reflection: I couldn't see that people didn't know what to say. Didn't know how to handle what I was going through. So they made insensitive comments, which felt like they were minimising my experiences. I had no sympathy for those people, I make no apology for making them feel uncomfortable. It's avoiding the subject that keeps people victims. Self-worth can't be fixed with a plaster, or a new car, or physical health. Self-worth has to come from within, but I needed others to make me feel worthy at that time and they didn't and I didn't know how to obtain it.

Notes:

14.06.16
Today was the darkest of days I can barely write. I left work, returned to my car and had the strongest urge to self-harm. I called the Samaritans and she listened and she didn't judge and she waited until I was calm until she talked to me.
To all those people who expect me to be strong, I am sorry. To all those people who are tired of listening, I am so sorry. But that's how I feel about myself, but I can't get away from it. So if you're pissed off, you can only imagine how I feel. I am really struggling to cope. I need to find some inner untouched, but I can't. I just want to be held. I just want to get through this and feel something else that isn't on the end of a blade. I feel so afraid.

Reflection: That was a tough day. The pressure to 'get over it' when I couldn't. The demands from Alan to behave 'normally' only added to my frustration with myself. I didn't want to feel so bad, so trapped in a cycle of emotional trauma. Other people's frustrations frustrated me and I just wanted to cut out the poison. The only way I could think to do that was with a blade. The Samaritans were my saviour that day.

Notes:

15.06.16
Another night of nightmares, that's every night this week. I am so tired, so very tired today.

Reflection: People need to understand that nobody chooses to be traumatised. Nobody chooses to have flashbacks, feel suicidal. Expressing their impatience is so distressing. When somebody is traumatised like I was, they can't just walk away from it when they get tired, they can't put it down and come back to it when they feel stronger. Trauma drags you down when you are awake with flashbacks, when you are asleep with nightmares, when you are tired and you have to go to work, maintain a family. Trauma drags you down on a good day. Trauma drags you even further down on a bad day. It interrupts your life, your conversations, your breathing when you have a panic attack. When I was experiencing that trauma, that's exactly how it was for me, it never left me alone. And when it did I was numb, so I felt nothing anyway. So, impatient people, think on!

Notes:

16.06.16
My Mum called to say she has an appointment to make a statement on Sunday at 3pm. She also commented on the police saying she appeared reluctant to do so, she dismissed this as concern for my Dad. After I spoke to her I felt anxious. I believe she is going to let me down for the last time. She will either be open and honest and tell them she remembers little about all the time I spent there, despite only meeting Emily once. Or she will cry, make it all about her to distract from the reality that she was so disinterested she doesn't remember. Either way will make her look bad and me feel worthless all over again.

Reflection: She chose the former. She didn't cry. If she'd have cried it would have meant she felt something. She didn't. She told them she remembered little and made no apology for it. Her disinterest in me was very apparent. She didn't believe it made her look bad. She couldn't understand why this was being dragged up as it had all happened such a long time ago. She succeeded in making me feel worthless.

Notes:

17.06.16
I saw Jayne today and really had to hold it together. Not because I didn't feel safe, but because I felt like I was going to completely fall apart and knew I had to go back to work, but I also knew I wouldn't be okay in an hour.
I feel exhausted.

Reflection: I felt like I was carrying the weight of the world on my shoulders. I felt like I was being pounded into the ground. Nobody who I believed should love me did and I felt I was fighting to be heard. Fighting to be validated and my own Mother couldn't even do that. I felt beat.

Notes:

18.06.16
I have been reading about grief. Ever since my Sister died I have been angry with her. Angry that she left me and I was sexually abused because my mum didn't care anymore. Today I thought about her as me, the adult, who would look at an eight year old little girl who had to go to hospital so many times, who had to wear nappies at school because she couldn't control her bowel and bladder. Who was often in pain. Today I felt overwhelming compassion and grief and cried solidly alone this afternoon.
We made a pact the week before she died to be friends, not fall out and we did it. The day she died she was angry with me and I have always looked at that as rejection through my seven year old eyes. Today I saw it differently, maybe it was fear, maybe she knew, maybe she just really didn't want the pain to be happening again and me telling made it real. I grieved and cried so much for my Sister today, for the first time ever. And after the tears stopped I felt so close to her, so connected, not abandoned and scared, but very, very sad. I miss her so much and I feel frightened for the fear she must have felt.
I wish I had honoured her memory, her birthday, the anniversary of her dying, but I never have. But I will always honour and remember her now, because she was a part of me and now she always will be. I will hold and cherish her in my heart every single day, my poor frightened Sister. I will always hold her close.

Reflection: That was a real moment of insight. I was able to acknowledge my own childhood feelings and then see how my Sisters life might have felt for her. I was then able to rationalise those feelings as an adult. It was a really poignant day and I continue to carry my Sister with me.

Notes:

19.06.16

I was really anxious today. My mum was making a statement to the police and I'm gutted, distraught, dismayed by her lack of insight. Forty minutes after they were supposed to turn up I told her to call them and it turned out she has the wrong week. My head is all over the place. Then tonight after 8pm she calls me. My Dad is punching her. She says he is walking out and starts screaming at him *"Stupid bastard"*, at which point I hear him come towards her and she's screaming *"Get off me, Get off me"*. Charlie and Elizabeth heard as they were next to me on the bed and were so scared. I called the police and Alan ran to their house. I didn't let my Dad in when he called because I am so angry with him and her.

The police picked him up and took him home. He agreed to a hospital admission. That scream down the 'phone took me back to when I was little and he battered her. She was screaming and shouting and so was he and they wouldn't let me through the door.

I hate them both for game playing.

Reflection: My Dad had Alzheimer's disease. My Mother called me to tell me how disgusting he was because he had vomited in the conservatory. He was looking for his wallet and he had vomited. He wanted to come to my house because they had been there earlier in the day and he thought he might have left it. She told me on the 'phone that he was a *'filthy pig'* because he had vomited. My Dad got angry with her and he tried to leave the house. She was on the 'phone all this time to me and she shouted at him asking him where he was going. He told her he was coming to mine, so she shouted at him *"Go on then you stupid bastard go!"* She started screaming as he came back and started punching her. I shouted Alan to go and I called the Police. My Dad in the meantime walked to my house as it was only a short distance away. It was about 7pm and Charlie and Elizabeth had just been showered and they heard it all on my 'phone. They were really frightened and asked me not to let my Dad in. He knocked on the door and it was pouring with rain. I didn't let him in and the Police arrived. They brought him inside and I explained what had happened. I called a neighbour across to mind the children and I went with the Police and my Dad back to his house. My Mum was crying and I hated her for what she did next. She told the Police she couldn't live with him any more and they forced my Dad to agree to go into hospital. He eventually agreed and I knew it would be the end for him. Domestic violence is deplorable, it went on between the two of them, no doubt throughout their relationship, but the cruelest act of all was to use his vulnerability against him. She did that just like Stewart did to me and Alan did to me.

Notes:

20.06.16
I didn't sleep last night. Alan said he would stay at there's but he didn't. I was so afraid my Dad would attack her in the night. I called GP and CPN and a hospital admission has been arranged for tomorrow. She has finally got what she wanted! The world revolves around them, always has. I hate what they do!

Reflection: I knew once my Dad went in to hospital that he would never come home again. Domestic violence had finally destroyed them both. She didn't know it then, but I did. I took the children round to see him to say goodbye. I was crying on the way home. I told the children that grandad would not be coming home again.

Notes:

21.06.16
My Dad has been admitted to hospital for assessment. She has finally got what she wanted. It turns out that she called him a filthy pig for vomiting in the conservatory. That's what kicked it all off and she was telling me this because she cannot believe he would do such a thing. Thirteen weeks in hospital and she has destroyed him. I am overwhelmed with anger, distress and frustration. I hate it all.

Reflection: My Mum and Dad had always put me in the middle of their violence and they had done so right up until the end. I hated them both for that.

Notes:

22.06.16
Too much stimulation today. Had to attend an autism awareness workshop 10am-12 noon. Got home, Alans Mum was there, went to parents evening and then out for a meal with a friend. It was much too much! I just want quiet.

Reflection: I needed time to process what had happened to my Dad. I needed to grieve for him, but I couldn't. That had been my life up until that point. Not being able to express emotion, or feel emotion, or even process an event and it was still happening. I didn't have the strength at that time to express my needs and I wouldn't have for fear of them being ignored. My Son has autism and attending a workshop was a requirement for getting additional support. I attended the workshop, but the additional support never materialised.

Notes:

23.06.16
My mind is still over stimulated - very busy at work, sports day at school. I managed to fall asleep, too much going on. I just need quiet. Too much stimulation, I can't cope.

Reflection: I was so overwhelmed, I was in fact coping really well, I didn't have the tools, the self worth to look after myself. I was running on empty.

Notes:

24.06.16
I saw Jayne today. Last appointment for five weeks and feeling anxious about it. Not having anybody to talk to when emotionally I feel overwhelmed feels really scary.

Reflection: This felt like a very challenging time for me and my only support was being taken away. I didn't know if I could hold on with so much going on I felt like my head was spinning.

Notes:

25.06.16
Saw Melvyn and Rachel tonight. We had a lovely evening, but my heart feels heavy.

Reflection: I felt like I had been left to cope with everything on my own. I had nobody. I was balancing on a tightrope.

Notes:

26.06.16
Saw my Dad in hospital, scruffy, not wearing his own clothes. I feel angry at her. The man has no dignity in here and it's all her fault.

Reflection: Seeing my Dad destroyed by her, dehumanised with no dignity broke my heart. She had done it. She had completely destroyed him and I was angry and I was determined from then on that I wasn't going to let her destroy me any further. The results of her cruelty was standing right in front of me. What a despicable woman she really is and I was beginning to see that.

Notes:

27.06.16
Went to Wimbledon with Alan today. What I loved more than anything was that despite how I feel, I was able to just be in the moment. I didn't feel anxious about how we would get there, what would happen throughout the day, I just experienced the day. Usual anxieties began to creep in at the end of the day, but I was able to put them aside and enjoy the day to the end.

Reflection: Although I enjoyed the day at Wimbledon, we went as two separate people. Alan barely spoke to me, or acknowledged me. He was very distant. The anxiety I experienced towards the end of the day was being on my own with him on the journey home. He didn't speak to me and I felt so alone.

Notes:

28.06.16

Attended a ward meeting about my Dad today. During the meeting I felt more and more angry with my mum. My Dad is never coming home because she won't care for him. He has deteriorated so fast because of her. I have tried my best to protect him, but in doing so has resulted in me and the kids losing him from home forever. My feelings are indescribable.

Reflection: Watching a human being destroy a vulnerable human being was heart breaking. I couldn't believe what was happening to my Dad and she was so cold about everything.

Notes:

29.06.16
So low.

Reflection: Nothing to describe here. It's in the journal to mark time.

Notes:

30.06.16
Can't lift my mood. Feeling so trapped, out of control with everything. I wish I could shrug it off but I can't and then I feel frustrated with myself and the cycle goes on!

Reflection: Being at the mercy of other people and their decisions was so difficult for me. I felt trapped, just like I did when I was being abused. I had no voice, no say, no influence over what was happening to me. It was torture.

Notes:

01.07.16
Feeling alienated at work, isolated and totally overwhelmed. I want to scream to make it all stop!! I am tired of games, manipulation and control. I feel like I want to press a reset button. Just to start again. I want to scream and shout and fuck everything off, but something is holding me back.
I am all alone and tired of this ache inside. I wish I could begin again. AAAAHHH!!

Reflection: I felt alienated and isolated at work because I couldn't feel part of what I perceived to be irrelevant, unimportant, worthless conversations. I had so much riding on the CPS decision. I felt the direction my life was about to take hinged on this decision. Then there was my Mum destroying my Dad and Alans ongoing attempts to destroy me. Work chatter just annoyed me. Inconsequential conversations irritated me and because I couldn't immerse myself into work culture I became isolated.

Notes:

02.07.16
Today was a better day. I just felt grounded and felt determined to be in the moment. It does work. I just need to be given the opportunity to just be with me. That happened today.

Reflection: I had renewed energy. I was stronger than I ever believed at the time, because despite all the desperation and hopelessness at times, I kept trying, when I had the energy I just kept trying to feel better. I couldn't give up.

Notes:

03.07.16
Today was okay.

Reflection: Enough said.

Notes:

04.07.16
My Manager told me people had noticed I'm quiet at work. It's difficult to explain feeling overwhelmed, powerless and trapped. At the mercy of other people deciding my credibility, my worthiness. So difficult.

Reflection: I remember her talking to me. I told her how not getting the Safeguarding job had dented my self-esteem. She explained to me that the person who interviewed answered better on the day. I pointed out to her that I had sixteen years midwifery experience, four years as a specialist midwife and qualifications at Masters Level in Safeguarding. All that hard work, loyalty and determination counted for absolutely nothing, because my personality didn't fit. I couldn't get my head around it at all. If hard work didn't help me to achieve my goals, then how could I keep going with this. This was the hardest thing I had ever done and what if it didn't work? What if after all my hard work I didn't recover? I really questioned every about my existence based on that rejection.

Notes:

05.07.16
Being sexually abused, as a kid really messes with your head. Especially when you try to bury it and function as a normal human being. Letting it out last year in a violent flood of emotion fucks with your head and destroys you to your core. Having people treat it like an event, such as the police, is unbearably difficult to cope with. It wasn't an event like a holiday, or a house move where you remember, but have moved on. This is a poisonous virus that lies in the body, always waiting there for me to become vulnerable, then attacks and overwhelms me.
Nobody can understand me, something in the present has to have happened for them to understand. It was this time last year I saw the GP and told him I was suicidal. He gave me medication and advised me to tell those close to me. I told Alan, he didn't want to know. I told Carol, I told Daryl and Melvyn. We were going on holiday with Daryl and his family so he said I could talk to him if I needed to.
I was shaking inside and out, I didn't know what was happening to me. I knew everything that had happened was very prominent in my mind and I was struggling to hold it back, hold myself together. We went on holiday on 14th July last year and by this time I had already started having panic attacks. I was shaking inside and out, I couldn't control it and images and flashbacks were beginning to consume and dominate my thoughts and I could no longer control it, no longer push it away. I was terrified because I couldn't control anything any longer and I could almost feel it was going to erupt in a violent, overwhelming rush of flashbacks and uncontrollable emotion.
I went to Daryls tonight because I wanted to try and explain how I felt. We are going on holiday on 13th July and it all feels like Deja vu. I can vividly recall how I felt and whilst that doesn't make me anxious, it makes me feel uneasy, like I am watching it all unfold again, but this time I know what is going to happen.
I feel very tearful, insecure and lonely, but I can't explain it in a way that anybody understands. It's so difficult to explain. Watching a film for the second time, so you know what's coming. Of course I don't feel like that now, but the events remind me of this time last year, so I'm watching it unfold and I just want to cry. I feel so alone.

Reflection: What happened to me in July 2015 was absolutely life changing. In the sense that it was make or break time for me in terms of whether I lived or died. Having that time come round again, although I didn't feel the same, catapulted me back to those intense feelings. It was an overwhelming time and I felt overwhelmed again remembering it. An incredibly significant time in my life. I just wanted to be with somebody who would understand how I felt. How I looked back on that time a year ago and the impact of what I had decided to do still had on me. It was incredibly emotive and I had nobody. I was so, so alone. So isolated at that time, it was really devastating.

Notes:

06.07.16

I met a friend, Sara today, she has had a heart scare and her Mum has just died. We talked together for a while and just before she left I felt and overwhelming urge to tell her how I feel. And she got it! She really understood. Her Mum has died and they've had the funeral and everybody's getting on with life and she feels in a bubble because she is grieving for her Mum. It's like being on the outside with all your painful emotions going on and nobody can see it, yet you think they should.

People expect, or assume just because the 'incident' is over, then you must be back to normal. She recognised I am in this bubble of emotion, full of very poignant memories about this time last year as well as the emotion of being sexually abused. I couldn't believe it!! She understands. I cried all the way to my next appointment, but was able to cover it because I have a cold. She told me I didn't need to explain myself to anyone and if I need to be in my bubble for self-protection, then I was entitled to be there.

I can't believe I'm understood. I said if we weren't going on holiday at exactly the same time, it might not be so powerful. I didn't want the same event this year. I wanted to re-write this time with a different experience. Now this might actually happen because we are going to get a puppy and today is Wednesday and we are going to see it on Friday. And the day we are picking her up hopefully, is the day I went off sick last year 24th July. I would love it to become a positive memory. But for now I am happy to feel understood.

Even though Daryl was with me right from the start, he didn't get it because he said for him it was just a normal holiday, but now I am not alone. I am understood.

Reflection: Sara was a friend who I had got to know through work. We met up because she had heard I had been off sick and she wanted to offer me her support. She had also suffered a loss and she understood how it felt to be experiencing grief and not ready for her world to keep turning. She needed to step off and have that time. She understood that that was what I needed too. Suddenly I no longer felt alone. I had spoken to somebody who completely understood that for them time just needed to stand still in their world, in order to process. I had been craving that for as long as I could remember.

Notes:

07.07.16
Today I woke feeling okay. What seems to haunt me is feeling an emotion and feeling guilty about it. I still need that validation that it's okay. Just writing that makes me feel angry. I have battled for years to be able to feel how I feel, no I can, I should.

Reflection: I had always been denied my emotions. If I expressed emotions when I was a kid I would be told off for behaving out of turn. I would be ridiculed, even told by my Mum that what I was feeling was wrong. Growing up like that as a child, I believed this must be true and I learned to deny my own feelings, even get angry with myself when I couldn't. When I met Stewart, my emotions were completely ignored. His emotions dominated everything. His violence, his rape, he expressed it all. I was nothing. I wasn't even there to him. He used me like a rag doll and any emotion was met with violence, or total disregard. Being ignored is soul destroying. And it did destroy my soul. With Alan however, it was the opposite. He expressed very little emotion and I was expected to do the same. If I was upset, I was silenced, if I was angry I was mocked and laughed at and if I was sad, or overwhelmed I was crazy. I had to suppress every emotion, or there were consequences.

Notes:

08.07.16
Met with the guy who interviewed me. It was my personality. Well fuck that. I am never ever changing for anyone.

Reflection: Good for me. That was a strong day. Every strong day was a step forward, but I couldn't see that.

Notes:

09.07.16
We saw the pups yesterday and chose one. Elizabeth is so excited. The boys are happy. I feel nervous.

Reflection: Elizabeth had been pleading for a puppy for months. She had taken to writing on her white board that she would feed it, train it, look after it. Alan worked from home and eventually I gave in to pressure. The puppy would not be left alone all day. I don't know why I felt nervous.

Notes:

10.07.16
Saw my Dad in hospital today. When we were leaving he asked me for a hug. I felt sad for him because I am a good person. I felt subdued for the rest of the day, but can't put my finger on it. Except to think when I am scared and lonely - when I was scared and lonely. Where was my hug?

Reflection: I saw real fear in my Dad's eyes when he asked for a hug. The Alzheimer's was not there in that split second and I wanted to cry for him. I wanted to take him home with me. It was like he knew his fait. It was heart breaking. Then later when I reflected upon it and realised, I didn't have hugs when I was a child and I was scared and lonely. I didn't have hugs now and I was still scared and lonely. I felt confused inside. I wanted to be angry with my Dad, but I hated to see him suffering, even though he had been more than happy to watch me suffer when I was a child.

Notes:

11.07.16
Sitting in clinic today working and feeling confident. This very day last year I was trembling and experienced a panic attack. My head felt foggy and I couldn't control the words coming out of my mouth.
I could hear myself speaking like there was a time delay. Very, very frightening. But today it was okay.

Reflection: Now I was getting flashbacks from that same time the previous year. As if the initial traumas weren't enough, I was now traumatised by my trauma. I felt slightly removed from the day. Almost like an out of body experience.

Notes:

12.07.16
Going on holiday in the morning. It has been emotionally challenging these past few months. I am not building big hopes, but I do hope I can rest, re-charge and come home more focused, rational and stronger.

Reflection: What I would do when something positive was happening, was I would spend all my emotional energy believing it would lift my mood. A positive event, must mean positive moods and much better wellbeing. The problem with that was, I was taking my mind with me and my mind wasn't taking a holiday. My expectations were way too high, but I was still desperate to feel better.

Notes:

20.07.16
Having been on holiday for a week, I knew better than to think everything would be okay. But even so I think my emotional expectation was set too high. I felt down, flat and even recognised I wasn't present, but even then my mind kept drifting. I slept badly all week, had nightmares about Jack. Was so body self-conscious. I am eating healthily and not exercising obsessively, but I felt so big, especially my stomach, the part of me I have always tried to keep small. I hate it being touched, I hate it protruding. I really hate it, but the only way to make it small is to exercise obsessively and not eat enough. I really hate it. I'm finding it so hard to accept and cope with.
It's funny though, I do feel healthier, with more energy, and the kids say they love having a chubby Mum. My mind is so split.
I had a call from Fern today, I rang her back as soon as we got home. Jack has been charged with two counts of indecent assault!! I am so shocked. When she first told me, I felt a bit scared about what is going to happen, but as the day has gone on I'm starting to think, finally, I am going to be listened to.
After thirty six years I have been heard. My horrible, sick feeling inside me has been listened to. I know I won't go to Court until next year, Fern told me that, but my God, all those years of crying on my own. Crying so hard, wishing somebody would hear me. All those years and finally I have been heard. Little me, growing up me, adult me. ALL OF ME! Has finally been heard and I am beginning to feel the enormity of that. It started as fear this afternoon and gradually it is growing into elation, from shock, disbelief and now THIS! This is what I have always wanted. That bastard ruined my life and I am fucked if he is going to ruin it any more. I am going to do the scariest, ballsiest thing in my life. I am going to stand up in Court and tell the whole room just what that scum bag did to me and how he destroyed me. Bastard Jack, You Bastard!! You will NEVER hurt my life again. You absolute Bastard. You have robbed me of everything. YOU WILL GET WHAT YOU DESERVE. I HATE YOU, YOU BASTARD I HATE YOU!!! TODAY!!!!

Reflection: I have always been self-conscious about my stomach because Jack started off tickling it and it always felt like it was protruding after that. I hated it being touched, ever. My body image was so bad.
Now receiving that news when I arrived home I was so elated. I had so much energy inside me, I wanted to scream from the roof tops. Alan offered no response. I was elated and it had nowhere to go. There it was, my emotions shot up, really high, I'd had that hit again, but there was only one way that was going and when it crashed later, it crashed hard.

Notes:

21.07.16
Today we got a puppy, so everything has changed. I hardly think about Jack. It's like it still hasn't sunk in, but I don't want to tell anyone until it has. I need to/want to understand my own feelings before anybody else expresses theirs.

Reflection: Our Tiny puppy, Penny was a Bichon Frise. She was the cutest thing I had ever seen. She helped everything to slow down temporarily, as I watched her slow timid moves when we got her home. She had a really calming effect.

Notes:

22.07.16 Shattered - new pup.

Reflection: Okay, so nobody told me puppies cried. Oh boy, did she cry and she was loud. None of us got any sleep that night.

Notes:

23.07.16 So tired I can't think

Reflection: What had we done buying a puppy?

Notes:

24.07.16
Alan really bollocked the kids tonight, he is so tired, but they were so upset and confused. I felt sick in the stomach, I went upstairs with them. I hate that scared feeling.

Reflection: I don't remember what Alan was shouting about, but the kids were frightened, I was frightened. He shouted at them and then verbally abused me. We all went upstairs and left him downstairs to sleep with the puppy. I tried not to show the kids that I was scared, but I was. This wasn't about being tired for Alan, this was the mask coming off, because nothing was right after that. He became nastier and nastier and I was really frightened.

Notes:

25.07.16

The most destroying night. Alan and I argued about his attitude towards the kids, then he verbally battered me. I felt I could hardly breathe. He was so angry I was scared. But he mocked the way I talk, how I talk, what I say, then I was back there all over again. In Jacks living room when he sniggered when I told him I didn't want to play anymore. I was with my ex-husband when he would humiliate me, mock me, laugh at me and tell me I looked like a freak. The flashbacks were so powerful they made me feel sick.

I hate myself, I am rubbish, I am just an object to be battered, my feelings don't count. I wanted to hurt myself so bad so he couldn't hurt me anymore. Just like I did when he was raping me. I would send him out for snacks, then when he was gone I would binge on biscuits until I was so full I thought my stomach would burst and my heart would explode, it was thumping so hard.

Elizabeth was sat on my knee and came to bed with me. So I didn't hurt myself, not this time.

Reflection: I needed to call on what tiny resilience I had developed. Being emotionally battered to the point that I felt like I couldn't move without being mocked was terrifying. He destroyed me with his words and all that abuse, all those times it had happened before were right there in that room that night. I resorted back to previous beliefs. I couldn't understand how this could all be happening again. I believed all those things I said about myself. Inspite of all that, I knew what I needed to do to keep myself safe. Alan slept downstairs with the puppy. I felt so frightened.

Notes:

26.07.16
Shaking all day. Frightened, shocked and overwhelmed by the massive flashback. Afraid when he got home he would start again. So very afraid.

Reflection: I was frightened to come home from work. Everything I said or did Alan mocked. My mouth was so dry, I didn't know what to do. I was trapped all over again.

Notes:

27.07.16
Stunned at work, shaking and afraid. No sleep last night. He's working from home today and I'm so scared to go home. The flashbacks have consumed me, the feelings have destroyed me. I can't stop crying. I'm terrified of what might happen. I eventually got home after 6pm and he stays out, but that feeling of dread came back when he came home. That feeling that I haven't felt since waiting for Jack to come home. Terrified that something was going to happen. God I feel sick, the flashbacks are destroying me.

Reflection: It is indescribable the extent of the fear I was experiencing inside. I was exactly how I had been waiting for Jack. I was trembling inside, my mouth was dry. I was shaking, I felt cold, I felt this incredible sense of dread. I was terrified of him coming home. Waiting and waiting, not knowing what time that would be and what would happen when he got back. I was beside myself with fear, it was horrendous.

Notes:

28.07.16
Shattered at work, but thankfully he's out from when I get home until 9pm. I don't know what to do. I am so weak, I am angry that I am not stronger, but I am drowning in flashbacks. I have not felt so bad for so long. The terrified feeling. Terrified of the trigger and terrified of the flashbacks.

Reflection: This was all consuming. Not only was I feeling the fear of Alan, I was experiencing the fear on top of that of all the abuse, the rape, the assaults. I didn't know how far he would go. I was horrified. The flashbacks were there because my mind couldn't process what was happening. All my boundaries had been destroyed, so in my mind Alan could have done anything and I had to wait for whatever that might be to happen.

Notes:

29.07.16
I am talking at work, learning to talk and getting support. This stops the self-harm thoughts and the feelings of worthlessness and self-hatred. We talked a lot about feelings, coping as a family and personality. I opened up about me. From the support I have had, I have a bit of me back. If I am open and honest, then I am genuine. I have to risk the response and if it's negative, I don't know how I will cope. I am so very frightened. I don't want the flashbacks to carry on, they are so destroying. I don't know how much more I can take. I am so scared.

Reflection: Beginning to talk at work helped me to feel less isolated. What I wasn't prepared for was those who listened because they wanted to support me and those who listened for the gossip, the story. When people ignored me after I had talked, I felt rejected and hurt. But I didn't own my own feelings at that point. Yes I wanted to talk, but I wanted to talk to vent and to get validation. When that didn't happen, I felt exposed, vulnerable and robbed. Robbed because I had given my story and they had taken it away without care or consideration. I still had a lot to learn.

Notes:

30.07.16
Feeling very lost, very tired. Two weeks of nightmares about Jack.

Reflection: Well I'm not surprised by this entry. I had nobody at this point. I was shouldering the lot.

Notes:

31.07.16
Feeling very lonely and isolated. Can barely write. Nightmares again last night.

Reflection: I was holding on by a thread. I had nothing and nobody. My resilience was weak.

Notes:

01.08.16
Really need to talk to Jayne. I was hoping I would be feeling more positive, but I feel so shaken up after the argument. Almost like I don't know how to be. So anxious and edgy. God I hate this.

Reflection: I didn't know how to be because there was recovering me and all my new found feelings and emotions, that were emerging into beliefs, then there was the old me, or injured me that was so very familiar. The old me could have got drunk, gone crazy, screamed and shouted. I knew that me, but I also knew from the old me what the consequences of that would be and that would be more abuse. I was torn, really torn. I didn't know what to do. Half of me was vulnerable and the other half of me was really vulnerable.

Notes:

02.08.16

I saw Jayne today and we talked and talked. I talked about how down I have felt about coping on all levels with sexual abuse. Living with it, coping when it erupted last year and coping with people trying to intellectualise it. Unbearable.

I talked about how I am finding it so hard to cope with my personality. It's coming up fast and I don't know how to respond. It's like I've been given a new brain and told to get on with it. I don't know how to manage it.

Jayne tried to reassure me that this is not going to come in a couple of weeks when I have suppressed it for thirty six years. She is also reassuring when I talk to her about Jack being charged with two counts of indecent assault. She hugged me and told me she was delighted for me. A truly spontaneous response that matched my emotion. It felt so good to be responded to after very measured, but positive responses. Warm genuine contact I crave so much.

I read a quote tonight *"Do not waste time trying to get somebody to love you, spend time with people who already do."* Oh God, I wish I had that. My children do of course, but I feel so alone. I want to be cherished emotionally, wrapped in love. I just want to be loved, not asked to be loved. My heart aches so much.

I spent the whole afternoon with my Dad, just being with him, giving him the love and compassion he needed. He was so angry and agitated and I know deep down he was scared. He was moved from hospital to care and I spent all afternoon helping him to re-focus. By the time I left he was calm and happy to stay. He even viewed it as a Hotel. I am so drained. Hungry and tired. The Care Manager praised me, she had watched me all afternoon, but when I got home, I wanted to feel wrapped in love. I crave that safe, loved feeling. I am so drained and so very, very on my own. I just want to be loved. Shown love, but held, cherished and cuddled. I have been craving it all my life. What have I done wrong?

Reflection: Despite all of my efforts and hard work, I still believed I had done something wrong. I wasn't doing anything wrong, I was rebuilding my life in the face of adversity. The only thing I was guilty of was being new at it. My personality, values and beliefs felt like they were changing really fast and not on a conscious level. I was responding differently to situations and I didn't know where it was coming from. It really was like I'd been given a new brain and pushed out into the world. I didn't know from one situation to another how I was going to respond. It was good, but scary because I didn't feel in control of anything.

Notes:

03.08.16
I slept badly last night, I just can't get my mind to relax, even with meditation. Last year memories, flashbacks, erupted like a volcano. Now my thoughts, feelings and opinions are erupting the same way, like a box has been opened. Jayne tried to reassure me it will calm. I am reacting, not responding. She pointed out that thirty six years of suppression released in a couple of weeks is not going to level out.
I know I understand, but feeling out of control is horrible. Too many flashbacks. I just want to be wrapped in love. I don't want to be lost.

Reflection: One of the awful things about all of this was everything erupted at once. It was very violent, very aggressive. Once I could no longer contain the memories, the flashbacks, they erupted so violently, now my thoughts, feelings and emotions all wanted to be heard at once and they were violent and aggressive. I felt betrayed by my mind. I had surrendered to it, I had stopped trying to suppress everything, or control it, so I couldn't understand why it had to erupt so violently. But as Jayne pointed out to me 36 years of suppression was not going to come out quietly. I had been flooded, completely flooded with it all and I had no control, I thought it was going to consume me. I wanted that hand to hold, to save me, to stop me from drowning, but it wasn't there.

Notes:

04.08.16
Very tired, but gone to bed unhappy. Why does he prefer an unkind word to a pleasant one? In relation to my Dad, I am struggling to articulate my feelings, other than to describe a huge build-up of tension in my body. My Mum treated him so cruel, he ended up in hospital. He has finally been placed in a lovely home near to us, but he want to go home. He is so distressed and agitated, the staff can't care for him. So he is going to be moved back to hospital to be assessed again. How cruel and awful is that and it's all her fault.
She did this to him and I have to bite my tongue again so she can support me in Court. I want to yell and scream what a hateful, cruel bitch she is and I want to cry for my Dad.
Then tonight he (Alan) just has to be unkind again. Why do people get off on making other people's lives miserable. I am trying hard to cope and then I get shit from him. Why?

Reflection: The answer to that 'why' was because he was an abusive person. I wasn't worthless, or bad, or cruel. Alan was and he was because he could see I was getting stronger and he had to knock me down by ridiculing me and mocking me because he knew my self-esteem and self-worth were fragile. He felt threatened by my strength and he needed to destroy me. The stronger I became, the more abusive his behaviour. He was trying to overpower me. He was trying to keep me a victim because then he could continue to control me and abuse me.

Notes:

13.08.16
I haven't written anything for a while because the difficulties I have been facing have not been specific to my recovery, but on reflection, maybe it has. On Friday 5th August, my Dad was returned to hospital and I think I was more bothered than him. I have lost my Dad, he has gone. He is so confused and disoriented, angry and agitated, but in his own world now.
I feel so sad, but I have nobody to turn to. I have such mixed emotions. He never looked after me and protected me, but he was a practical man and he helped me in that way. But he's gone and I feel such grief.
I haven't felt the same way about Alan since that big row a couple of weeks ago. I have seen a cruel, hard, cold side to him and I feel that's how he really feels about us. Then last night confirmed it. He walked away from a conversation which annoyed me, then accused me of being provocative when he asked me what was wrong and I told him. Again he felt angry and defensive, but told me it was my fault for arguing in front of the children.
He began the conversation again later in the evening, then accused me of not letting it go. Character assassination was what my ex-husband used to do and I have that same tight feeling in the pit of my stomach as I did with him. Wanting to defend myself, but knowing in doing so will lead to more character assassination. I felt sick last night, but spoke to a friend who reminded me I am better than this. Then I realised.
He told me he didn't love Sam, he sat in the conservatory reading a magazine when we had a major flood. He told me he didn't want to marry me and I begged him to try. He commands respect, but gives none and all this time I felt guilty and bad and believed it was all my fault. I wasn't good enough. But now I realise after eleven years. It's obvious he no longer loves me, if he ever did. He no longer cares for me, or he wouldn't be cruel. He certainly doesn't fancy me as he rarely come to bed with me, when he does he's plugged into a device.
And now I realise, it's me that's been needy. It's me that's been desperate to be loved, because that's what I never had. I just want to be loved, cared for, respected and accepted for who I am and I have spent my whole life trying to be what people want so I can be loved. (This doesn't apply to my children, my relationship with them is so different). This is therefore all my fault, because I have been trying to make something work that was never destined to work because I am so needy. I don't want my marriage to die, but I have finally realised I can't make somebody love me for who I am, even if I love them dearly.
I just wanted to be loved.

Reflection: I had developed insight into my relationship and in doing so I had realised that all the time, all the abuse I'd endured was because I wanted to be loved. Yes okay I was needy. I was needy because I hadn't had the foundations of love from my Mum and Dad, so I had spent a lifetime searching for love. And a perpetrator can sniff out a vulnerable person at fifty paces. I just wanted to be loved. Of course I did, we all do. But being rejected, ridiculed, mocked and abused, just led me to believe I had to keep getting better to be loved, so I tried to mould my personality to suit that person. I gave every part of me to meet the needs of that person and they could all see it and they all abused it. None of that was my fault, but I still couldn't see it, not yet.

Notes:

16.09.16

I have desperately missed writing in this journal. I hadn't realised how much of a companion it had become. I couldn't write because Alan, my now ex-husband, read my most personal entries. He used it to humiliate me, demean me, mock and laugh at me. He made me feel sick to the core. I sought help from the Police, Domestic Violence Unit and colleagues at work. And I had to cope with him attacking my character, slating me to the kids, calling me names, just because I refused to engage in conversation with him. He called me weird, bizarre, unstable, suicidal, unsafe. I was advised to keep my mouth shut so as not to aggravate him. I was and still am devastated by what he has done.

How could he stoop so low? To think he has such little, even no regard at all for what he was doing. He must really hate me. Since he has left Charlie and Elizabeth have wanted to sleep with me. I understand they want to feel safe and secure, I really do and I love Sam, Charlie and Elizabeth so much it makes my heart ache. But I desperately need just a little bit of time to myself. I just need a tiny bit of quiet.

Jack appeared in Court on the 13th September. Fern (Police) called me the day after to say he will be appearing in Court on 11th October, therefore I have to complete my witness impact statement. I started today and I felt so sick. The raw emotion is so powerful and I am frightened of the impact it may have, this has all emerged so recently, it scares me so much and I feel so alone. I just want to sit with my head in my hands and cry. Why did Alan have to hate me so much to do what he did? What did I do wrong for him to want to hurt me so badly? I feel so terribly alone. So sad and so, so wrong. What do I do to make men want to hurt me, break me down to my core. I am so destroyed by Alan. Why? Why do men hate me so much to want to destroy me?

I read a quote earlier:

"You don't know pain until you're staring at yourself in the mirror with tears streaming down your face and you're begging yourself to just hold on and be strong." That is pain. God, that's how I feel today. I am so tired of being alone. I am carrying so much, I feel I have a mountain to climb and I feel so very, very alone. Whatever I have done, I am so, so sorry. I have never meant to hurt anybody, I have only ever tried to be good, but what have I done to be not good enough? What have I done to make men hate me so much they want to destroy me? I don't know who to turn to, but please whatever I have done, I am so, so sorry. Please make the pain go away. I beg whatever is out there, please make it stop. Please.

Reflection: Alan left on 01/09/16 and we all breathed a sigh of relief. No more abuse, no more fear. Alan turned out to be just another perpetrator from a long line of perpetrators. I blamed myself because the behaviour kept repeating itself, but the behaviour repeated itself because I was still vulnerable and perpetrators can see that. I kept being abused because I was vulnerable, neglected and desperate to be loved. None of that was my fault, but I kept apologising for it and at that time I still didn't know who I was apologising to.

Notes:

17.09.16
Today was a better day.

Reflection: Even amongst the bad days there were good. Maybe it was because I had my journal back. My companion that didn't abuse me at all, except when I abused myself, then read it back and it reflected in my face.

Notes:

18.09.16
Feeling very down. Writing my witness impact statement. Talking about how Jack has destroyed me, is destroying me.

Reflection: Writing a witness impact statement is very difficult. I had to write how Jack had affected me physically, emotionally, psychologically and financially, and during my life generally. Family, relationships etc. It meant I had to really pick apart every aspect of my life that had been destroyed. If that wasn't rubbing my nose in it what was? It was incredibly challenging.

Notes:

19.09.16
Feeling very low and so very, very alone. I have exposed my raw emotion, an emotion that has always threatened to destroy me and now I'm exposing it again on my own. I wish I could be held, just to feel safe and never feel scared again.

Reflection: I couldn't remember the last time I had felt safe. I felt totally exposed and vulnerable. So raw.

Notes:

20.09.16
Feeling very overwhelmed. Really sinking in hard, the impact Jack has had on my life. Feeing trapped, like I can't breathe, like it's happening all over again. I am living it all over again.

Reflection: This was bound to happen after writing the Witness impact statement. It took everything he did to a whole new level. I was absolutely distraught. Tormented and overwhelmed, but I held it together, I cared for my children and I went to work every single day. If that isn't strength, then I don't know what is.

Notes:

21.09.16
Really disconnected today. I am telling people I am struggling and they are not listening again. What do I do?

Reflection: This was something I had feared since I'd been suicidal. Talking to people and them not listening. I didn't realise then, that it wasn't only me that wasn't listened to. That in fact anybody might not be listened to and needs to really speak up. But I had such low self-esteem and self-worth, that was a real barrier. Low self-esteem and self-worth was a real danger for me in terms of being able to seeking help and support and not turning in on myself.

Notes:

22.09.16
Feeling slightly panicky today. Scared that what I have exposed writing in my witness impact statement is going to overwhelm me so much, it destroys me again.

Reflection: My resilience was low, but I was hanging in there. I had inner strength from somewhere.

Notes:

23.09.16
I saw Jayne today, talked about how every association made me feel like I can't go on and scared those feelings will come back. I need to get rid of this witness impact statement. I need to not feel so exposed, so overwhelmed, so vulnerable. I really need this to not get the better of me. When I write my book, I will include my statement, so it makes sense. Right now I feel very vulnerable, very scared.

Reflection: See Glossary.

Notes:

24.09.16

Little by little I am getting stuff done. It feels like I sort half a dozen things, then a dozen more things need to be sorted, but hopefully it will slow down. I get the bed to myself too, which is also good. Fern called me today about my statement. Now I just need to sign it. I really hope he pleads guilty on the 11th October, I really do. I want this thirty six year nightmare to end. Please let it end. Please, I will be the best I can possibly be, please, please just let it end.

Reflection: When I feel overwhelmed even the smallest of tasks feels like a chore. It was difficult to function on any level when I felt like this, but I did it.

Notes:

09.10.16
Today has been a bad day. I dreamt about Jack last night, I was crying and looking for help. I woke up feeling very sad and looking for help. I feel so very alone. Why have I always been alone? I plead that Jack pleads guilty on the 11th October. I just want this to end. I have to stop feeling so alone, but I feel so disconnected from real life. God this hurts!

Reflection: Jack was appearing in the Local Magistrates Court on the 11th October to enter a plea. I have never wished so hard. I just wanted him to plead guilty so it would end. I was ready for it to end.

Notes:

11.10.16
I have felt a wide range of emotions today. Jack appeared in Court. I felt powerful, powerful that I have put him there. But then I felt strange, so very strange, thinking that people who don't even know me are talking about me and what Jack did to me. All that going on in Court whilst I am 100 miles away. Then I got the call and I was told Jack has pleaded not guilty. I expected that, but desperately hoped he would. The I was told the date for trial is 25th September. I can't believe 12 months. Fern said it would be six months.
I can't believe I pinned so much on Jack pleading guilty. I just want it to end. I am trying so hard to stay strong, but I'm constantly pulled back. I need space to get strong, but I can't have it. Alan, my mum and Jack holding me back and I desperately want to move forward. I feel trapped all over again. I don't know what to do.

Reflection: I was at work when I heard that Jack had pleaded not guilty. I was helping some colleagues move into a new office and I was actually washing down some tiled walls. I couldn't react. There were people around me. I just wanted to scream "*no*" and fall down on my knees, but I couldn't. At least I felt I couldn't. that was exactly how I had to behave when all the abuse was happening. Not react, carry on as normal. Even now at home, I was not able to let my emotions out, because I had to be there for my children and they didn't know anything about any of this.

Notes:

04.11.16

If I'm not careful I am going to pin all my hopes on Jack pleading guilty. And then I might not get the relief I have been wishing for all my life. I don't want to live just waiting for the outcome, I want to live and move forward. I don't want the next twelve months to become a blur.

We have a shed in the garden and Elizabeth wanted it for a play house. We spent the whole day decorating it, painting it, we put lights up in it. For the whole day I was totally absorbed in something. I thought of nothing except what we were doing. I stopped being on the outside, worrying about consequences, spilling paint, getting cleaned up. I enjoyed my time and it was incredible. I suggested things I would never have thought of, like putting tiles on the floor to keep the blanket on top of them dry and putting wrapping paper on the ceiling. I feel as though my brain has started to wake a side of itself up that has previously been consumed with feelings and emotions and thoughts left by Jack and those who came after him.

Reflection: Being able to allow myself to be absorbed in enjoying this time with my children was a welcome retreat from everything that was happening. I felt safe, I felt like I was hiding from the big monsters. I also surprised myself with my creative ideas, I didn't know I had it in me.

Notes:

10.11.16

If I didn't have my kids would I still be here? Honestly, no. I saw Jayne on the 4th November and I talked about feeling more present. At the end of the session I told her about somebody who talked to me about their trauma. I felt very present. But then she ended it by saying she couldn't have got through it without her partner by her side. Then BANG, a switch went on in my brain and suddenly all the abuse and loss I have experienced alone hit me – bang again! It's enormous and I can't shake it off.

At the moment I can't comprehend how I can even put one foot in front of the other. We went to the cinema and I have no recollection of the film. I was consumed with flashbacks. I have very little recollection of the whole week. I spoke on the 'phone to Jayne and she pointed out that at least I am aware that I'm not present, when previously it would have scared me. I also realised how easy it is to not be present and how much work it takes to be in the moment.

I just want to be able to talk without fear, just to let it go, but I can't and the pressure builds and the thoughts of cutting come back. I don't see it as self-harm, I see it as a release. I just want to talk and talk and talk, to release the pressure. Life is so hard, I just want the pain to stop. I don't want to be alone anymore.

Reflection: I don't even know what the name of the film was. Later my daughter asked me what I thought was the best bit. I reflected it back to her and asked her what bit she thought was best and when she told me I told her that was my best bit too. I had no idea at all what happened throughout the entire film. Being aware that I wasn't present was definitely progress and made me less afraid of those black holes in my memory. I wasn't scared that it might happen randomly anymore, because I knew why they happened. Self-harm was always buzzing about in the background, because I hadn't developed a sense of myself and I hadn't learned self-care.

Notes:

26.11.16
I have been completely overwhelmed for the past two weeks. Overwhelmed with being sexually abused, overwhelmed with getting divorced, overwhelmed with responsibility and I couldn't see a way forward. Then one night last week, I fell into an exhausted sleep and as I drifted off a voice told me *"Paula, this is your journey."* Now it wasn't my voice, Jayne's voice, or a schizophrenic voice. I don't do the word 'journey', I find it cringing. What I did wake up feeling though, was I have always reacted to other people's actions, because my thoughts and feelings have always been ignored. I have reacted and tried to cope emotionally with what other people have done to me. I woke up feeling that whatever happens around me, whoever has an effect on my life, either positive or negative, I am entitled to express my very own emotion, right there and then. Without reacting to how I think somebody might want me to react. I have done this for as long as I can remember because I have always had my feelings ignored, sometimes laughed at, mocked, belittled, or humiliated. I have finally woken up and realised I am allowed to feel. I am allowed to express myself. I am allowed to be me. It is okay for people to disagree with me, it doesn't mean I'm wrong, or I'm being ignored, or I'm worthless.
I am worthwhile, I am valued and my voice does deserve to be heard. I don't have to put up with anything I don't like. My feelings count. I don't have to live with other people's hurtful behaviour. I have a choice. I can live with things I don't like, or agree with, but never to the detriment of my own feelings of self-worth. I never ever have to do this ever again and I have just realised it. I can be me, I can speak, I can express myself and I can be heard. I can't believe I have just realised I can be me! It's okay to be me, think about what's best for me and never again be worthless, used and disregarded. I am going to look after me. Only I can look after me. I can be real, be congruent, BE ME.
Nobody can ever destroy me again, now that I have found me. I am me -yes I am. I haven't been me since I was ten years old and Jack took me away and I became the property of everybody else. I am me! And I will be heard. This feels absolutely incredible. It's like I'm meeting me for the first time. Like I've been given a brand new me – To Keep. Oh God! I will make mistakes, finding my feet and I might get it wrong, but I am good and kind and honest and I love people and will never intentionally hurt anyone.
I apologise to anybody who might be reading this book, please forgive me, but I am finding my feet and I love it. I have been given me, back to me. Last seen age ten. Ooh! What a big hug to me. I have found me.
I am so excited. "Hello me." My organismic me!

Reflection: Dreams can be incredibly powerful and this dream certainly made a difference to me. But who would it have been that was talking to me?

Notes:

30.11.16

"With congruence comes great responsibility." That should have been the quote.

I think I am beginning to understand what is going on. I am flitting from feeling completely overwhelmed and scared of very powerful emotion, to enjoying and feeling very, very different being congruent. My brain if flitting back and too, just like a light going on and off actually. I am experiencing many different feelings. Feeling very calm, having vivid dreams, but then not remembering them in the morning, but dreams I am not familiar with.

Then I am feeling incredibly emotionally overwhelmed, scared and feel like I am drowning. What I understand from this is, how can I be congruent, present and an emotionally aware person, yet not be acknowledging or be emotionally aware of everything that has happened. Of course the two cannot be separate. I don't know if this makes sense, but I hope writing it down makes it clearer.

I am enjoying new awareness, awakening one minute, then absolutely terrified the next. I am not going mad, I am not going mad, I am actually seeing things much, much clearer. I think the last two weeks, being totally overwhelmed was the beginning of me dropping my guard, dropping my barriers to everything. My brain, my mind, does not want to hold on to the trauma, does not want to ignore, or suppress it any longer, but as usual it comes out in violent emotional outbursts.

Earlier this week a friend was messaging me about some problems she was having with her Sisters and ended her message saying it was alright for me being a singleton, as I would never have to put up with the emotional drain of siblings. Two weeks ago I would have thought, of course it's alright for me. My Sister's dead, so what have I got to worry about! I would have had a knot in my stomach and felt anger and self-hatred for everything that happened. Instead what I did was I messaged my friend back and explained that my Sister had died when I was seven years old and if she hadn't have died none of what had happened would have happened. And that on reflection, I would prefer to have my Sister with me, even if she had turned out to be a bitch.

Of course I blame Jack for what happened – at the start anyway, but then what happened was I suddenly became overwhelmed with grief for a Sister I desperately wish I still had. Grief for little me who was left to fend alone at seven years old and an overwhelming realisation of the awful path I went down which started with Jack. I became completely overwhelmed with grief, horror and devastation about what has happened.

That's the bit that really scares me, like I'm really feeling it for the first time and it hits really hard. Taking from this – I didn't have the knot in my stomach, I didn't have the self-hatred, I was heard by my friend who went on to explain how she really did love her Sisters, but they gave her a hard time at times. And I didn't have that disgusting secret eating away at me again, because her comment had reminded me of Jack and every disgusting thing that has happened since.

I am so very up and down and really need to talk this through. Sometimes I feel like my mind is running away with me and I can't keep up. My mind is behaving like an excited child that has just found itself, it's racing through all emotions and dragging everything along with it.

Going back to my quote at the start, I suddenly feel very, very emotionally responsible, not only for myself now, but for myself then and it's all happening so very fast and it's all so overwhelming.
This feels like a monumental breakthrough for me. I have sent this to Jayne as an e-mail to talk it through further, but I feel like a key to my mind has been unlocked and there is a huge clear space just flooding with brand new emotions. I couldn't feel more strange if I'd had a head injury. Everything I thought I knew for the past thirty six years is now being re-written. Colossal.

Reflection: This entry itself is a reflection and an amazing step forward.

Notes:

15.12.16
For the past week I have been receiving nasty text messages from my ex-husband. They have hurt me deeply and scared me so much I cannot sleep and I am trembling inside every morning when I wake up. I have had a panic attack for the past two days. First thing in the morning as I come round. I am absolutely terrified and I am with Jack all over again, Jason and my first husband. Trapped, knowing I can't do anything to stop what's happening and knowing he can violate me whenever he wants and I can't do a thing about it. I have felt physically sick to the point where I have started retching and my mind cannot cope with anything except the essentials and that scares me. It's like living it all over again.
I have tried so hard to meditate. I think "*I am not my thoughts*" and I have been able to take a step back and think, what is it that makes me scared? And it's this – He is saying I am asking for it (Alan)! He is saying he can get to me and there is absolutely nothing I can do. He is saying everything I believed to be right was wrong all along. He deceived me, betrayed my trust. That's why I feel scared. I have repeated the same thing all over again. I've been in a situation I thought was safe, with a person I believed I could trust. He abused that trust, used it to humiliate me, blame me and let me know he can do it again if he wants to.
I have contacted the police in order to gain some control and they have advised me to make it clear that he only needs to contact me to arrange access to the kids if he becomes abusive again. So I feel sick, waiting for him to launch his tirade again. Waiting to be abused again I can't bear it. This has to stop! I can't cope! Help me, I really need help!

Reflection: Being threatened by Alan was exactly the same as when I was with Stewart, my first husband. Being told he could get to me whenever he wanted to terrified me. I felt I couldn't do anything to keep myself safe. I felt like I was waiting for something terrible to happen, just like I had to with Jack. It was that waiting and not knowing that made me feel like I couldn't cope. I was going through those torturous emotions all over again.

Notes:

02.01.17

So Christmas came and went. Being at home with the kids was brilliant. My love for them has swollen my heart so much, it feels like it might burst. This is the fantastic side of feeling true emotions. My panic attacks have stopped and my ex-husband has crawled back into his shell. My heart felt very heavy at times and I felt like I wanted to cry. So for the first time I thought about why I might feel like this and I concluded it's because I am lonely. I am so very lonely and I don't want to be any more. I understand why I am lonely is because I have always been closed off, because I was afraid to let people get to know me because I was hiding this terrible secret. But also because I didn't trust people, I've always been at the mercy of other people. Now I am beginning to develop a sense of myself. I am beginning to trust myself, value myself and accept myself. My thoughts and opinions are valid.

During this time I have also come to realise how I develop relationships. I have embarrassed myself in the past because I believed if somebody was kind to me then that must mean we are friends, or they must want to be in a relationship with me. I discovered this over Christmas. I have three very good friends who are kind, trustworthy, caring, wise and sensitive and I couldn't understand why I believed I was in love with all three of them.

I looked up unrequited love and a paragraph within a text illustrated that sometimes we think we are in love with somebody because they display an aspect of their personality that we are attracted to. However, we have no real idea what they are really like in the rest of their life. Suddenly, for me the penny dropped. Of course I love these friends as my friends because of their qualities that matter so much to me and my needs! I have yet to understand what my qualities are because I have attracted people who have abused me. I am learning to develop relationships with people who don't want to abuse me.

I finally believe I am beginning to develop healthy boundaries for the first time in as long as I can ever remember. It feels like my brain has had a complete clear out. It is being renovated to a healthy brain. I am also developing so much more self-respect. My Mum has always been disrespectful towards me. Portraying this victim mentality, but I snapped and told her I was not going to tolerate it any more. I stood up to my Mum for the first time in forty seven years and as I rather vociferously articulated how she made me feel, I felt I could see myself growing. I no longer feel held down, or pandering to her emotions.

Reflection: These insights made me feel brilliant. However, despite telling my Mother how she made me feel, she showed no emotion, displaying instead only a cold disregard for what I was saying. It wasn't the last time I told her how she had made me feel and the response was always the same.

Notes:

08.01.17
I talked all this through with Jayne. It feels very exciting, very new and like a breath of fresh air. I feel like I can breathe again. When I left her I began to feel nervous. So I thought about why I was/am feeling this way, then once again I realised. When you pass your driving test, or learn to ride a bike, you feel so happy, so excited, so fresh that you have acquired a new skill, achieved something so exciting. Then when you go out on your own, you suddenly feel nervous, because although you have acquired this skill, the reality of your inexperience hits you and you realise you know very little about what you are doing. How to deal with a skid, how to avoid a crash. How to get petrol. So with this in mind! I feel I have acquired a whole new set of perspectives, beliefs and understandings. They are so new, so exciting and at the same time I am anxious that I will be able to cope with challenging situations without resorting to old patterns of behaviour. Now I recognise this and I am aware of this, I am already less anxious.
I can't believe that when I am struggling with an emotion, I can actually sit and think about it and then come up with the solution. I have NEVER, EVER been able to do this. My emotional stresses have always lead to experiencing trauma, despair and self-harm. After forty seven years I am beginning to find my own solutions to my own emotional difficulties. Incredible.
And all the time this is going on I have not forgotten that Fern has not called me about Jack!

Reflection: More insight, bigger steps forward.

Notes:

19.01.17
I have just finished reading the Velveteen Principles loaned to me by Jayne. It's about becoming 'real'. Experiencing real emotions, irrespective of external influences, such as other people, or material items. I have for as long as I can remember, been completely 'unreal'. I have developed a personality based solely on survival since the age of ten and being sexually abused and emotionally destroyed by Jack and all that followed. But since November when I felt completely overwhelmed with emotion, I believe that is when I started to become 'me'. I have rediscovered me. When I begin to feel sad, lonely, vulnerable, angry, I am expressing it to people like I have never been, or felt able to before. I don't wait for that emotion to build, I don't wait until I can't control it and I don't try to ignore it.
Last week Jayne and I were talking and we began to talk about when we first met and how overwhelmed I felt and absolutely terrified. Jayne told me she understood my terror, my fear of talking about horrific stuff. But I looked at her and said "*no*." The reason I was terrified was because I had given up. I had called the centre repeatedly because nobody had answered. When somebody did answer and offered me an appointment the following week, I told them I couldn't wait that long. I told them I couldn't/didn't believe I could be helped. She told me to hold on. I told Jayne the reason I was terrified was because I knew if it went wrong I was going to walk out of there and step in front of a bus. I had the image crystal clear in my head. Round the corner from McDonalds the double decker buses go and I would step right into it's path. Talking to Jayne I felt the real intensity of emotion and I looked at her and thought "*my God, you had no idea.*" Right there and then I wanted to give her a hug. She is another person to have saved my life. I felt an enormous energy in the room. A very poignant moment and writing this I now understand why I have felt subdued all week. It's the absolute sadness.
Yesterday a very good friend helped me with a Johari window exercise to help me to understand my emotions and how I am seen by others. Whilst we were doing this she told me that she wouldn't be able to do the exercise herself as she didn't feel too well herself. She began to describe how she was feeling and it mirrored what had happened to me. Waking up at night, not being able to sleep, beginning to panic when particular emotive topics are discussed and identifying with clients whose experiences mirrored my own. I felt that rise of anxiety for her and for me for that awful, most terrifying time of my life. A time when everything felt like it was out of control and I completely lost the ability to suppress or control horrific feelings from years of being sexually abused. It has been an unearthly, other worldly, unusual kind of a week. I called Fern today, but she has heard nothing from Jacks defence lawyer. I feel like I have a guardian angel!

Reflection: The atmosphere in the room with Jayne that day was so heavy. As I talked to her I wanted to cry, because she hadn't realised how close I had been to ending my life. It made me also acutely aware that if the conversation had gone this way instead of that. If she'd made any comment that gave me the slightest inkling that she would struggle to help me I would have finished it. Ended my life. Even though I knew it at the time, seeing the reality of it dawn on Jayne's face almost overwhelmed me. It was that mirror reflection again. I had really been that close to dying that day we met. It showed me how fragile I was and just how much responsibility I put onto Jayne. How much I was investing my life in her ability to hold on to me. If I had committed suicide, it wouldn't have been anybody's fault, except my own. But sometimes a counsellor can be holding a life in their hands and a word, just a single word can be the difference between life and death.

Notes:

04.02.17

So many epiphanies. I have just read "*The Discovery of Being*." It helped me to understand that to resolve emotional trauma, whatever it is, has to be done by breaking the emotion right down to it's route cause. I have spent most of my life thinking about, being afraid of, contemplating and attempting suicide. I always believed it was because Jack sexually abused me, because I was raped. But it wasn't at all. I became suicidal because I truly believed I had no worth. I truly believed I was only alive to be used by other people, but reading this book has helped me to understand I wouldn't have done everybody a favour by killing myself, I wouldn't be better off dead. I truly, truly believed I was worthless because I took responsibility for all their actions. Jack didn't sexually abuse me because I was worthless, he sexually abused me because he is a sick, depraved specimen of a human, who got his kicks out of sticking his fingers in my knickers.

I wasn't raped because I was worthless, I was raped because sick individuals could see my vulnerability, could see I believed I had no worth, so used my vulnerability to meet their needs. My God! I was never worthless, I was born into this world as equal a human being as any other baby. What went wrong was I was neglected by a mother who was incapable of seeing my worth. She was incapable of nurturing me, and saw my strengths as some kind of threat to her sense of self-worth.

My Sister was physically disabled. She was very strong in character, so my mum could fight for her every need, but didn't need to care for her in a nurturing way. I am not physically disabled, so I didn't need her in that way, but I did want to be nurtured, loved and emotionally cared for, but she couldn't do that. She did and still does see emotional need as a weakness. So she rejected my emotional needs repeatedly, telling me I was strong and independent and because I am not physically disabled then repeatedly she will tell me it's alright for me. Whatever struggles I have had, her response has always been to say, it's alright for me, or there has been no response, or I have been rejected because I am not disabled. Her rejection nurtured a strong belief that I am not good enough. Eventually I grew tired of being/believing I am not good enough and I gave up.

Introduce suicide as my get out clause. Reading this book has helped me to understand that I am as equal as anybody else. What I have done is accept the responsibility that people gave me. I am not responsible for my mum's perception of me. She is responsible. I am as equal as anybody else. I am not responsible for Jack sexually abusing me. I was looking for love, I was not looking to be sexually abused. I also realise it was because I believed I was worthless, that I was raped. I walked off with this man who took my hand, because he talked to me, he took my hand. I wasn't responsible for being raped. He took my hand and he was nice to me. He was nice to me and I like that he wanted to hold my hand. I felt worthless, I had nothing to lose, somebody was being nice to me, talking to me. Why would I not want that? Of course I understand now why I felt so guilty, why I allowed myself to go with him. I was thirteen years old, I didn't go with him so he could rape me. I am not responsible for being raped.

Everything that has happened to me has happened because of my sense of worthlessness. Cruel people can see vulnerability and will always use it to their advantage. Kind and compassionate people will try to protect and strengthen vulnerable people. I have been rejected by people all of my life. It is only now I understand why. What I have to begin to learn is rejection is not associated with self-worth. What this amazing, fantastic epiphany has taught me is that I am not responsible for the actions of my abusers and I no longer believe I have to take responsibility for why it happened. I am me and I have every right to be loved and cherished and none of it was my fault. Can you believe that. <u>None of it was my fault!!</u> I feel like a huge weight has been lifted off my chest. Moving very, very fast, I can also see now what an impact my behaviour has had on others, especially my children. How easy it is to screw people up without being intentionally hurtful. I am beginning to love being me, because I am beginning to be me. I am rediscovering me. It's absolutely amazing. It's an incredible feeling. Like I have been gagged all my life and the gag is coming off.

I was out this afternoon with two of my children and their friend and a voice inside my head/my mind said *"I forgive you Jack."* What he did to me destroyed me and set me on a path of more destruction and abuse, but he is so deluded, so sick, so morally reprehensible, so, so very condemnable, so mixed up, so screwed up and wrong. He sexually abused me because he is sick and not because I felt worthless. He is so sick he did not and still does not know what he is doing is wrong. He has to be forgiven for that, because if he did know what he had done and is still doing it, he wouldn't be able to live with himself. I am free. I am finally free.

Reflection: These reflections are getting smaller, because I am developing a deeper understanding and reflecting more and more in each entry.

Notes:

05.02.17

Today has been a great day. I have felt liberated, I felt fresh, peaceful and completely unburdened. I feel like I could fly. Not in a high way, but because I feel so light. My mind has been so clear and untroubled all day. I had to be careful I was so quiet and at peace, even thought I had visitors. My mum and Dad spent the day with us, but I had nothing to say, but also held no anger or tension. It's like I have fully accepted I don't need to take responsibility for anybody else's feelings. It's amazing. I only meant I had to be careful that I didn't appear rude, or unwelcoming. I was totally and utterly relaxed. A great day.

Reflection: That realisation that I am only responsible for my own feelings was so uplifting. I could almost feel the physical weight lifting and I developed new insights over and over again.

Notes:

09.02.17
I continue to feel lighter, less troubled. I have been met with challenges along the way, but I have faced them and not ignored my feelings. Even when something annoyed, or upset me, I have taken time to think about why I am experiencing these feelings. This has made me be able to consider and value my thoughts and feelings, understand why I feel like I do and then accept why I feel like I do. This is completely the opposite to ignoring why I feel emotions, which I have done all my life due to my perceived lack of self-worth. I have self-worth. I own my feelings, which is making challenges and difficulties so easy to cope with. I have been smiling all week, without really thinking and a little voice in my head is saying "*I never thought I would smile again.*" But another little voice was asking "*What about me?*" And I must listen to that voice, it's not ready to let go just yet. It doesn't stop me smiling, but it does take me back to July 2015 when I fell apart and this all began. I need to listen to that little voice, it has only just started. I need to look after it.

Reflection: I was riding on the crest of a wave, enjoying all of this new understanding and feeling great. I didn't want to listen to that little voice, that little voice was still hurting and I didn't want to think about that hurt. I was enjoying not hurting, I was enjoying the 'new me'. That little hurt voice was dragging me back and I didn't want to look at it. But I didn't know who it was just yet.

Notes:

11.02.17 - Suicide

We talked about suicide yesterday in counselling. This is my last taboo. My relationship with suicide, my experiences have lasted almost as long as my sexual abuse experiences. I feel very emotional even just writing about my most personal experience and relationship with suicide. It is as familiar as my experience of sexual abuse and rape, yet my least ever talked about. Every time I have been suicidal, I have felt exactly the same and I am going to try my best to expose it.

I first remember feeling suicidal after being sexually abused by Jack when I was 10 years old. I don't know that I actually knew what suicide itself meant, then, but I do know that as time passed I hated how I felt every day and night. Unable to sleep because of feeling terrified that Jack would come into my room and sexually abuse me again. I was terrified he would climb through my bedroom window and it was a real possibility because we lived in a bungalow. I was distracted day in, day out by images, flashbacks and constantly trying to understand why he abused me. I don't know why I decided this, but I did decide that by the time I was 14years old I was going to die. Why 14 I don't know, but it was an obsession. By the time I was 14 I had decided I would have had enough of this constant torment, I would be so sick and tired of the stuck record, the constant reliving, the ever compounding belief that I was worthless, no good, not good enough, a bad person. Reliving and reliving that agony day after day after day. I gave myself a deadline. A real deadline. I would live until I was 14 and then I would die. Then I watched an episode of Fame on television. I loved Fame, it was a fictional American TV show about teenagers at a performing arts school as I remember. In one particular episode the story was about a suicide not found amongst vandalised lockers. During that episode the teachers and counsellors were trying to find out who the note had been written by. A young girl appeared to be distressed and disclosed that she had contemplated suicide. The advice she was given was that whatever is causing so much pain, however bad it feels now, will not be present in 10 years time. In 10 years time the situation will be gone, no longer exist.

I searched for that episode tonight and found that episode listed as "*Help from my friends*". It says it was aired on 10th March 1983. Nine months before my 14th birthday. I watched that episode at that time over and over again. I believed I had hope, I believed what it said. It was the first time my life was saved. I really believed it. I was terrified to turn 14, I had convinced myself I was going to die and now that I had found hope, I didn't want to die. I was terrified that I had been so fixed on something happening, that I really was going to die.

I had given myself another chance. But then things got worse, I was raped when I was 13 years old and I was raped again when I was 16years old and then I went on to marry a man who emotionally destroyed me and raped me so violently and repeatedly that my only escape was suicide. I have given myself a reprieve, convinced myself that I still had something left in myself that hadn't been got to, that there was hope and something to hold on to. Now that was gone. I had nothing left. Nothing left of me. I was physically, emotionally and sexually violated. I was destroyed. I had nothing left. I hated myself, everything about myself because I attracted violence and destruction. I had to take control, I had to destroy myself. I had to die, I couldn't take any more. I had to destruct myself, but be in control of how that destruction worked and I knew exactly what to do. I wanted to disappear. If I disappeared nobody could hate me anymore. And so I began to starve myself, so very gradually and so very controlled. I slowly, slowly cut down what I was eating, so slowly so my body got used to existing on less and less each day. I started exercising to help the process along, to lose weight quicker to get smaller quicker and I was drinking alcohol, so much alcohol, as much as I could to block out the rape, to block out the pain, to hopefully block it all out for good. I would go to bed every night, look at my wrists and whisper "*Please let it be tonight. Please let me be thin enough to die tonight.*" But I never did. I would exercise so hard my heart would be thumping out of my chest. And I would whisper "*Please give up, please give up.*" But of course it never did. I escaped that marriage alive, but I had given up. I had been destroyed. When my ex-husband and Mum and Dad found out that I was anorexic, because of course they didn't see it, they saw me every day, but didn't care to see it. When I told them, they humiliated me. Ripped me apart with demeaning, cruel, humiliating comments. So even when I escaped, I still wanted to die. I was tired, so very tired, I had had enough. I just wanted it all to stop. I needed my torment to end. I was 27 years old. But then Melvyn, a colleague I worked with saw right through to my soul. The façade I held day in, day out did not fool him. He began to talk to me, but I only really disclosed the tip of the ice-berg. I had made my decision, I was going to commit suicide.

He came to see me one day and he just asked me outright if I was going to kill myself. I told him I was and he asked me how I had planned to do it. I told him I was going to drink a bottle of neat Vodka and just before I passed out I was going to take a load of tablets and wash them down with poison. He asked me if I had written a suicide note and I told him I had, he asked me for the note and I gave it to him and he read it. Then he looked at me and said "*Please don't die, I don't want you to die.*" In that moment I was stunned. Somebody had asked me not to die. I was shocked that he appeared upset that I should die. He said if he promised to come and see me the next day, would I promise not to commit suicide. I made him that promise and he took my suicide note. It was a poem and it wasn't written to anybody, but I still remember it.

If I was a suicide what colour would I be
Shiny bright and orange for everyone to see.
If I was a suicide what clothes would I wear
Anything expensive, tres chic and debonair.
If I was a suicide everyone would know
This girl has had enough of life
And now it's time to go.
Goodbye.

For the first time I could ever remember in my life, somebody actually wanted me to stay alive. Had told me they wanted me to stay alive. Had said their life would never be the same again if I died. I processed this in my mind over and over again.

Finally, there is what lead to all this coming out now. And it all began with an 'innocent' Advanced Communication Course which lead to two episodes of deliberate suicidal intent. I was 45 years old. What lead to these episodes was overwhelming emotional rupture of all the abuse I had experienced. This was triggered in a role play scenario where an actor disclosed to me that they had been raped. My distant Professional, Practical response was immediately shut down by the Tutor who stopped me and said *"Somebody has just disclosed something to you, you need to asked them more about it"*. Immediately the lid came off and all the sexual abuse I had experienced came crashing through my head and I was completely overwhelmed and absolutely terrified.

However, how that manifested was I began trying to explain to my Manager that I was stressed at work. I told her I was identifying with my client group and I asked her for support. Her response was to dismiss my concerns as too financially costly. I was requesting Supervision. I gave her examples of how the job was stressing other colleagues and the response was maybe they were not up to the job! This made me feel guilty and desperate to try and put a lid back on to this massive eruption of emotion. I was panicking, asking for help, being ignored, I was terrified. Flashbacks, emotions and feelings continued to explode into my head. I was becoming more and more distracted. Identifying more and more with the sexual abuse in my client group.

I started to feel more and more removed from life. Like I was continually being sucked back to being 10years old, 13years old, 16 years old. Being raped over and over again. Feeling trapped, held down and suffocated. I tried to tell Martyn, my Tutor that I was struggling, but that just came out as struggling with the course and being stressed at work. He referred me back to my Manager for support. I was screaming inside, screaming for help, but I started to believe nobody was listening. I was asking for help and nobody was listening. I started to feel more and more removed from real life. I was being sucked back and completely consumed. I was starting to live another life. A life surrounded by flashbacks. I couldn't reach out, I couldn't get back to my life, I was trying so hard, but I couldn't get back. I was trembling, shaking, completely swallowed up. I was back there, terrified. I was trying to get back, I was grasping at my life, I was screaming for help, but nobody was listening.

I started to lose all focus, I became withdrawn and I could barely speak. My head was swirling and I needed to get out. I had lost it! I had lost my life and I couldn't get back. I was no use at work, I was no use to my husband, I was no use to my kids and nobody would listen to me. Nobody would help me get back. Suicide, the pull of suicide began to get stronger and stronger.

There was something very calm about the Advanced Communication Course. Martyn was very calm, my group, there was only 6 of us, was very calm. One day we were talking about difficult conversations, difficult emotions, people in desperate states. Our classroom was on the 6th floor, the sun shone through the window, it was hot. We were asked to open the window and as I opened my window I said to the person next to me "*God, doesn't that just make you feel tempted to jump out.*" She looked at me and asked me if there was something she should know and I laughed and sat back down. I'd made my decision, it was perfect. They would all understand how desperate and emotionally overwrought people could get. It was calm, it was warm. I decided the very next time we were back in the classroom, when everything was calm, I would climb on the window ledge, push the window open and just slip out. So quietly, so calmly, so peaceful at last. I was no use to anybody and I couldn't get back. I was finally finished.

I was in a complete daze and a couple of days later a colleague at work asked me if I was okay. I could barely speak and I just looked at her and said "*I don't know.*" She then asked me if I was thinking of doing anything silly and again I said "*I don't know.*" I felt rooted to the spot, almost catatonic. She talked to me quietly about what, I don't know, but she said she would speak to my Tutor, which she did quite quickly and he called me and asked me to meet with him the next day. I did meet Martyn the next day and he just listened. For the first time in my life I was sat with someone who was calm, listened and he didn't try to take anything away. He listened and he listened and he listened and I felt like he was holding on to my life. He held on to me emotionally and I didn't feel alone. He didn't judge, he didn't panic, he didn't blame me. He was calm. My head was racing and he was so calm. He gave me that flicker of hope. He didn't rush me, he didn't take anything away from me, he was just with me and my head stopped spinning for a few minutes.

I found enough strength to find help, enough strength to hold on. He had no idea that he had saved my life that day. No idea until much later. The intention returned very soon after. Counselling was not working out, I was desperate. Martyn had given me hope, but whilst well intended, my belief returned that nobody could help me. I was still clutching to hope when I contacted my current Counsellor, clutching, but not believing. The pull of suicide was so strong now. This was going to be my last ever attempt. When I called I was told I could be helped and the person on the 'phone sounded so sure. Something about the calm confidence in her voice made me believe that she believed I could be helped. But I couldn't take the risk. I couldn't carry on being strung along again. I was at the end of the road for me. I was so very tired, this was it.

The image of suicide was all I could see and I was terrified. Terrified to go to the appointment because I've reached the end. The bus, the double decker bus that comes round the corner, he wouldn't have chance to see me, he wouldn't have a chance to stop. It would all be over in an instant, no more suffering. I was terrified to go, because I was terrified it would go wrong. I was tormented, the pull of suicide was so strong. So strong, but I was so scared, scared to be dead, but also at the end of the road. I knew I couldn't go on any longer. It had to stop. I was nothing any more. I was at the end. I was finished. The pull of suicide is terrifying. The pull of suicide is so strong. Like if you are dared to jump into a pool. You so desperately want to do it, but something pulls you back. The pull of suicide is torment, all consuming torment and so incredibly strong. When it's so strong the only thing to think about, the only image is suicide. Nothing exists outside it's torment. It's a battle of strength and when I have no strength, it pulls harder, so hard that I can think of nothing else. It's torture. I am terrified of suicide, but suicide is my friend, my constant, my relief. Suicide is my enemy, my demon, but suicide is my friend. It sticks by me through thick and thin and will always be there to help me out should I need it. I don't know my life without suicide, but I need to let it go. Being suicidal is letting everybody know how being abused has destroyed me.

Suicide tells everybody just how awful, just how devastated I am to have been sexually abused. Being killed in a car crash is catastrophic. Being violated physically, sexually and emotionally is catastrophic, so to show people just how catastrophic it is, means committing suicide. Committing suicide shows people I am destroyed, because I am destroyed. I have no physical scars to show. I am terrified of going to Court in September. Not because Jack may be found guilty, or not guilty, but because exposing what happened, exposing what he did is catastrophic and how do I tell people how destroyed I am, without committing suicide?

Thoughts of self-harm are associated with obtaining a physical scar. A physical scar that I can look at and know it's the scar representing what I've been through. Other people will see the scar and I will know why I have it. The last few weeks I have felt I have been getting stronger mentally, emotionally and becoming more rational. A little voice in my head is saying "*What about me*?" That little voice is my suicide. My suicide that has been with me all these years, loyal to me, ready to take me when I'm ready. I have to listen to my little Sui, my little Sui is saying everybody should know I'm destroyed by what happened and if Sui doesn't stay how will anybody know how catastrophic and devastating being sexually abused and completely violated has destroyed me.

I am terrified of being suicidal again, terrified of that pull and it's strength, but I am equally scared to let it go. I thought I would never smile again, but I am and Sui doesn't like it. Sui is holding on to the pain. And sometimes I feel real pain. Sometimes I hurt so bad inside, but the only person I can talk to is suicide. I want to be devastated and live, I want to feel pain and live. I don't want suicide to be the only time I get help. I am terrified that one day it will pull hard enough. I need to listen to my little voice, so she never has to pull at all. Even writing that she has to go scares me. Because without suicide, how will people know when I am in pain? What if there is nobody to help? The pain I feel is so strong. When it comes it overwhelms me and there she is waiting to take me.

Reflection: That is a very powerful entry and I think you, the reader should reflect on that entry. That little voice wasn't suicide, but I couldn't see it yet. I didn't have anything that existed between elation and suicidal feelings. Yes I was developing a sense of myself, but there was still a gaping hole inside of me. That little voice wasn't suicide and it was really dangerous to think at that time that I believed it was, because that still left me very vulnerable and feeling very unpredictable in terms of taking spontaneous action against myself.

Notes:

03.04.17

This has been the first break in this journal. I suppose I stopped because other life events have overtaken, but I am back now. Alan I have found out has been physically abusing my Son. The Police have been informed, social care will eventually talk to him and since I found out, none of my children have had any contact with this awful, awful individual.
So, up to speed: I am supporting my children as best I can, but I feel sick to my soul. The only thing I care unconditionally about is my children. They are my reason to breathe and he has shown me I cannot protect them. He knew I deplored violence and child abuse is my overwhelming emotion of abhorrence. And he abused my child. My own flesh and blood, by beautiful, but vulnerable souls. That bastard cut right through me and he hit it. He must have felt so powerful knowing he was deceiving me, knowing how much he was hurting my Son and me. He knew if I knew what he was doing I would have battered him, reported him, brought him to justice. That bastard has to be held to account for his actions and my Son will get his voice. He will not suffer.

Today I went to renew my car park permit at work. I was forced to disclose why. I felt very vulnerable, both being forced to disclose in a public place and to the hospital police. I was humiliated, embarrassed and belittled, all for the sake of a car park permit. How dare I be judged for being sexually abused. How dare they make me stand and have to explain myself to a bunch of tactless, insensitive, uncompassionate nobody's. How dare they look down and me and insist on speaking to Fern (The Investigating Officer) to ascertain if my anxieties are justified. How dare they belittle me in this way! I cried when I walked out of the office, both with distress and anger at being forced to disclose and then have my feelings dismissed. I will do something to change peoples' attitude, I will. Writing this book is only the beginning, but I will make sure nobody EVER ignores, or dismisses me and my children EVER again.

Reflection: I decided to keep this entry in the book because my children being abused felt like an extension of my abuse. The emotions I felt when my Son disclosed that he had been physically abused by Alan took me right back to Jack. The fear, the isolation, the dread, the difficult behaviours. I was devastated. The one thing I believed I could protect, my children and he showed me that I couldn't. I felt like I had been violated again, through me children and I was determined that they were not going to grow up like I had, unheard and neglected. The guilt about what they suffered hadn't kicked in yet for me. That came later.
In terms of the work car permit. I felt objectified all over again. Was my sexual abuse enough to warrant a piece of paper. The abuse that had almost killed me, destroyed most of my life. That was the question being asked. Was that deemed by people who didn't know me, serious enough to warrant giving me a car park permit, so I didn't feel vulnerable walking great distances to work. Absolutely disgusting.

Notes:

05.04.17

Why can't I stay angry? I couldn't sleep last night. I am overwhelmed with anxiety and so anxious about protecting my children, anxious about threats that might happen. I am so scared all the time, I am shattered. Why can't I stay strong? Why do I get so tongue tied and my mind abandons me when I want to get my point across and defend myself. I am so anxious, my chest is so tight. Why can't I stop it? I can get angry about that, but not angry about how I am treated.

Reflection: I was very frightened for my children' s safety and my own. It was that dread, that unknown threat that was causing me so much anxiety. I felt backed into a corner.

Notes:

15.04.17

I realise again today that no-one is completely on your side. Daryl, somebody I considered to be a friend, who supported me through some very dark days has destroyed our friendship by concocting a story in his head that I had feelings for him. I think he used it deliberately to end our friendship. He treated me badly and I feel both sad and angry. My children were also upset when he betrayed our friendship. Today he sent my daughter a card and voucher for her birthday. She accepted it stating he had not upset her. I realise now how absolutely loyal I am as a friend, mother, daughter. What you see is what you get. But having never had unconditional love, I still search for it. I crave it because I have never had it. Nobody has EVER displayed unconditional love, or loyalty to me EVER. I feel a huge hole inside of me. I feel so empty and alone. I feel so lonely, so sad and worthless. I really do despair. If I never did anything so bad and I try to stick up for myself and not be a victim, then why am I constantly betrayed? Why do other people including my own children not value me enough for me to feel I have any value?

Reflection: I was so upset, I couldn't see at that time that children have different perspectives of adults than adults do of other adults. My children were upset by his betrayal, but happy to receive a present, because it was a present. It was really as simple as that. But I couldn't see it then and I felt let down by my children, because they were the only people who I gave unconditional love to. I protected them and they loved me. I felt betrayed by my daughter. I'm not perfect.

Notes:

22.04.17

Anger appears to be the prevailing emotion at the moment. Anger has always frightened me. Other peoples and my own. My efforts to stay in control are being challenged now by this anger that has crept in. I have been saying for a while now that I am tired of being scared all the time and I am tired of being scared all the time, but tears are being replaced with anger. He (Alan) is taking me to Court to get access to the children. I now know that he has been seriously physically abusing at least one of the children. The ONLY thing I hold any attachment, unconditional love and feel sentimental about is my children. Knowing what he has done is beyond comprehension. Abhorrent, sick and depraved. I didn't protect the one thing, the only thing I am whole heartedly attached to. When I think about him I feel physically sick. Gut wrenchingly sick. Nobody will help. I feel utterly powerless. As the Mother of my children I should know what to do. I should be able to protect my children and get justice when they are hurt. I cannot comprehend that that is not happening and it is messing with my head. My Solicitor is playing the long game, but I don't play games. I am screaming inside.

Reflection: After Alan left in September 2016 the children had mutually agreed access with him. However, what happened over time was the children would complain of feeling unwell towards the end of the week, or when they were due to see him. More often than not I would be messaging him telling him that one child or the other didn't feel well enough to see him. He didn't like this and he decided to take me to Court to force them. When I asked him why he would force the children to see him if they didn't want to, his response was *"Well it wouldn't be me forcing them to see me, it would be the Judge."* It was that word force that made me feel sick. My children were distressed by the idea that they were going to be forced to see him when they didn't want to and he was absolving all responsibility of that. Being forced. Being forced to wait to be sexually abused, being forced into rape, being forced to wait for food. Being forced to starve. That word brought all of those sensations and flashbacks back to me. I was frightened and angry at the same time. I was determined that my children would never experience the emotion of being forced to be abused like I was.

Notes:

25.04.17

I know what is wrong with me. I have been experiencing my children's emotions as if they are my own. One of my children is terrified that he is going to be forced to do something he doesn't want to do. This makes me feel sick, being forced to touch Jack. Being forced to perform oral sex. Being forced to have sex, being forced to wait for Jack to come home.

My other Son is angry about not being listened to. Nobody listened to me telling them I was lonely. Nobody listened to me telling him to stop, I didn't want to play anymore. No-one listened to me say I didn't want him to walk me home. No-one listened to me say it's hurting me, I don't like it. No-one listened to me say I can't cope anymore.

I am very anxious about going to Court. I am being forced to think about stuff I don't want to think about. I am going to have to defend my children. If I don't do it well enough I will be letting them down. I don't want to let anybody down. My children trust me, I can't let them down. Two people helped me today. One person at work helped me to navigate a computer package for travelling expenses. Another was an Electrician. He bought my oven for me, came after work and fitted it. I was supposed to buy it, but I think he could see I just couldn't make a decision. I don't think either knew how much I really appreciated their help, even though I thanked them. It made all the difference in the world to me.

Reflection: That old chestnut. You might not be able to change the world, but you might be able to change the world for somebody. Those two people did on that day. You never know when a simple act of kindness could make the world of difference to somebody.

Notes:

02.06.17

I'm divorced! I haven't written for a long time because this journal is about me and my recovery, not my children. Having to protect my children from major threat has brought horrible feelings to the surface. Feelings I had waiting for Jack to come home, dreading something bad was going to happen and it did. Feeling trapped, helpless and powerless, exactly how I felt trying to protect my children. So many nightmares, so many flashbacks from my first husband. Waiting for the next time. The next time I was going to be raped. That waiting time was so suffocating, at times I felt I couldn't breathe. Being divorced is an amazing feeling. No connection to him anymore. I'm finally free.

Reflection: I never saw Alan as part of a future mistake, a repeated pattern of behaviour, I saw Alan as part of my past. I met him in 2005 and we separated when I was re-building my life. He was just another perpetrator from the past I needed to disconnect from. Being divorced was great. Not out of spite for him, or the marriage, but because I had gotten rid of another toxic part of my past.

Notes:

09.06.17

I had a dream this week. A cathartic dream. Since I wrote about my deepest relationship with suicide, it has released its grip. Throughout the stress and flashbacks I have been experiencing over the past few weeks, it has never factored in my thoughts. The voice in my dream said *"You no longer think about suicide, because you are no longer angry with yourself."* I have forgiven myself for my mistakes. I have come to terms with what happened and put the blame exactly where it belongs – with my abusers, including Alan. I recognise that for anybody to be heard, they have to scream, shout and rant. It isn't because I'm worthless, or not important, it's because I'm no different to anybody else, no more, or less important. I just have to rant, scream and shout like everybody else who is valued, important and worthwhile. Realising this is so freeing.

What makes me sad and angry is the disgusting lies that are being told about me. I realise now that he brainwashed me into thinking I was weak, mentally unstable. He has on more than one occasion made libellous comments, slander and defamation of character. What he says is irrelevant, but other people judging me because they believe him really hurts. Not because they judge, but because what I'm being judged on is untrue. But I will continue to rise above it. I have found my pride and self-respect. I know who I am and I will keep reminding myself of that. Karma will come to those that wait. I am important to me and my children are my world. I am strong and will continue to move forward. Alan, his abuse and my abusers are all part of the past. I am allowed to be vulnerable, emotional and strong. Just like everybody else.

Reflection: Any dream analysts reading this will probably understand the importance of dreams. I didn't care at that time, I was happy that they were giving me guidance, but I still didn't recognise who they were coming from.

Notes:

16.06.17

Feeling emotionally charged tonight. I had one glass of wine, my usual Friday evening glass and I felt quite tipsy. I also felt very emotional. A young character on EastEnders had been raped, she was crying and devastated by her realisation. I just wanted to scream and throw a tantrum, throw my wine glass against the wall.

I spoke to Jayne today. I am ready to talk about what Stewart did to me. Not to relive any trauma, but to try to put to bed the emotions, associations and flashbacks that have become my life. But a part of my life that I am recognising as something I don't want anymore. I didn't notice it before, but now I do. She said we have to do it in stages, because if it consumes me then I lose the ability to process anything. Instead of a memory, I am left with a black hole. She recognised that this was what happened to me before. I disassociate so much that I have great voids/holes where I have no recall at all. A black hole, as if that time never existed. I'm glad she told me, because now I know how to recognise it happening again, then I know to slow down, or take a little break, or just stick with and deal with what's causing it. I feel so grateful that she pointed it out to me. Shocked really that she saw it. A recognisable sign that I am struggling too much. She saw. She sees me. Nobody has even known me well enough to see me. She really sees me. How I would love to be able to trust somebody, love somebody who really sees me. Who loves me enough to be able to check out if I'm okay. Who will see I am starting to have black holes and just know I am so distressed, so overwhelmed, so traumatised that they will hold me, love me and care for me. Help me get back, help me through it. Love me enough to help me come back.
Jayne saw me, I can't believe she really saw me. She saw what I have never seen, but now I know what happens to me, maybe I will see it too. If there was ever a wish I had, just one wish, it would be to be loved so completely that they see me. I just want to be loved.

Reflection: Jayne really knew how to keep the pace safe. Whilst she worked at my pace, within that she guided it so I didn't become overwhelmed, rush too far forward. It wasn't me that wanted to rush it, it was the force and speed of the flashbacks, memories and emotions. They were so powerful, so full of energy, they did not want to sit inside me a minute longer than they needed to. Unlike Vicky, Jayne never paced it by changing the subject. Jayne paced if by focusing on a particular experience, or emotion. Jayne is absolutely incredible.

Notes:

15.07.17

I went out the other night for the first time in months. My Mum looked at me up and down and said *"You're not going out like that are you? Your hair isn't even dry."* And the rug was ripped from under me again. But then I realised, maybe a short time ago that comment would have reinforced why I hate myself. I would have wanted to self-harm, been very angry with myself and loathed myself for even existing as an individual who is not good enough and I wouldn't have gone out. Instead I felt very sad, very hurt, very self-conscious and thought to myself, well I thought I looked okay. I liked my dress and how I looked. My feelings were hurt by her comments and not how bad I felt about myself. I didn't feel bad about myself. The rug was pulled and I fell over, but I got up again. It wasn't ripped from under me, it didn't destroy me, I felt sad and confused because I thought I looked okay.

Somebody paid me a compliment that night, but I couldn't accept it. So although she didn't destroy me, she managed to influence how I felt I presented. It's progress, big progress. I need to get to the point that my self-belief is concrete, so when I get knocked back, my self-belief remains intact no matter how hurtful, or personal other people's comments are.

Another big step for me is at 47 years old, I have felt like a child in an adults body. Cognitively and emotionally. I have functioned as an adult, but when faced with personal and emotional challenges, I have felt like a 5 year old. So that's another reason my self-confidence and self-esteem hasn't grown. In the past few months, I feel I am beginning to develop emotionally and cognitively. When things have gone wrong for me I have always wanted to hide, cry, curl up into a ball, block everything out. Even throughout talking about all my disclosures I have felt like a tiny child. Now I am beginning to feel more like an adolescent. When I am challenged emotionally, I strop and pout inside and want to 'kick off'. But I have recognised that I am doing this, so I am seeking help from appropriate people to help me when I am struggling with life challenges and I am getting results. And people are being kind. It is really difficult because my brain just wants to 'kick off', but now I am recognising it, it is like trying to manage a stroppy teenager. Regulating emotions in an appropriate manner is very difficult when they have been suppressed for so long, they just want to go wild, not be suppressed. Which they never will be again, but I need to learn to express them appropriately. I feel very, very angry sometimes because I just want to let it all out, whatever the situation. I have suppressed emotions that so strongly want to rebel. It's so, so hard. I am due to go to Court on 25th and 26th September to give evidence against Jack. But now also it would appear that the Court Case with the family Court is also going to be in September. This is too overwhelming. My focus after all these years is Jack. Both of these together is too much. I don't know how I am going to cope.

Reflection: It felt like emotionally I was beginning to grow up. My mind had been 10 years old for so long, but now it felt like it was beginning to start the process of catching up. During that time, I felt like emotionally I was like a teenager. I felt selfish, spontaneous and stroppy.

Notes:

28.07.17

Sometimes things start to begin to make sense all at once and I have no conscious understanding why it suddenly happens. Maybe it's because I am tired of trying to be, or wondering all the time how I am supposed to be. I have spent my whole life trying to be what somebody else has wanted me to be in order to be loved, accepted, not rejected, not ignored. Now, and I don't know why now, but now I think that actually I'm okay. I am okay. I am me. I believe it is okay to be me and trying to be what somebody else wants me to be is irritating, because I don't need to do that anymore. Being me. Not having to say 'how shall I be' to myself is incredibly liberating. I feel so high. The energy, the effort, I can stop it all, because I am okay! I've looked at this before, but even though I understood what it meant, I've not been ready to let go of the other me's. Maybe because I didn't think it was okay to be me at that time. I'm also getting pictures in my mind when recalling memories, I have no black holes. No maybe that's not entirely accurate. I do have things that I don't remember, but that's when I'm overwhelmed, or distracted. The difference to before is now I know I am distracted and I know when I am not taking things in. Before, I didn't have that awareness. I didn't recognise that I was overwhelmed, I just wasn't there. My mind or my brain feels like it's expanding, opening up. It feels like a light is on. When I recall a memory I see a picture. I look at the picture and I remember. It feels like it takes ages for me to recall a memory and re-count it, but I think that's just my perception. Is this what everybody does normally? I don't know. I'm so used to holding on to something so as not to forget, but now I am actually able to recall something. I am becoming more present.

Being present more and more each day. Being present, being me, means I might be embarrassed or experience embarrassment about things I have done in the past. Being embarrassed about it or not, just not being defined by it. No longer living down to everyone else's expectations. The crazy one, the silly one, the stupid one. I was mocked and laughed at by Alan and his friend for not being clever. The truth is I never skived a day off school. I just couldn't take anything in, I couldn't remember what I did take in. I was either reliving the abuse over and over again, or I was living in terror and disbelief about what had happened. Nothing was ever going to go in. I left school in a haze and I have lived that way since I was 10 years old, that is until now. I have lost so much of my life reliving the abuse I was subjected to. I never felt embarrassed when they were putting me down, because I was with them putting me down. Full of shame, self-hatred and loathing. I believed I was stupid because I was incapable of learning, so of course it was my fault. Only now I know it wasn't my fault at all. None of it was my fault, none of it. I'm not embarrassed now that I didn't learn , I'm embarrassed that other people know more than me and they know that. I feel embarrassed that my kids ask me questions that I can't answer. If I'd had an illness or a brain injury I could explain and people would understand, but without being able to explain, I don't know how else to stop feeling embarrassed. I don't want people to put me down and I'm not going to put myself down. I'm not sure what to do.

I was sent a fantastic quote today:

Free to be me: With good mental health I am no longer afraid to tell you who I am, even if you don't like me, I am free to be me.
Diana Hayes.

And there is my answer. I don't need to be afraid to tell people who I am. Look out world – I'm coming.

Reflection: Another reflective entry. I will leave it to you to form your own opinion.

Notes:

29.07.17

I'm surprised after yesterday's big revelations that I feel really down today and I'm not sure why. Really out of sorts. I guess that's just one to think about, but I genuinely have no conscious idea why everything feels wrong. Maybe it's because everything is coming right. Being present means I am not thinking about anything except what I am doing now. I think my brain is a little bit agitated by this because it's so used to planning and worrying and being hyper alert. I'm not thinking too deeply about this, I'm just accepting it. I just don't like being in a bad mood.

Reflection: Or perhaps it was just a bad mood day.

Notes:

30.07.17

I woke up dripping with sweat this morning. I dreamt all night about being in Court with Jack. I wasn't anxious, I wasn't frightened, I was just in it going through it. I felt very calm, but my body had other ideas I think. I genuinely didn't feel anxious. I still felt irritable today though and I was about to say I still don't know why, but I do. My brain and mind are re-routing and my emotions are trying to sort themselves out. It's like the house has been renovated, but now the furniture is being brought in, but is still being moved around until it fits in the right place.

Reflection: I couldn't really explain that any better, except to say everything was transitioning inside me and my mind was working hard to regulate.

Notes:

31.07.17

I felt confused and irritable today. Probably pre-menstrual. I always feel a little anxious or tearful before a period. The relevance to this small and insignificant change in mood is, I have never acknowledged or accepted that my mood is influenced sometimes by external factors. I have only recently allowed myself to show emotions during television programmes. But admitting my mood may also be influenced by hormonal changes is really huge for me . It means I accept my different emotional states, instead of being this cool, level, unemotive person who never displays anything other than this trance like demeanour. Also accepting my femininity. I have denied my periods since they began. Ignored cramps, pains, even getting to the point of being annoyed with other people when they showed emotion at this time. I wanted to completely disconnect from anything that made me female, which I perceived to be a beacon for men to abuse. A sexual object to be used and abused. Hated by men. An object, nothing more than an object. So I have behaved like any object. Denying everything about myself. That's why I'm irritated. I'm no longer denying myself. I am feeling everything, but it irritates me and I don't know why. I'm tired of not feeling, but I think it just makes me feel vulnerable and being vulnerable makes me feel more vulnerable in relation to being open to attack.

I need to work this one out next.

Reflection: Accepting my femininity was a big thing. Periods meant I was a female. I started my periods when I was 14 years old and my Mother made a big deal out of it telling me I was becoming a woman. That terrified me, as for the previous 4 years I had been introduced to what it meant to be a woman and I was frightened that there was worse to come. After all, if I'd been sexually abused and raped by the age of 14, what else was in store for me? I denied my periods as much as possible. My Mother said they should only last 5 days. Of course mine went on for many days more and she told me that wasn't possible. So I would put tissue in my knickers, or have nothing there at all. I would ignore the pain, the emotions and I hated the bloating a period brought because that made my stomach protrude and a protruding stomach made me think of Jack touching me, tickling my stomach. My stomach felt huge and I hated anything touching it. I didn't want to associate with anything that made me female. I hated that my breasts were growing, I didn't want to wear a bra. I had been touched and fondled when I had no breasts, so then growing was a bit like the protruding stomach, it magnified the place that men were going to abuse. What they were going to touch to violate me. I had my hair cut short, but I was teased for looking like a boy and that gave me more unwanted attention.
Starting to recognise and accept that I had hormonal related emotions, as well as period pains that I could acknowledge was a really big deal. It made me want to care for myself in terms of pain killers for the pain, finding a place to be quiet and peaceful when I felt irritated. Just acknowledging it all and feeling compassion towards myself was brand new to me.

Notes:

01.08.17

Today was the shittiest day. I had a day off work and a social worker came to take a history of emotional abuse, then concluded by saying a judge may expect me to encourage the children to once again be exposed to emotional abuse. Well fuck that!! That stupid bastard has no idea what it feels like to be subjected to emotional abuse and the damage it does. There is no fucking way that having escaped emotional abuse I am going to be subjecting any living thing to any abuse. It makes me so fucking angry. Why am I never left alone to get on with my life?

Reflection: I was really destroyed by this visit. It brought all those emotions and sensations back again of having to wait to be abused. Of acknowledging the devastating impact abuse had had on me and terrified that my children's lives would be destroyed just like mine had. I felt trapped, cornered and my chest felt tight. It felt like I was trying to get away from the sensations and emotions of abuse and circumstances were dragging me back to it. I just wanted to scream.

Notes:

02.08.17

Still playing the meeting over and over in my mind. He reminded me of Alan. He didn't like it because I didn't agree with him. He kept pressing the point and in the end he decided that I didn't understand the point he was trying to make. I understand perfectly and I will never allow anybody to force my children to do what they don't want to do that causes them the high level of emotional stress that he did.

Reflection: This social worker sniggered at me and that reminded me of Jack and Jason. He told me that it wasn't my decision about the children seeing Alan. He said it was the Judge's decision. I pointed out to the social worker that it wasn't his, mine or anybody else's decision whether they saw Alan and stated the decision lay firmly with the children. He told me again it was the Judge's decision. So I asked him if he was going to manhandle my children into his car. When he told me he couldn't do that I asked him what was the point of him even doing this assessment. He backed down, citing it was his job and I told him it was my job to safeguard my children from abuse. I felt like a lioness. I would have gone to prison for my children, because they needed to know I would never have allowed them to be forced to be abused. Thankfully it never came to that, but I didn't know that then.

Notes:

03.08.17

Still playing the meeting over and over. Meditation eludes me, it's so frustrating. I have woken up in the early hours every day since the meeting. I hate it! The anxiety, the stress, the anger that he causes. I just want to get on with my life. At least the kids don't feel stressed now.

Reflection: I had done a good enough job in reassuring the children that they wouldn't be forced to do anything they didn't want to do. They knew the door was always open to see Alan if they changed their mind. However, my reassuring them just helped to land a whole lot more stress onto my shoulders. They believed in me 100% when I was only just learning to believe in me.

Notes:

04.08.17

Decided to read this morning. Reading works, hurray, finally something to stop the incessant thoughts whirring round. So I read from 5am until I got up at 6.40am. I saw Jayne today and talked about the meeting. That helped me to feel stronger. Then I saw my friend Sara and talked about the meeting. I feel so much better. My children have made it very clear that they don't want to be exposed to any more emotional abuse. They have told Alan, the Social Worker, me, their teacher. They have told all these people that they don't want anything to do with him. I will do whatever I have to do to protect that. Nobody protected me, nobody. Whatever my children need I will support. Always!

I spoke to my Mum about going to Court today, she told me she feels frightened about going to Court. She feels scared she will let me down. She has no idea that the reason all this is happening is because she has always let me down. I felt no anger towards her, I didn't feel anything. Instead I just told her to say what she remembers and not try to say something she doesn't. She told me she doesn't remember much because it was a long time ago. She doesn't remember because after my Sister died, she told me nothing was special anymore. She kept telling me that 'it was alright for me'. She didn't bother to get a babysitter when they went out drinking every weekend, they didn't consider me when they were having violent arguments, or violent sex. They didn't consider me at all. But Jack and Emily did. They made me feel so welcome and loved and part of a family. Emotional neglect - such damage beyond any comprehension.

Reflection: Something inside my Mother clearly died when my Sister did, but I was 7 years old at the time and not responsible for her feelings. She let me down the minute she said nothing was special anymore. She let me believe I was nothing and I was 7 years old and when everybody else treated me like I was nothing that validated those words she had used.

Notes:

05.08.17

Today has been a much better day. Not being able to talk about the social work visit really played on my mind. As soon as I was able to it left me and I ended up laughing again.

Reflection: So nothing changed in terms of what happened, but I was learning to talk and although talking doesn't always change a situation, I was learning that talking could change the way I coped with a situation.

Notes:

06.08.17

This book was never about anybody else, it is about me and how I have come through the worst experience of my life. But sometimes I have to include others to give context to what I am experiencing, so I try to keep this to a minimal, but this is what happened yesterday.

My eldest Son needs new shoes, but fashionable shoes because he's at an age now where image matters. When we were in the shop he suddenly commented that that's what made him confused about Alan. Alan had bought him the latest trainers and that had made him happy. Yet he felt justified to intimidate him, swear at him, punch and strangle him. I told my Son that that's what perpetrators do. They give you just enough to keep you okay, so when they do despicable, abhorrent things, you feel confused. That's when they have you. That's one of the reasons people stay in abusive relationships. And suddenly this morning, in the shower, the answer came to me. Yes I am being congruent, yes I am being real. Now I am beginning to understand how absolutely vital it is to trust your gut instinct. No matter how many people disagree with you. If you don't trust your gut feeling, then you will never be okay. I trust my gut feeling, for the first time I can remember in my life, not only am I trusting my gut feeling, but I'm not afraid to act on it.

Now I understand how I can never let anybody abuse me EVER again. If it doesn't feel right, no matter what anybody says or feels, then I won't do it. Oh my God – another epiphany. I can't believe these answers keep coming to me. Trusting my gut feeling means I will always be alright. Because even if my gut feeling turns out to be wrong, I will never feel abused again. Because I will always have felt alright. If somebody hurts me again, it will be about them not me. That's why I have always felt guilty, because I didn't trust my gut feeling.

I knew it was wrong to be on my own with Jack but I didn't listen to my gut. I knew it was wrong to take his hand in the park, I knew it was wrong not to scream at Jason, I knew it was wrong to let him walk me home. I knew it was wrong to be with somebody who raped, humiliated, physically and emotionally abused me. I knew it was wrong to ignore my feelings for somebody else. Deep down I always knew all these things were so very wrong, but I ignored my gut feeling. I ignored it because I was told I was worthless, I was told I wasn't important and I was completely emotionally neglected. I knew it was all wrong, but I was screaming inside to be heard. I wanted to matter, I wanted to be valued, but I was nothing and I was treated like I was nothing. And deep, deep down I know that's why I feel guilty, because I knew it was all wrong, but I ignored my gut. That's why I 'let' it all happen. I couldn't stop it because I knew I was nothing. I meant nothing to everybody. I hated it all, hated myself for letting it happen, because deep, deep, down in my gut I knew it was wrong and that's why I feel guilty.

I am so, so sorry I ignored my gut feelings. I had no strength, no value and a destroyed soul. It had been ripped out with my heart and I was an empty shell, just wanting to die to escape the horrific torment I lived every single day. I didn't feel guilty then, I felt pure self-hatred. A hate so powerful it destroyed anything good inside. Now I know why I felt all of this. Now I understand why I have had this obsession with suicide. I have been running on empty for so many years, terrified of the next 'attack' that I would 'let' happen because of my complete lack of self-preservation, or self-belief.

Oh my poor, poor mind, I have tortured for so long. I feel so, so sad and I am so sorry for everything that has happened. You see it wasn't my fault at all, none of it was. I was just broken. I was destroyed and broken to my very core. Life has been so terrible, so utterly devastating and my Son's comment suddenly made me understand why. I am so, so sorry for all the victims who have been abused, I now understand the whole reason behind self-hatred, self-loathing, suicide and guilt. We are just broken souls who have had our souls ripped away. I am so, so sorry that I didn't get it, I didn't understand. I am so sorry for everything. This is just so sad. I am so sorry to everybody that I hurt, because I just didn't understand.

This realisation is truly devastating, completely overwhelming.

Reflection: And it was devastating and overwhelming, not least because I hadn't made the connection to who I was apologising too.

Notes:

07.08.17

I felt really sad today. A little disconnected too. Probably not helped by another night of poor sleep. Yesterday still sinking in. Maybe this is just another layer of the grief I feel for a lost childhood, a lost life. It's incredible that I understand and that's amazing. If none of this had happened I would never have understood. I just hate feeling sad. I realised that understanding means I have to feel embarrassed, guilty, angry, but sad I don't like. Sadness frightens me because I have felt sad inside most of my life and I have always had to pretend not to be sad. When I feel sad now I am frightened that it won't go, that it will stay and I have to pretend all over again. I have to trust my gut, I want to trust my gut that I accept being sad and I trust when I have come to terms with it that sadness will lift.

I was so trusting when I was a child, I didn't know how I had to protect myself , so my 'self' was destroyed. After all this time I have got it back. I have learned to believe in myself again, but this time I know I have to protect it. I can do this by trusting myself and how I feel and not allowing anybody to take that away from me. I have spent a lifetime giving myself to everyone else, trusting them with my heart and soul. Children do this because they are so trusting and don't believe anybody wants to hurt them. That was me and I became nothing. No wonder I believed suicide was the only way out. That's why I feel so sad. I was that innocent child and I still feel like that innocent child inside who has just realised that my life was stolen. I was stolen, my soul destroyed piece by piece because I didn't even know I had to protect it. I didn't even imagine anybody would try to take it. But now I do and it all seems so simple. I gave myself away because I just wanted to be loved. I wanted somebody to love me, but I was used and thrown away. All my life I have been used and all I want is to be loved. I feel too sad today to think I can be me and be loved. I feel too sad for all my wasted life.

Reflection: A day of grief, another day a step closing to healing.

Notes:

08.08.17

I slept for 10 hours solid last night. I fell asleep looking at sadness. I cuddled down into it and fell asleep feeling it, I had to. I woke up shocked at how late it was and sadness had lifted. I had a lovely day with my children and we laughed and enjoyed the day. I dreamt last night, but unfamiliar dreams that I didn't remember when I woke up. I lived with sadness, then it went. At least for now. Maybe when I become less frightened of sadness I will be able to fully accept it with all my emotions. I continue to live one day at a time for now. Accepting myself feels good.

Reflection: Apart from being afraid of sadness because I had lived with it all my life, I was frightened of it because I still couldn't see where it was coming from. Yes it was the experiences, but inside of me I couldn't see where it was coming from.

Notes:

09.08.17

Today was a better day again, until I received an upsetting text message. People condoning child abuse makes me feel sick. People who are trying to force my children back into an abusive relationship makes me feel sick. I will do whatever I have to do to protect my children. I will never let what happened to me, happen to them. EVER. My desire to be loved took me back to Jack and Emily. I was terrified of being sexually abused again, but my desire to be loved was greater than that. The guilt I hold is massive. Yes I know it wasn't my fault, but I had lost my gut feeling My gut feeling was terror, danger. But my need to be loved, accepted was even greater and horrifically damaging. I will never allow that to happen to my children.

Reflection: My new strength, my past experiences were giving me good armour and insight into how to protect my children.

Notes:

10.08.17

Today my mind gave me a rest and I was so lucky to be given time back at work to be able to spend time at home with my children. I feel very, very protective of them.

Reflection: Another one of those days where my mind bailed out. That must have a physiological or psychological term. I would love to know what it is.

Notes:

11.08.17

What a hugely emotional day. Today I saw Jayne and she talked back to me what I had written on the 06.08.17. Hearing her reading it back to me made me feel so, so sad. But it also helped me to understand what I was saying and who I was saying sorry to. It was me! I have felt so sad all day, but because I wanted to. I have thought a lot more about my new insight. I understand now why I couldn't name him. I couldn't name him because of the horrific abuse and complete same I feel. All consuming shame, embarrassment and absolute humiliation because I gave myself to him and because I hated what I had done, I punished myself for doing it and then carried on doing it. I tried so hard to starve and drink myself to death when I was already hurting so much. I am so, so, sorry. His name was Stewart Watts. He destroyed me and I was an adult and all that he did I feel utter shame. I know it wasn't my fault, but I knew it was wrong, I knew it was horrific, that's why I wanted to die. But instead of stopping it, I punished myself over and over again. I have never hated anything more than I hated myself. I hated myself because he made me feel worthless, I hated myself because I allowed him to do it, I hated myself because I knew it was wrong and I didn't stop it. I hated myself because I couldn't punish myself more than he was punishing me. I couldn't make me feel worse than he did. I hated myself because I couldn't even do that. He caused me more physical and emotional pain than I could ever imagine was possible and I hated myself beyond anything imaginable for allowing that to happen and not being able to do worse to myself. I couldn't even kill myself.

He had absolute control over everything and the whole time I felt a failure. A disgusting, worthless failure. Even now writing this I feel angry. Angry because I am feeling right now how I felt back then. I wanted to scream, scream and fight and destroy that bastard, but all I could do was destroy myself. I am so, so sorry. I so desperately wanted to go. I so desperately wanted to die. I so desperately, desperately wanted to go, more than words can describe. I just wanted it all to stop. Physical and emotional torment day after day after day. I hated myself so, so much and I am so sorry. I am just so sorry. I haven't been able to talk about him because I have been devastated with guilt. But I'm not that little girl any more. I'm not that little girl who was raped, injured, bruised. Not now, but I was then. I was only a little girl who had no idea what to do. A tormented, frightened little girl. A little girl who didn't deserve to be punished by anybody, not even me. I was the only person I had and even I destroyed me. I am so sorry little girl. Ever so sorry.

Reflection: Finally, I recognised who I was saying sorry to all that time. It wasn't suicide, it wasn't suicide who was my friend, my enemy, my soul mate. It was little me. It was the little girl inside of me and I had finally recognised it. It was 10 year old me, 11 year old me, 13 year old me and 16 year old me. But I was still 2 people.

Notes:

12.08.17

Today I was exhausted. I'm so emotionally drained, it's been a really tough week. I'm so tired, too tired to be sad. I feel defeated, I feel like I've been running for so long trying to get away from it. But I couldn't do it anymore. I've been caught out, exposed and I can't hide it any more. I have to face what happened and come to terms with it all. Now is the time to come to terms with what happened. I have been horrified by it, lived it over and over again, I've been sickened by it, even denied it. But in order to come to terms with it I have to face it. Face what happened and face myself when it was happening. This is absolutely devastating me, but if I can face it then there is nothing else to destroy me. I will have looked at what happened from every angle and it won't be able to hurt me anymore, it won't be able to destroy me because I will have picked it apart and put it back together from so many different angles that t will have nowhere left to hide, nothing left to destroy. I really believe after 37 years, that I have almost destroyed the demon. The demon that almost destroyed me. But today I am just so tired. Stewart can wait 'til another day. I'm so brave.

Reflection: I was conscious that Court was coming up and I was too frightened to take the lid off Stewart. I felt like I was needing to hold myself together, to develop my resolve, so I could be as strong as possible for Court.

Notes:

13.08.17

I woke up this morning and began to cry. I talked about my fears around sadness and Jayne suggested I try a technique whereby I invite sadness in to sit down and have a cup of tea. I dreamt that I did this and sadness swiped that cup off the table so hard it smashed against the wall. He wants exposing, my mind doesn't want to let it out a bit at a time, it wants him out and it has erupted. I woke up this morning, not feeling a part of this world. Abject sadness has consumed me. It's so overwhelming, it's so sickening. The absolute horror, the absolute guilt. It this why victims commit suicide, because the horror, the guilt is just way too much. Much, much too much.

Reflection: Sadness to me represents calm and reflection. I did not feel calm and reflective about my experiences with Stewart. They were violent and horrifyingly painful and my memories were the same, the flashbacks were worse. There was nothing calm and reflective or sad associated with Stewart at that time. The experiences needed to be aired, before I could feel anything else.

Notes:

14.08.17

Today was so hard, I feel so low. I wanted to be busy to avoid flashbacks, but the effort to do anything was so incredible. Then as soon as I was alone, flashbacks. I'm so tired.

Reflection: I was trying hard to avoid them because I wanted to be able to focus on Court and Jack, but flashbacks don't care about what else is going on in your life. When they want out, they want out and the worst thing to do is to try to either suppress them, or ignore them. Doing so just intensifies them, sends them into a fierce rage. I was consumed.

Notes:

15.08.17

Feeling so very disconnected, very, very traumatised by flashbacks, constant and sickness and feeling trapped, like I can't breathe. I e-mailed Jayne tonight. I get to talk tomorrow and I feel sick.

Reflection: This is what happened to me when I tried to contain them. Physical symptoms appear. The mind I have since learned is incredibly powerful and needs to be respected, but I didn't know how to do that yet.

Notes:

16.08.17

This is the e-mail I sent. I was too low to write another thing last night.
I am not suicidal, I have no thoughts of self-harm. I have no faith. I have no 'go to' coping mechanism any more, even though the ones I had were negative. I no longer hate myself, I no longer want to hurt myself because I have a very new sense of self belief. But that doesn't make the impact, the sudden rush of flashbacks, feelings and sensations any less destroying and overwhelming than they were two years ago. Like two years ago when the lid came off with massive force and I don't know why it does that. It is so terrifying and I have no 'go to' way of coping and I am completely overwhelmed and in such a dark place. I understand now why I couldn't name him. I couldn't name him because of the horrific abuse and shame I feel. All consuming shame, embarrassment and absolute humiliation, because I gave myself to him and because I hated what I had done.
I punished myself for doing it and then carried on doing it. I tried so hard to starve and drink myself to death when I was already hurting so much. He destroyed me and I was an adult and all that he did I feel utter shame and revulsion. I know it wasn't my fault, but I knew it was wrong, I knew it was horrific, that's why I wanted to die. But instead of stopping it, I punished myself over and over again. I have never hated anything more than I hated myself. I hated myself because I knew it was wrong and I didn't stop it. I hated myself because I couldn't punish me more than he did. I hated myself because I couldn't even do that. I hated myself because I hated what he was doing and I felt dirty and injured and disgusting. He caused me more physical and emotional pain than I have ever felt, than I could ever imagine was possible and I hated myself far beyond words for allowing that to happen and not being able to do worse to myself. I couldn't even kill myself. He had absolute control over everything and I felt a disgusting, worthless failure. I wanted to scream and fight and destroy that bastard, but all I could do was destroy myself.
I so desperately wanted to die. For 6 years I was fixated on ending my own life to escape the torture. I am consumed with guilt and shame. I was really only a little girl. I was only 10 years old and subjected to despicable violent sexual acts and emotionally destroyed. But in reality I wasn't. I was a 20 year old woman and my mind was blown. In my mind I was 10 years old and being raped, being expected to do grown up things, but I wasn't, I was a woman and the flashbacks and the feelings and the sickness are for a 10 year old girl.
I feel exactly how I did then. Trapped, sick, horrified all over again, but absolutely disgusted and ashamed and I can't get rid of the flashbacks. I don't know how to change the ending. Suicide and self-harm have always been my 'go to' place when I have had to face this complete violation of my mind and body. Stewart Watts destroyed me. He completely destroyed me and I have never got my head around that and now it's out I feel so exposed, because I don't know how to get my head around it.
When Jack sexually abused me I really was a child, but when Stewart did I wasn't. I feel like I have to take responsibility for what happened. I have to look at it and come to terms with it, but I don't know how to. Self-harm and suicide have always

been there and now they're not and I have to look at it and it's destroying me because it always has.
How am I ever going to be able to look at this? I'm so frightened because it was going to kill me. I don't know what to do. The lid is off and I have to deal with it, but I never, ever have. After Stewart I had no relationship with men 1996-2005, until Alan. My way of dealing with it was to shut it out. The threat of death went when he went. The anorexia continued for years after, but the threat going meant I was able to put a firm lid on it. Protect my life by not allowing anybody in, but just punishing myself enough to remind me what a disgusting person I really am. Having Sam re-booted my mind, because my desire to have a child and be healthy enough to get pregnant became very powerful. Now like with Jack and everything else that erupted 2 years ago, this has too. And I'm so frightened.

Reflection: I was about to confront what Stewart had done to me. As in the entry, I had only ever had two coping mechanisms. Self-harm and suicide. My mind had healed, recovered enough to understand that they were no longer 'appropriate' thoughts and feelings to have. However, I had not replaced them with anything else. So Stewart and his experiences were ready to erupt, but I had no coping mechanism, no alternative thought processes to help me through it. I was really frightened, it was like I was on a tightrope and somebody had removed the net underneath, but there was no option but to walk. I had no option but to walk back through my life with Stewart. My mind was determined to do it, I felt I had no control over that, but I had no safety net, at least that how it felt, so I was really, really frightened.

Notes:

17.08.17

Too exhausted to think about anything.

Reflection: Another one of those days.

Notes:

18.08.17

I was very apprehensive about talking to Jayne today after my e-mail. But today we talked about attachment. It began because I was talking about my new garden and my mixed feelings. I really like it, but don't want to feel it in case it gets taken away from me. This isn't about material things, this is about my lack of attachment. I need to find a way to be able to accept and come to terms with what has happened. I have been thinking about what has happened and my response to it. Hopefully this will begin to make sense in a minute. I begin with the first event.

My Sister was taken away from me = I am told nothing is special anymore and she is never spoken about.

Jack took my innocence = I then hate all men and it is never spoken about.

My Cousin Jason Jones violated me = Confirms I hate men, never spoken about.

I married a man Stewart Watts who abused me = Confirms I hate men, confirms I am here to be used, I have to die. Never spoken about.

I stay away from men to protect myself, then 9 years later I get into another abusive relationship = I have not changed.

I have an ectopic pregnancy, never spoken about so I disconnect from future pregnancies in case they are taken away from me.

I have 3 children, but struggled emotionally to let myself go, let myself connect with them, in case they are taken away from me.

I lose my first marital home, so I don't get attached to anything I own in case it gets taken away from me.

I am so lonely, isolated and disconnected! It has been postulated that it was Albert Einstein who said "*doing the same thing over and over again and expecting different results is a definition of insanity*". I have been doing just that. Something goes wrong and I shut that emotion right down. So, going back to the house analogy. Yes I might lose my house, yes something might happen and it gets taken away, but equally it might not. I have moved house so many times. I buy a house, get it how I like it, then sell it. I sell it before I admit to, or start to feel safe, secure and settled, just in case it gets taken away. Yes I have had this experience, but to completely disconnect from any material attachment means I never feel safe, secure or settled, because I am always running.

I loved being pregnant with my first child. I loved my growing bump, it made me feel he was getting stronger, healthier and I loved that I was doing that. After the ectopic pregnancy I disconnected from my other 2 pregnancies, just in case they were taken away from me. I hated my growing bump, I had no control, I hated feeling the baby move, because I was terrified they would stop. I had no attachment whatsoever, I hated it until they were born.

Had I been allowed to grieve for my loss, talk about it, share my anxieties and my feelings, I could have had emotionally positive pregnancies. Now that will never ever happen.

I didn't have a relationship for 9 years to protect myself from men, but when I did, I went straight back into an abusive relationship. I had not changed! I have felt alone, sad, isolated, disconnected all of my life because my response has not changed. Not only that, but because I have not been allowed to express myself, I have not been heard. I think and I have reflected a lot on this today. Instead of focusing solely on self-preservation to the exclusion of any emotional attachment to anything, then I need to try to balance an element of self-preservation with some different responses. Such as allowing myself to feel emotional attachment. I have to change if I am to feel connected. I can't change the past, but I can respond differently to how I feel about it. Plus I will never not be heard ever again.

This brings me on to Stewart and my fear of expressing the overwhelming attachment to what he did. In order to be heard, in order to 'give it back' I have done a few things. I have written complaint letters, I have made a statement about Jack and I text my cousin. I have tried to give the responsibility back to my abusers, so I am not left with it. It has given me the ending I needed. Now with Stewart I was suicidal. I gave myself that ultimatum. Nobody forced it upon me, nobody told me I had to kill myself because of my complete belief that I was worthless. I have a voice that I will never lose again because I have developed self-belief. So I don't need to keep punishing myself for what Stewart did. What I need to do is stop being defined by what he and everybody else has done to me. I need to stop responding to other peoples' behaviour and start living the life I want to live.

What Stewart did was depraved, horrific, disgusting and any other adjective that describes what he did. By continuing to live in response to what all my abusers did, I am continuing to punish myself. I am continuing to be defined by that experience. All my coping strategies have been negative. Suicidal tendencies, anorexia, alcohol abuse, emotional detachment, self-harm. None of these coping strategies have been positive, or helpful. So to continue to do those things is to continue to demonstrate and element of self-loathing, blame and responsibility.

The opposite of this is to live life to the fullest, eat well, not abuse my body, allow myself to experience and allow emotional warmth. And to forever forgive myself for my mistakes. But most of all to validate myself and to continue to believe in myself. Of course what Stewart did is horrendous, but experiencing it and talking it out means I will be able to let it go. I don't need to 'give it back' there is nothing to give back. He has gone and it's time to stop carrying him. Reporting Jack was the logical next step. He had committed a crime. Texting Jason had to be done, because he was in my life and I didn't want to pretend any more. Stewart is not in my life, he never needs to be in my life. There is nothing to give back, just me to stop living by the consequences of what he has done. Negative punishments are no longer an option, should never have been the option, but I was made to feel worthless, so I knew no different. Now I do and it's time to begin to live by my values and beliefs. I need to keep thinking about this.

Reflection: It never ceases to amaze me as I reflect on all of this, that I can go from feeling hopeless, exhausted and defeated to having amazing insights. Perhaps that really is what happens during those 'numb' days. My mind is doing some research of its own, going to its own library and figuring out some answers, because I have no idea where they come from.

Notes:

01.09.17

I haven't written because we have been on holiday. I needed a break, time to switch off. But now! Now is the lead up to Jacks trial. Fern from the Police has been in touch a few times, but yesterday! Yesterday I had to recount everything other than Jack. The man in the park when I was 13 years old. When I was 16 years old and even Stewart. Using words like forcing me to have sex until he ejaculated made me feel sick. Seconds after saying his name out loud. I felt so sick after that 'phone call. But everything is out now. She knows everything and in a way that feels like a relief. It puts everything into context around Jack. He did what he did, Jason did what he did, the man in the park, then Brenda Smith sealed my fate by saying *"these things happen"*. So being cajoled into being walked home following comments such as *"what's wrong with you, why don't you like men?"* Being made to feel guilty, abnormal, so going along with it, then being raped - "These things happen."
Too much was exposed in one 'phone call and I felt so shocked afterwards and for the rest of today. I was shaking, almost panicking that the lid was being lifted off again, but more violently. But it's not like before, because as sickening as I have felt, I talked it out with Jayne and Carol and thankfully I had cancelled appointments at work today, so it gave me a little head space to slow everything back down. I calmed later this afternoon and then I just wanted to cry. But even that passed. I will be okay.

Reflection: That was one of those experiences where what happened to me was reflected back to me. Made it real. I don't know if I have explained this properly so I will give an example of somebody I looked after at work and hopefully this will clarify those times I have referred to this.
I cared for a young person who only found out she was pregnant weeks before her due date. Anyway, just before she was due to give birth she developed pre-eclampsia and became very unwell, very quickly (I will let you look pre-eclampsia up yourself if you don't know). To put it in lay terms, she had tubes coming out of pretty much every orifice, she was monitored in intensive care and had to have her baby delivered by emergency caesarean section to stop the condition becoming life threatening.
When I went to see her postnatally, she was recovering really well. She was loving being a mum, felt she was recovering physically and was really happy with how her experience had gone and how she had been cared for. I saw her several times and she went from strength to strength. When I saw her for her last visit ready to discharge her, she presented really differently. She was very low in mood, tearful, pale and completely different to how she had been during previous visits. When I enquired about her mood, she told me that her and her Mum had been talking about the birth and her Mum had told her that she had been seriously ill and she had thought she was going to die.
This to me illustrates what I have been referring to when people have reflected back to me my experiences when I had talked about them. Just like this young person, I had given her the opportunity to de-brief about her experience. I talked to her about her understanding of her experience, however, her Mum told her what had hap-

pened explicitly and although she had lived the experience herself and accepted it. Being told explicitly what had happened caused her an incredible amount of trauma. Every time somebody used words such as rape, forced ejaculation, horrific abuse, or expressed concern that I was going to die. It had that same hard hitting impact and I felt absolutely traumatised, as if I was hearing it for the first time. Going through all of those experiences with Fern on the 'phone left me feeling traumatised. She needed to do that she said, so there were no surprises in Court. But she used those words and I didn't realise it then, but whilst I was learning to understand more about my experiences I hadn't come to terms with them, so every time I heard them it was a punch in the stomach to me. It was a horrific shock.

Notes:

02.09.17

I'm exhausted today. I didn't go to sleep until after 1am. I began to read my journal from the beginning. I don't know why. So much pain. Unbelievable heartache and such loneliness. I never ever want to be in that place again. At the same time it was like reading about somebody else. The most terrifying time of my life these past 2 years. In 21 days' time I am going to be standing in Court giving evidence. Evidence about not only being sexually abused by Jack, but everything I am going to be asked about and every question I answer will tag along a line that goes on for 37 years. So being 'touched' by Jack has left a sensation I have experienced over and over again for the last 37 years. Feeling trapped by Jack has left a sensation I have experienced over and over again. All roads lead to Jack. Never being able to forget it is one thing, but talking about it, reliving it is more intense. Doing it with emotional support is incredibly hard. Doing it cold and matter of fact is sickening. Like it's being forced out of me aggressively. No gentle questioning, no allowing me to take a breath, or take my time. I feel like I am on a tiny platform surrounded by hot lava and on that tiny platform I am expected to be a Mum, run a home, go to work and all the time hot lava is raining down around me, forcing me to face it, watch it, be aware of it and be burnt by it. Always there. Jack has always been there, attached to everything do. After the trial I have to let him go. Guilty or not guilty. How am I going to do that after 37 years? He destroyed my life, he is being brought to justice, so there is nowhere to hide him anymore. He has been exposed, he will have been brought to justice. There will be nothing left. It will be like a grief.
He has been hiding inside me for so long. He has touched every significant part of my life, affected everything. He's been like a constant pain. A constant emotional, often physical pain that nobody could get to. I have exposed him and Court will get rid of that hidden pain, because he can't be hidden any longer. But what if he doesn't go? What if he continues to haunt me, tap me on the shoulder, remind me that he is still there? The few close friends who know what's happening have said this will give me closure, they have said I can put it all behind me and get on with my life. But I have lived with Jack for 37 years, what if he won't go? Or I don't know how to let him go. I can barely remember life before him. I have made a mistake, a massive mistake. I have believed Court will be the end, I have believed I will feel completely different, I can't believe I have allowed myself to believe this. A door will close and all gone! Oh God! What if it's not? I'm expecting to feel a massive relief. Guilty or not guilty. I need to feel a massive relief, I have to, I really really have to, because right now I am consumed by him and everything he has done and everything he has caused and still causes me to feel. Oh please, please let him go, so I am not in pain any more. Please!

Reflection: It was beginning to dawn on me the impact Court would have. Remember when I believed 'giving it back' was all I needed to do. I suddenly had this realisation that whatever the verdict I might still not be able to let Jack go. That was a really frightening insight. Not least with the pressure of those well-meaning around me telling me I could put it all behind me when the Court case was over. As if I was deliberately holding on to it.

Notes:

03.09.17

Today I am subdued, but focused. No longer panicking like I was yesterday. I slept well. I saw my Dad today and him and my Mum were reminiscing about their younger days and I could feel my irritation grow. My stomach churns when my kids ask me to talk about when I was growing up. That is how I carry Jack. Every childhood memory is considered before, or after Jack. Before Jack I lived, I loved, I felt safe until my Sister died. Then I felt sad, lonely and scared. After Jack I felt loved, I lived again, I felt safe. Then he sexually abused me and I felt so sad, so lonely, so scared, but I also felt worthless, unloved, terrified, horrified confused and stuck. Stuck feeling trapped, touched, fondled and those feelings live with me right now. The wrong touch, the wrong environment, the wrong look and it's happening all over again. 37 years of it happening again and again and again. I feel so sick, I could vomit. That touch! That creepy, sickening trapped touch. Please let it go away, I can't stand it anymore.

Reflection: I was angry that they could reflect on their youth. I had nothing about my youth that I wanted to reflect on and it was all their fault. I had been robbed of my youth and it was all their fault. My children would often ask me to talk about my childhood and all I would see was Jack and all I would feel was sensations of being sexually abused. It made me feel sad, it made me feel angry, it devastated me. I had to make things up, I had to pretend to my children. How dare they have a youth to reflect on and I didn't.

Notes:

04.09.17

I'm really frustrated, I need the Court date for Alan to be moved from the day after the trial. I've been told it could run over. Instead of saying she'll sort it, my Solicitor tells me she needs to get his consent. Well bollocks to you all. I'm not asking anybody for anything. 37 years of a life fucked up by Jack Kilbourne and finally my voice will be heard and he will be brought to justice. 37 years, I'm not asking, I'm telling. Nobody is ever going to push me around EVER again! Sadly though I took my energy out on my daughter. I shouted at her because she was frightened of a spider in her room. A fear she has inherited from him. I got angry with her because she is still affected by him 12 months after he has left. And here's me 37 years after Jack still being affected by him. How dare I do that! I apologised so much to my daughter. I wiped away her tears, we cuddled and then we laughed together. How could I ever be angry with my baby girl for being scared, whether it's irrational or not. And what right do I have to be angry that he still affects her. How dare me! I can't even stop Jack from affecting me. I'm so angry with myself and I haven't been that for a long time. I'm just frightened. So frightened that this won't all go away after Court. I'm tired of being frightened and I'm tired of living in Jacks shadow. I'm angry about it, but I don't know how to change it. I feel so helpless. Somebody please help! Please help me I am so alone.

Reflection: Despite being angry with myself there was a lot of insight in that. Yes how could I not expect my daughter to be affected by Alan 12 months after he left? I was angry with myself because I still wasn't whole. I still hadn't made that connection inside.

Notes:

05.09.17

I was so down today, so low. I could barely talk. Every action is an effort. Nobody is helping me. My Solicitor, my GP Surgery being obstructive with my medical records. All I want to do is focus on 25th. I am ready and I don't need people to be difficult. All the abuse is out now and I am consumed with flashbacks about Jack. Particularly that trapped and being sniggered at feeling. Everything is going to come to a head in 3 weeks' time, all of those memories are floating around. They are ready to be talked about. Fern from the Police is the only person who is bending over backwards to support me. I hate where I live so much. I want to go home, but I don't know where home is. I'm so lost, so alone. My children are my everything and they are so kind, so thoughtful. I am so, so proud of them. I love them with everything I have. I am so tired.

Reflection: This was all about stress. My Solicitor was being less than helpful in moving the family Court case and resorted instead to putting pressure on me. Pressure I didn't need to absorb as I had no control over how long Jacks trial was likely to last. My GP surgery were being difficult about getting my records to the Police. All these people were taking their frustrations out on me and I was only going to work every day, caring for my children and preparing myself, or at least trying to prepare myself psychologically for Court and I was doing that all on my own.

Notes:

06.09.17

I felt so sick today I could vomit. My heart has been racing and my hands clammy as well as the delightful diarrhoea. I met my friend Sara today, she is a lovely, warm caring friend. I feel okay when we are talking. I felt very panicked at work and looked for somebody to talk to, but there was nobody available, I just needed help to be grounded. I just need this to be over.

Reflection: This is just pure stress. Nothing to reflect on except all this was going on around me, people knew, but I felt so alone. I really needed a hand to old. Sara was understanding, but I needed more. I can't believe how strong I was. Good for me!

Notes:

07.09.17

4am appears to be my wake up time this week. I an get off to sleep okay, but my appetite has gone and I feel so sick. Since Fern talked about Stewart I can't get the images out of my head. I have to talk about what happened again. She reflected back to me what I was telling her and that made it happen all over again. And it keeps happening over and over again. She also sent me crime report numbers for what happened when I was 13 years old and 16 years old. Seeing it was a shock. All of this together is what completely overwhelmed me 2 years ago. Seeing it reflected back somehow validates the horrific flashbacks and the horrific nature of it. Particularly talking about injuries and knowing that they are documented in my medical notes which have now been requested. With the exception of Jack, everything feels like it's been blown wide open and it's going to be talked about in Court. I know I can't rush any of this, but I need to work hard to make this as manageable as I can for Court. The flashbacks are so vivid I can almost feel the physical pain, because I know what that pain felt like. Pain like nothing I have ever felt before or since. I feel like I need a whole day to talk about what it will probably take 5 minutes to say, but that's because the flashbacks are on and off all day and when they are not happening I can only think how horrified I am that they are happening. Sometimes I wish I could just sit with somebody whilst they hold my hand. Just so I'm not watching this horrific video on my own, because it's just so lonely. It was 5.11am when I sent this e-mail to Jayne, then I lay in bed and I cried. I couldn't wait to get up, for it to be morning. I went to work, went about my day, but was looking at people and wanting to scream "help me! I don't know how to cope with this."

Reflection: Nobody prepares you for Court, or how it's going to be. Because Fern had asked me about all of my experiences, I believed that all of these would be brought up in Court. I was frightened because I hadn't even nearly begun to come to terms with Stewart and I didn't know how I was going to cope with that. My mind was thinking about all the abuse and I was trying to stay focused. On top of that, knowing that my GP records held evidence to my physical injuries and anorexia and more recent mental health. I believed they were going to rip me apart in court. I was beginning to panic.

Notes:

08.09.17

Today I spoke to Jayne. We talked about Stewart and how I become completely overwhelmed by what he did. My anxieties about Court and how I'm worried that they will talk about Stewart and I won't be able to cope. I was googling quotes about suicide. Suicide marks the intense destruction of a person who cannot bear to live with pain another second.
Stewart destroyed me, what he did still horrifies me. I wish I could talk about him, what he did. If I could come to terms and move forward. Suicide was my 'go to' because that marked complete destruction. Stewart completely destroyed me and I had my way out. I don't know how to come to terms with what he did and have no closure. No mark of the destruction he caused. We talked about A;am and his recent behaviour. His behaviour and Stewarts behaviour were exactly the same. I can objectify Alan. I have no feelings towards him in regard to myself. I see him as a behaviour. Everything he does is typical of a 'behaviour' and emotionally abusive behaviour. I am not denying my feelings about Stewart, I am not suppressing them, but he can wait. I have to focus on Jack in Court. Stewart will have to wait. To be able to cope with this for the next 2 weeks I have to focus on him as a behaviour. Just to make him manageable should I have to discuss him in Court. For the next 2 weeks Stewart is just a behaviour. He was just a behaviour type.
Dear Soul, if I promise to look after myself as best I can, please keep me strong. Please be with me, hold me and be my strength when my hands are shaking and my legs are wobbly. Please let me feel your warm glow inside that makes me feel solid, so solid I feel stronger than I have ever felt. When I feel hollow, fragile and ready to crack, please ignite that warm glow and let it rush through my body making me solid, making me so strong. Please soul, I have nothing else.

Reflection: I was praying. I don't think I have ever prayed before in my life, or since.

Notes:

09.09.17

Today has been a better day. I slept well last night and I felt okay today. I went out for an hour tonight for somebody leaving work. I was very anxious about going out, but it was okay. I'm glad I went out, it was just long enough, but I was very happy to get back home. I hope I can sleep well tonight.

Reflection: Another mind knitting together day I hope.

Notes:

10.09.17

Today was okay again. Keeping busy is good and It's my Son's birthday tomorrow. Heard from the Police again asking me for more information, but it was okay. I need to return a statement Recorded Delivery. This will be all over soon.

Reflection: My mind was working hard behind the scenes, I guess.

Notes:

11.09.17

So this is what it means to cope. Two years ago I went off sick from work when a trigger brought back horrific flashbacks of sexual abuse which spanned 16 years. When I felt stronger I returned to work in February 2016. Shortly after, I reported this to the police, more for closure than anything else. Eighteen months later and he has been charged and I am due to appear in Court up north to give evidence regarding his crimes in 2 weeks time. Thirty seven years after this all started and I am about to face my abuser. When I began this process my ex-husband became abusive and 12 months ago we separated and are now divorced. I have since found out that he had been abusing my kids and he no longer has contact. Police and social care have been involved. I have a counsellor who I speak to one hour a week, she is great and is helping me to process my emotions around a lifetime of neglect and abuse, but one hour a week doesn't even nearly begin to cover it.

My ex-husband is taking me to Court for access to the kids and this has caused them untold levels of stress and anxiety. For the past 12 months I have supported my kids, rebuilt their confidence and helped them to feel safe and secure, both at home and within themselves. During all of this I have continued to come to terms with what has happened to me, continued to work full time and have only one hour a week to be me.

The Court date is looming and I am contacted by the Police almost daily now, to clarify points and make further statements. I cannot remember a day that I haven't had flashbacks in the last 2 years. I am focused at work and do my job well. As a consequence of being strong other than being able to talk to a few friends when they are free, I have absolutely nobody. I am so consumed with flashbacks that I must allow in, in order to be focused in Court, but I am so lonely it's indescribable. My Mum has to go to Court to give evidence, but she neglected me and she remembers very little. As soon as she has given her evidence she will be leaving and coming home, she has no interest whatsoever and her behaviour never fails to cut me inside. Even though I have come to terms with her behaviour, her repeated rejection still has the same impact. I have nobody, I have never experienced unconditional love (other than my kids) but this is not appropriate for them.

I am so focused on Court, but afterwards the real work begins and I have to learn to have a life without him over my shoulder and what if I can't do that? What if he won't go? I use everything I have to make myself stay strong for probably the scariest experience of my life. I sleep because I meditate, but I can't control the nightmares I have and I wake early full of anxiety and I just need the day to begin. My job helps me to focus on something else, but as soon as I am not with my clients the flashbacks and anxiety return. I feel like I am on the outside looking in. Every daily routine feels trivial and is such an effort, but I carry on and I function. But I really feel like I am on the outside.

The Court date with my ex-husband has been scheduled the day after the trial is due to finish and my Solicitor is being awkward about it being adjourned, although the Police are supporting me with this. It's incomprehensible to believe that I could switch off after a trial and focus on something completely different. Nobody appears to understand, or care about the massive emotional experience I will be going through whether he is found guilty or not. This is massive for me, this is marking the end of an almost destroyed life. A landmark that says it really is time to move on. But nobody cares, I am nobody's priority. I have never experienced unconditional love, but it doesn't mean I have ever stopped looking for it. I am not important to anybody, everybody wants a piece of me, but nobody can see me. I am strong, I am so strong, but that's because I have to be. I feel like I have the world on my shoulders and I have nobody to pick up the pieces if I crumble. Not without an appointment at least.

This is not self pity. This is utter, utter loneliness and absolute isolation. I look forward to nothing, because all I know is dread. This is something I have to go through, nobody can go though it for me, nobody can stand and give evidence for me and nobody can take this away because it is going to happen. At the moment I can't see past this trial date, I can't look forward to anything because this is so massive. Thirty seven years of an affected life and it's all going to come out in Court. That's more massive to me than the word massive. It's truly overwhelming. Everything is coming to a head and every day is torture. Every day is a day closer and it's absolute torture.

Reflection: So that was what I wanted to shout to people, anybody. I just wanted a hand to hold. I just needed somebody.

Notes:

12.09.17
Today I spoke to a colleague at work and tried to explain how I feel. It really helped to be able to talk, tomorrow I go to my local Crown Court for a pre-trial visit. I am absolutely exhausted.

Reflection: At least I had an outlet that day.

Notes:

13.09.17

Today I went to Crown Court and it changed my whole perception of the trial. Seeing the layout of the room really helped. Being told where people stand. Even standing in the witness box. It suddenly dawned on me that those addressing me will be wearing wigs. And suddenly it all seemed comical. I have been through a horrific experience and men, or women are going to be asking me serious questions stood in fancy dress. It really has taken the fear out of those people.

Also my witness support person asked me how I would cope with a Barrister disputing what I am saying. I said I would respond by saying *"well there really isn't anything I can say about what you think, if you don't believe me that's your problem not mine"*. He was a kindly gentleman and laughed and directed me to a more appropriate response. Such as *"What I have already told you is the truth"*. He made me feel comfortable and relaxed and as the day went on my mood lifted for the first time in a long time. People in wigs! Do me a favour. I am ready for you Jack! And after 37 years I am coming for you.

Reflection: It really helped going to see a Court room. Apparently the lay out in Court is the same, so the witness support person told me where everybody would be sitting and who I was supposed to look at when I was giving evidence. It did allay my fears, but it felt like another world. I told the person with me that I wanted to sit and listen to everybody else's evidence and he told me I would have to sit in the public seating area and that might include sitting with Jacks family. I wasn't sure how I felt about that, but I wanted to hear what people were saying about me, so I needed to think how I would cope with that.

Notes:

14.09.17
I received a call today, the trial has been moved to another Crown Court. I also received the Court Report from the social worker. Alan has repeated that I had a breakdown, I made a suicide attempt and now he has added drug misuse. He is a sick bastard. How he can make up such dreadful shit does prove what a disgusting low life piece of scum the really is. And he will be sorry for what he has done. If there is ever going to be Khama it will be him it happens to. That sick lying bastard is going to look foolish and expose himself for the sinister evil bastard that he is.

Reflection: I really couldn't deal with Alan and his stuff at that time, I was focused on Court.

Notes:

15.09.17
I am ready now, so ready for Court. I don't know what else I can say.

Reflection: I just needed it to happen. I had waited so long.

Notes:

16.09.17

Two years ago I would NEVER have dreamt I would be here preparing for Court. I was destroyed, at the end of the road, I had nothing left. Thanks to all of you who have supported me. I am re-built, I have a voice. Okay I'm terrified, but my God am I going to use it to my strength. All those years of desperation, crying for help and being ignored, dismissed. Well not any more. This is my life and everybody is going to damn well know it. I just wish my brain would rest a while. It's so pumped, but I need to rest before next week. Please come on now!

Reflection: I was focused, really focused. The wait was exhausting.

Notes:

17.09.17

My anxiety levels rise and then I take deep breaths, meditate and bring myself back to the moment. I force myself to be present, then I look at the intrusive negative thoughts as if I am watching them in the television. Then I proper tell myself *"You're doing it again and if you can turn the thoughts on, then you can turn them off again"*. Courage, come on now courage. I can do this, I am mentally and physically strong. COME ON PAULA! COME ON! You have the courage, come on you are so much stronger than you think. One day at a time. Denial maybe, but I have a feeling this isn't going to happen. I am strong and I have courage and I will live in the moment. I will. I can choose what to do.

Had a great night tonight playing board games with the kids. I was living exactly in the moment. It takes discipline, but I love a challenge. I will do it.

Reflection: I was doing everything I could to get myself through those next few days, meditating, distracting, playing with the kids. But most of all I just wanted that day to come.

Notes:

18.09.17
Woke feeling much stronger today. I am totally focused on courage.

Reflection: I was in the zone.

Notes:

19.09.17
Spoke to Melvyn today. Made me realise how strong I am. This is going to be okay.

Reflection: Countdown to Court.

Notes:

20.09.17
Courage, courage, courage. My anxiety levels are really dropping. It's good.

Reflection: Meditation was a brilliant support then.

Notes:

21.09.17
Really focused now.

Reflection: I was.

Notes:

22.09.17
Feeling calm and ready.

Reflection: Nothing else mattered at that point.

Notes:

23.09.17
I feel very calm. It's dawning on me now. After 37 years I'm so close to seeing my abuser. Very strange feeling. Something very intimate went on between us and I will see it in his eyes. You know that look you give one another (whoever it may be) when you both know what each other is thinking and you see it in each other's eyes. He will give me that look and he will find it very hard not to nod. But I will see it and so will everybody else.

Reflection: I was focusing on Jack now. I was feeling very powerful over him.

Notes:

24.09.17

On my way to give evidence in Crown Court. There is an inevitability about it now. The Hotel I am in is right opposite Court. It's all dark inside and I think about tomorrow. Tomorrow I'm going to be in there and it's all going to be happening. Walking round the place I used to come shopping, or out for the evening. The Cinema, the nightclub, McDonalds, it's all gone. Shops empty, frontages boarded up. The town centre is like a ghost town and the drizzle. Fine drizzle, which just adds to the grim, grey sight. This all lead to feelings of despair, sadness, grief. Grief for the town I knew, that is no longer there. Sadness and despair for the memories I have of that time. I'm here because of Jack and the memories and feeling I had at that time consume me. I just want to go back to the hotel and hide under the covers. I hate this place and everything it represents. My Childhood, youth, bad emotions. Now I am back I have these past emotions as well as current emotions.
I had a bath at the hotel and climbed into bed. I slept so well.

Reflection: I travelled up with my Mother. We might as well have been on a jolly, for all she was concerned. We talked about nothing. We got to our Hotel and I had requested separate rooms, I didn't want to be near that women. I despised her and I knew after Court I would despise her all the more. I didn't want to leave the Hotel, but she insisted on walking through the town. Everywhere was closed and she was fussing about where to eat. I couldn't give a damn. I wanted to be in the Hotel, it was warm and I could be on my own and not next to her rabbiting on about the price of meals and how much the town we were in had deteriorated. It was all so irrelevant and all so her. No interest whatsoever.
The bath, my new comfort was really settling, the bed was so big and comfortable and I meditated. Cuddled myself down under the covers and slept better than I had in a long time.

Notes:

25.09.17 – Crown Court, the day the trial begins.
I'm awake early, a lump in my gut and chest pain. I meditate, focus. All I need to concentrate on is what I have to do and I calm down again. I go for breakfast and I'm ready for Court. I go in the back way at 0915am as instructed. Everybody is so kind. The man who walked me in. Witness support who sat and chatted and gave me drinks. I feel like I'm in a parallel world.
Court is delayed from 10.00am until 11.00am. Then 11.00am until 2.00pm. I go out for lunch, Jack is remanded into Court until 1.00pm to give me time to get lunch. I'm walking around the shopping centre in a daze. I feel like everybody knows why I am there. I have lunch. Soup, because that lump, that sick feeling won't go. I get back to Court for 1pm and wait. 2pm comes and goes and I'm told legal arguments are delaying the start. I have met my Barrister and he is lovely and kind. He apologises for the delay. I'm told we'll start at 3pm. 3.15pm and I'm told if we don't start by 3.30pm it will adjourn until the next day. At 3.50pm I am called into Court. The Usher walks in front and Witness Support walk behind. I feel like I am being taken to my doom. I sit outside for a further 10 minutes. I don't want to go in now. I feel sick, I feel emotionally saturated and I think I might faint. I walk to the witness box and I'm struck by how silent it is.
There is the Judge, Usher, Recorder, 2 Barristers, Witness Support sitting behind me. The Jury, Jack and security sat behind the screen. My Barrister begins with asking my name and I stammer as I'm asked to confirm. I had just affirmed and heard my voice for the first time in Court. There wasn't a single part of my body that wasn't shaking. I had to speak slowly, clearly and was asked to pause frequently. During the pause, I was living what I had just said. I was advised to avoid the temptation to fill the silence. But I was living, feeling and seeing what I had just said. I was glad for the pause.
Half an hour after beginning his questions, the Judge asked for the Court to be adjourned. Every sinew in my body was either shaking or sweating. I felt very exposed. I had just disclosed being sexually abused and it felt emotive, vivid and current and then suddenly it was stopped. I felt shocked, jolted and very sick.
Dinner that night was very hard to swallow. It was still grey and drizzling with rain. My body was aching with tension and I just wanted to hide under my bed covers and sleep. I wanted to block out all the grey, drizzle, the misery of my life growing up. I had a bath and went to bed and I cuddled myself around my pillows and slept.

Reflection: During that day I had 'phone calls from my Solicitor about family court and Melvyn who was minding my children with his wife calling me about my internet provider. These people had no idea and cared less that I was about to have my whole life of abuse laid out in front of me and discussed in cold blood. I couldn't believe how insensitive they were.
This was the day I met Fern, the Investigating Officer for the first time. She actually looked how I imagined her to look.
When the Judge adjourned Court that day he 'reminded' me that I was still under oath and I was not to discuss the case with my Mother who was yet to give evidence. I wanted to laugh. She was on another planet, she didn't give a shit about the court

case, she just wanted to go shopping and get home as soon as she could. You could not imagine a woman more cold, more disconnected, more disinterested than my Mother. She never spoke about the case before court, she never spoke about it during the trial and she never spoke about it since. I will let you form your own opinion about that. Some say it was too hard for her to face. She blamed me for being abused when I was a child, and she blamed me for bringing it all up again. I believe what I have always believed and that she thought I deserved it all.

Notes:

26.09.17
I woke up at 4.30am and my day begun. I am up, breakfast, showered and dressed. And the day is still grey. I walk to Court for 10.30am and I'm advised we will start at 11am. I had been given my statement to read the day before, but now I was part through giving evidence I was not allowed to read it. I didn't need to. I hadn't forgotten what Jack had done 37 years later. I didn't suddenly need my statement to tell me what I already knew. I was called into Court just after 11am and my Barrister began with his questions. It was about 12.00noon when he concluded and the Defence Barrister stood up. She asked direct, not open ended questions and I found that much easier.
During questioning a light malfunction halted proceedings for a minute of two, but I remained focused. A copy of a photograph was shown round at one point and I was asked if I had the original. After being passed round it was brought back to me and I did find that distracting at times, as the Defence Barrister continued with her questioning. The Defence Barrister, although challenging, was very respectful. Everybody was very patient and respectful and whilst I was no longer shaking, my hands were wringing wet.
After a short lunch break I was back being cross examined. This went on until just before 3pm. The Judge, both Barristers and all the Court Officials were very kind. The Judge addressed me before I left, but I have no idea what he said. But then the blow came. Oh yes I did look at Jack, I noticed he looked old, but also carried that air about him. That arrogant air. He didn't look at me.
At the end of the day my Barrister came and spoke to me. It was then that I learnt the case would not be concluding tomorrow. More witness statements needed to be heard. Then there would be a Prosecution and Defence summary, Judge summary, Legal aspects, closing speeches and then the Jury would be adjourned. I was told there would be no point in me staying. I was advised that it would be sensible to go home. But I didn't want to. I wanted to be where my life was being discussed. I met an old friend Jane who had given evidence. She was so sad and had suffered great personal loss. I felt so sad for her, so desperately sad, but even that added to the whole melancholic mood.
Under very different circumstances I would have wanted to hear about her life since we had last been in touch. But today, today she was a reminder of my past and I just wanted to leave. Boarding the train home I felt I was being taken away. Taken away from my childhood life. I had gone back to get closure, I didn't want to bring that back home with me.

Reflection: I had been told to look at my Barrister when he asked questions and then to look at the Jury when replying. However, my Barrister was stood in such a position that Jack was sat directly behind him in the box. I couldn't look at him, because that meant I would have to look at Jack. Nobody reprimanded me for that and I was relieved. By the time I had finished I had been stood in the witness box for over 4 hours. My back was killing me and my hands were very clammy, but I was determined and focused and I didn't sit down.
The blow came when I was told it wasn't in my best interest to remain in court after giving evidence. I was devastated. Fern had told me it was acceptable, the witness

care person who showed me round early in the ear had told me it was acceptable, but there I was told I could, but it could be detrimental to my case. Any body language, or facial expression I pulled, could be distracting to the jury. I was so disappointed. I wanted the opportunity to be able to listen to everything. To listen to Jack and his filthy excuses. I wanted to hear him squirm. I was told if he was found not guilty that he would walk right past me and I would find that really difficult. I felt like I was being held down again. I was being controlled, I was being stopped from doing what I wanted to do. What I needed to do to get all aspects of this abuse exposed.

When I left Court I was again sandwiched between the Court Usher and the Witness Support person and as I walked through the public area, there she was. Emily, sitting there on her own looking at me and I was looking at her. She had no emotion in her eyes, she just stared at me. I will never forget that look. It wasn't anger, it wasn't sadness, to me it was abject dejection. A look that told me she knew it could go either way and she would accept it.

Notes:

27.09.17
I have not slept all night. I have relived the trial and I still felt I needed to be back there. My childhood has been opened up and I need to be there to put it to bed. I couldn't stop thinking about what was happening today in Court. I should be there. I called Witness Support and they advised me that Jack was still giving evidence and this will continue until tomorrow.
A 4 day trial. I spoke to Fern and she understands why I need to be there. Even if Jack is found not guilty and walks out of Court in front of me. I was there at the beginning, I need to be there at the end. I have to see it finish. I just have to be there. This is my life! My childhood and I need to lay 10 year old me to rest.

Reflection: I had waited for my Mother to give evidence before catching the train home and as the train pulled away I felt like I was being dragged away from my childhood life. That period of my life where I had been abused and I needed to stay. I had instigated this. Or you could argue that Jack had instigated this. I had gone through over 18months of investigation to trial, been involved in one way or another answering questions and providing evidence, so I absolutely needed to see it to the end. Whatever that outcome were to be. It felt wrong, it all felt so wrong in my head. I wanted to hear Jacks voice, I needed to hear his voice. What they made me do coming away was wrong and it had a very negative impact on me.

Notes:

28.09.17
The verdict came in and I wasn't even there. Acquitted! I heard just before 4.30pm today and ever since then my brain has been spinning. It stops on a thought and feeling and then it spins again. It's desperately trying to find the one that fits. I sent this in an e-mail to Jayne. It's the only way to describe it. I cried tonight whilst the kids watched television. Thirty seven years I have carried that pervert and when I did report him he walked. But everybody knows now what he did. I was listened to, I was believed, yet people who knew absolutely nothing about me are given the responsibility of passing judgement. Jack Kilbourne, you disgusting slimy pervert - sleep well in your bed. And Emily Kilbourne, just remember the next time he has his fingers in your knickers, he had them in mine first!
I don't believe I'm the only one.

Reflection: I called Court and was advised that if the jury hadn't been returned by 4pm then Court would be adjourned to the following day. 4pm came and went and I rang a friend and asked her if she would go back with me. She agreed and I told Fern. I told her I would be leaving early the next day to attend Court. I needed to be there. I had come home and gone to work. It was all really messing with my head. But sadly just before 4.30pm, I was standing in the conservatory, with my kids near me when Fern called and told me he had been acquitted. I couldn't believe it and more to the point I couldn't react. This is exactly what I hadn't wanted to happen. I wanted to go to Court and get the whole disgusting mess over with in that place, so I could come home and leave it there. But I wasn't allowed to and I was stood in the dining room at home, listening to Fern deliver the verdict to me. I was broken, utterly broken. How callous to do that to me and I was all alone.

Notes:

29.09.17

I feel utter despair. I don't understand, I really don't. Waves of grief flood over me throughout the day. I'm at work, this is exactly what I didn't want. I am overwhelmed with emotion and I am on my own. Why do I always have to be on my own? I am so lucky to have my kids. Thirty seven years, I can't just switch off. I'm parked up, I can't go home, then my 'phone rings. It's Fern.

She talks me through what happened. It turns out that the Defence Barrister made a big deal of my friends' statements. Apparently when they were first asked, they said they didn't remember any disclosure. But then they later came back and said they did. It was this that put reasonable doubt in the heads of the Jury. It doesn't change anything, but at least I know it wasn't because of anything I did or didn't say.

I don't believe I was the only one and I don't believe this is the end. I have to give myself time. It's all over for me. I had one chance, one chance to bring him to Justice. At least I know I did that and it wasn't because of me that he was found not guilty. He will never sleep soundly in his bed again. He will always wonder if somebody else will come forward. Fern told me it had hit him too. His career is over and now everybody knows, there will always be doubt. I really believe Fern will be calling me again about Jack. But for now I don't know how I am going to begin to move forward. Today all I know is I did my bit and my bit was more than good enough.

I gave it back to Jack. I no longer own what he did to me. He has it now and everybody else knows it. So please make me feel better. I hurt so much inside.

Reflection: This had messed with my head so much. In my head the Court case was still going on. I couldn't get my head around the fact that it was all over. Jack had gone home with Emily, Emily who knew. It was the strangest experience, but all I could think of was Court and it still going on. I still needed to go back to Court. I needed to see the empty Court room. I hadn't heard the verdict myself and I hadn't heard Jack say he didn't do it, so it was still ongoing in my head. Everybody was still there and I couldn't make it be otherwise. That has got to have been the strangest thing, of all the strange things that my mind did. I knew what Fern said, but my mind absolutely would not accept that.

Notes:

30.09.17

I can't do this on my own. Today was so tormenting. Every bald guy I saw looked like Jack. Smells reminded me of Court. Conversations reminded me of both. Even Strictly Come Dancing had a Barristers wig as part of a costume that looked the same as my Barristers' wig.

I have had flashbacks of Court, flashbacks of being abused by Jack and him laughing at me. Because he is laughing at me I get a gut wrenching pain that he has got away with it again and he is laughing at me again. Then the next thing I am thinking is that I brought him to justice. He knows I know what he did and he knows it will always be with him. Back and forth my brain is banging and I am so tired and I cannot eat. This can kill people, tip them over the edge. Just because I am strong now doesn't mean I don't need the same help as those who are on the edge.

I need help so I don't go there again. Even tonight Elizabeth wanted me to play with her and I was back with Jack. I was told he was acquitted when I was on my own with my kids. I didn't want it to happen like that. I didn't want to be here, I didn't want it in my life, but it did and now everything around me is touched by Jack and Court and I didn't want it to be. It's real in my life now and I wanted to leave it in Court. I knew I didn't want to be here for that exact reason and now I don't know what to do to make it better.

The difference between now and before is I tried to make myself feel okay, not be affected. Now I am stepping back and allowing myself to feel how I feel. I talked to a friend today for the first time about everything. I am going to talk to another friend tomorrow again about everything. I can't make myself feel okay and I can't keep it bottled up. I won't pretend again for the rest of my life. But I can't do it on my own.

Reflection: Another very frightening experience was the smells and the images. Every single person I saw who was bald had Jacks face. I kept seeing him everywhere. The smells were of Jack and Emilys house. When a family has a baby, I always think the house either smells of fresh washing or baby sick. Jack and Emilys house smelled of baby sick. I could smell that baby sick everywhere I went. It was really frightening. I was seeing and smelling Jack and I couldn't stop it, it just kept happening. Every other stimulus either reminded me of Court, or Jack and the Court case was still going on in my head. The urge to return to the Crown Court wasn't lessening. I knew it had finished, but in my head it was still going on and I couldn't make it end. I needed to see that empty Court room. What was happening to my mind?

Notes:

01.10.17
I'm in Court and I'm shouting for the Jury to believe me over the Defence Barrister and I'm sure they are listening. I am going to win this, but suddenly something happened and I wake up. No! No! No! this can't be a dream, it can't be, it's just so real. And even though I have realised it's a dream, I still try to go back to sleep. I don't want to wake up and it's not real.
A friend came round tonight. She knew nothing about my past. I talked about being abused at 10 years old and the trail of destruction that left. Being raped, raped again, violently raped, anorexia and suicide. Jack being found guilty would have justified all that. Now I am having horrific flashbacks. I feel like I have seen Jack and Emily all weekend. Smells, sounds, vivid intimate images of being abused by Jack. Not being there for the verdict, it feels like it is still going on. I can't get rid of the train tickets in my purse because it still feels current.
I knew I had to be there for the verdict. I had to be there to see it end. I was panicking so much, I had to be there. But I was told at home, in the conservatory, with the kids at home. I didn't want that, I vehemently didn't want that. I needed to see it end and because I didn't, it's still going on in my head. Torment, torment, torment.

Reflection: I hadn't been listened to again and I was angry, so very angry. I had been persuaded to do something I didn't want to do, just like when I was being sexually abused and now that had happened again with Court. The bit that was supposed to end it all for me up there was now impacting those feelings of not being heard and being persuaded to do something I knew in gut would make me feel so bad.

Notes:

02.10.17
At work today, but not focused on what I was doing. I kept feeling convinced that Fern was going to call me and tell me somebody else has come forward. I have to see the end to this, I can't bear it. The Trial is still going on inside me because I wasn't there to see it end. God I don't know how to make it stop. This is torture. I need help to make it stop!

Reflection: It really was torture, because I knew on a logical level that Court had finished, but I couldn't stop it going on in my mind. So much so that it would almost convince me that it was still going on. I was so certain Fern was going to call me. None of Jacks family had been in Court, in fact there was nobody in the public gallery. Why had nobody been to hear what Jack had done to me? Where was his family? Where were the school colleagues, the parents of the other children he had abused? These thoughts were constantly going round and round in my head.

Notes:

03.10.17

I'm not thinking straight and I know I'm not. I was reading suicide quotes last night. Not because I want to commit suicide, but because the quotes describe how I am feeling. *"People who die by suicide don't want to end their life, they want to end their pain." "Suicidal people are just angels who want to go home". "Every thought is a battle, every breath is a war and I don't think I'm winning any more".*

I have thoughts of self-harm to feel a physical pain to justify my mental pain. Plus I am afraid I am becoming anorexic. Anxiety has left me with no appetite. But the past couple of days I have been hungry and ignored it, but felt the physical pain. I am asking for help. Last time I ignored it until I was suicidal, I was anorexic. I am asking for help now because I recognise it. Why am I feeling all this again? Because I am in so much pain. I'm living the nightmare that is Jack, I am living Court all over again and I can't make any of it stop. I want to be loved unconditionally. Loved and hugged. Allowed to express all emotion, but I can't.

I told people over and over again that I need to be there and now it's gone I can't stop it going round and round in my head, because the last time I was there it was still going on. I didn't see the verdict. And now it won't stop going on. I'm in so much pain. I love my children with every ounce of my body, without them I wouldn't be here. I don't belong here. There's nothing here for me.

Reflection: When I became suicidal I really believed everybody would be better off if I no longer existed. I was beginning to think like that again. Those quotes I could relate to, every single one. The last quote I related to particularly, because Court was the pinnacle for me and had battled through those thoughts, kept breathing when I didn't want to and Court was symbolic for me. The outcome was symbolic for me and that was taken away. I really didn't think I was winning anymore. Every time I tried to find something I could hold on to, it was taken away from me. I was giving up again, I felt I really was losing the battle for my life.

Notes:

04.10.17

Such an overwhelming powerfully emotional day. It comes in huge waves and one minute I feel like I'm coping, then the next I feel I am going to completely fall apart. I did fall apart a bit today in my car. I was talking to my friend Sara about how I feel, the pain I am feeling, suicidal thoughts. How feeling hungry gives me a physical pain I can cope with. I'm really not thinking straight, but I don't know what else to do. Fern e-mailed me today asking me for a statement about Jason. I gave it as well as explaining how I feel. It's funny, but (not funny) being explicit exposes everything. Although she only wanted a statement I expressed my feelings too. Being explicit really helps. I am so exhausted. I hope I can sleep tonight. What will it be tonight, Jack or Court?

Reflection: I think the previous reflection explains this ongoing emotion that was raging inside me. I was only hanging on.

Notes:

05.10.17
It was neither. I was so exhausted I fell straight to sleep. Feeling shattered today and just generally low.

Reflection: Great no Jack and no Court. That mind working hard on itself thing again.

Notes:

06.10.17
I saw Jayne today and talked about my fears of becoming anorexic again and how to end Court in my head.
Exhausted, can barely keep my eyes open.

Reflection: I have always had an issue with food since being anorexic. I never had any professional support to re-educate myself on my relationship with food. I had used it as a weapon of self-destruction, when attempting to starve myself to death. I had used it as a sense of control, when I had no control of anything else. I had used it to relieve the pain of being raped, by causing another pain much more powerful than rape. And now I had started using it as a tool to expose my emotional pain as physical pain. At first I had lost my appetite after Court, but when my hunger kicked in and I felt pain, the pain I was feeling was tangible and reminding me just how much emotional pain I was feeling. I didn't want to become anorexic again, but I didn't know how to manage the pain I was in and I resorted to the only behaviour I knew.

Notes:

07.10.17
Slept again last night. Absolutely shattered, but going through the motions.

Reflection: Healing, or deteriorating? I wasn't sure at that stage.

Notes:

08.10.17
My youngest Son talked to me today about his experiences of abuse and how that is making him feel. His distress and despair was heart breaking. I could feel myself begin to panic inside to think that a sick evil bad person could damage my Son who is so beautiful, caring, loving and clever. To think a low life piece of scum would to that to a genuinely good person broke my heart.
Then it dawned on me. I am a good, caring, loving and clever person. A low life piece of scum did break my heart when I was just 10 years old. And suddenly I felt broken hearted for myself. Scum bags are just that. They are lesser, weaker, disgusting human beings. Worthless. How can I let these worthless people destroy me? No! No more. Oh my God! An epiphany.

Reflection: It was healing.

Notes:

10.10.17
I'm hungry, so hungry. I can't eat enough I'm so hungry. Still sleeping so well, still shattered.

Reflection: I had started to eat. My epiphany just in time.

Notes:

11.10.17
Still feeling stronger, still sleeping, still eating. Twelve months ago today Jack pleaded not guilty.

Reflection: I was back on track. How absolutely incredible that when my conscious mind couldn't do it any more, my unconscious mind kicked in. This happens with physical survival too with the initiation of primal spinal centres. When a human is no longer consciously able to physically sustain life, primal spinal centres kick in and sustain life until support is provided, or eventually you will die. My unconscious mind kicked in because I could no longer consciously survive.

Notes:

12.10.17

Feeling angry today. Sick of people being disrespectful and I'm sticking up for myself. Feeling angry that my Son's physical pain is caused by emotional trauma. We saw a Consultant today Chronic sensitisation syndrome. I'm so angry, not at my Son, but so angry that that scum bag has caused this to happen. Angry and even more determined that my life to going to be affected no longer. Time to face everything head on.
Still shattered, still sleeping well and still starving no matter how much I eat.

Reflection: Emotionally I was continuing to recover. My Son, who was experiencing physical pain was told this was as a result of abuse and the trauma he was experiencing. I was so determined to overcome this for myself and my Son. I wanted him to heal, but I first had to understand how to do it so I could help my Son.

Notes:

13.10.17
Still feeling irritated, pounding headache. Slept well, still hungry, still eating. Glad it's Friday.

Reflection: Healing was never going to be easy.

Notes:

14.10.17
I dreamt last night, all night that the right thing to do is to allow Merseyside Police to investigate. This isn't about another crusade, this isn't about revenge. This is because I have continued to reflect on what I spoke to Carol about. I had a similar case at work and when you look at things objectively you see how utterly wrong it was. Why would my 14/15 year old Cousin want to have sex with 11 year old me? And why did he stick his hand up my skirt and fumble with me over my knickers? Dirty, disgusting bastard. And he laughed too. I e-mailed Fern and told her to progress it. Nothing will happen, but he will know that even at 14/15 it was wrong. I felt so elated after I had done it. I am looking after me! And I am never going to be used by anybody EVER again.
My confidence and self-esteem is growing at a very fast rate now. I spoke to Carol and told her. I am coming back. For the first time since I can ever remember, I am really becoming me. I still feel irritated and that doesn't feel like me, but my adrenaline is racing so I am trying to contain it until I calm down again. I am a genuine, loving, kind, caring and honest person, but I will not be taken for a mug. Never Ever again. It's like all the lights in my brain are switching on at once. No wonder I have a headache. I'm starting to feel brand new and it's so exciting.

Reflection: Fern had spoken to me just before Jacks Trial about Jason and taking it further. She had asked me afterwards if I wanted to pursue a case against Jason and I told her I did. Because Jason sexually abused me in my Nan's house, Fern originally referred it to Merseyside Police, but then after a made a formal report to her and explained the first incident where he was going to have sex with me was in another constabulary, she told me that her Police Force would keep it and that she would investigate.

Notes:

15.10.17

Still feeling irritated, but at least I recognise why. I shall just have to be patient. Tough times still ahead with Family Court, but I've had enough now. At least when it's over, it's over. I need to be a little more patient, but I have really had enough of being pushed around.

Reflection: I was getting fed up of being at the mercy of processes that I had no control over, because I wanted to start being in control of my own life. This felt like other people were still calling all the shots.

Notes:

21.10.17
Eight hours it has taken me to go through the Court Report and respond. It felt so good having my voice. Having my say and it even emphasised how abusive Alan was towards me. Absolutely horrible.

Reflection: The Family Court had requested a Report from Alan. It was given to me to respond to and I went through it sentence by sentence. Incident by incident and I was delighted that I could reply to all of the allegations he made against me to disprove his lies. I was finally going to have my voice heard in Court and that made me feel powerful and that I had regained some control. I'd had to listen to the lies he had told and that was very difficult. Particularly as I no longer felt bad about myself, I had to read lies that challenged that belief.

Notes:

22.10.17
Another two hours and I have e-mailed the Report to my Solicitor. I have responded to every malicious, sick comment. What a truly bad person he is. It shocks me how evil one person can be and still allowed to walk the planet. Why do people have to be so evil?

Reflection: I found it very difficult to read how somebody despised me so much. Despised me and was trying to destroy me. It no longer destroyed me, but I couldn't understand why men wanted to destroy me repeatedly.

Notes:

23.10.17
I feel free today and a big relief. Nothing to do expect focus on work. I have not had nothing else to think about in a long time. Actually, I was thinking about completing this book, but there is still a little bit to do yet. Stewart Kilbourne for one. And I'm wondering if the Police are going to get in touch, or if that's it. I'll leave it a bit longer, then contact them, just for closure. Bits left to tidy up.

Reflection: Yeah well, I underestimated the impact Stewart Kilbourne had had on me. Now quite a few bits left to tidy up.

Notes:

24.10.17
Sometimes when I spend a long time on my own I replay Court over in my head and it becomes so real I almost believe I can change the outcome. But of course I can't and when I realise I can't I feel so overwhelmed all over again.

Reflection: I was continuing to struggle with the Court outcome against Jack. I really needed to have been there to see and hear it all. There was too much unfinished business in my head.

Notes:

25.10.17
Today I got my Son's voice recognised. He was abused by Alan and I made a complaint because nobody wanted to hear what he had to say. It seems nothing has changed. I felt emotional after the Detective Inspector left, I fought and fought and now my Son will be heard. He will not experience what I went through. Maybe that's why I felt so emotional. It isn't easy I realise when you speak up people make you out to be a liar, or mad. But I'm neither and I won't be silenced by anybody, ever again and I won't allow my children to be silenced. I haven't heard anything yet from the Police, things are starting again, but it really is almost over. Just Stewart Kilbourne to clear, then nothing will be left. It will all be over.

Reflection: The Police had listened to my Son and the case against Alan was to be investigated. I felt good that I had gotten my Son's voice heard. I was determined that nothing was going to be dismissed and I would get justice from my Son, like I had never had. Still minimising Stewart Kilbourne, I had no idea.

Notes:

26.10.17
I was reflecting on yesterday and why I am so emotional that he is being heard. Because now I know he will never experience feeling worthless because he was abused and nobody listened. He will never feel worthless because his abuser felt it was okay to do it. He will never feel worthless because it affected him emotionally and nobody saw or cared. He will never feel worthless because when he spoke up about what happened to him it was minimised by others, because it wasn't. He will never know what it means to feel worthless because nobody listened, nobody cared. He will come to terms with what has happened as he is now a child. He will be able to work it out with all the support he needs so he can move on with his life. He will be okay and this will not be a shadow over him. That's why I feel so emotional. I felt worthless for all the reasons he never will. I am determined to make sure that he will never ever feel like I did. He will never end up writing a book like this and he will never waste a single moment on the ghosts that continue to abuse him. Because there won't be any – because of me!

Reflection: This is a reflective account in itself, if not a little over simplified. I didn't consider that all of the above is what would be expected from any supportive parent. My Son continued to be badly affected for a long time after and I was helpless to change that. That was very hard to accept. I put every ounce of effort into supporting my Son and accessing the help he needed, but in the end it is down to the person to work hard to overcome trauma. I didn't consider that at the time.

Notes:

27.10.17
Something doesn't feel right and I'm not sure just yet what it is. I still want the attention because of what happened to me. I feel like I want to tell everybody. Why? I don't understand it yet, but I'm sure I will. I saw Jayne today and talked about the last two weeks. I could have e-mailed her, so we could talk about Stewart Kilbourne, but I didn't because I am too scared to talk about my experience, but why? I don't know why and I feel frustrated, but more scared, more overwhelmed than frustrated and that stops me. He is the last bit, why does the thought fill me with utter dread absolute overwhelming terror? I don't know yet.

Reflection: I was beginning to recognise that Stewart, wasn't a bit of tidying up. But consciously I didn't know why.

Notes:

28.10.17s

I woke up this morning early and wanted to cry. I had been dreaming about Stewart and wanting to talk about him, but I couldn't because I need to know what's happened to him. So I e-mailed Fern this morning asking her why the sexual assaults, the violent rape has not been recorded. I need that validation. I didn't realise it until I dreamt about it last night. I hadn't realise how much having all the other crimes against me had helped in terms of recognising they were wrong and recognising they were crimes. I went back to sleep after I e-mailed Fern and woke feeling a bit better. I'd also asked if I was expecting to hear from the Police, or if it was just being recorded. I'm also still angry about having to fight for my Son's voice to be heard and angry that nobody did that for me. Nobody cared enough to be bothered to ask why I was failing at school, why I was drinking alcohol to excess as a child. Why was nobody bothered? Today has been a really hard day with no answers.

Reflection: Two steps forward and three steps back. I understood a long time before this why nobody was bothered and it was about them and nothing to do with me. But the rational, healing part of my mind was not always as strong and the injured part of my mind and self-doubt crept in at times.

Notes:

29.10.17
A Detective Constable from the Child Abuse Investigation Unit came to talk to my Son today. I didn't fully appreciate how upset I am still about what has happened to my Boys. My one thing has always been to protect my children and he proved I couldn't and I feel sick to my stomach. He is such a bastard. A wicked, evil, bastard.

Reflection: It was that mirroring thing again. Yes the children had told me what had happened, but hearing them talk to the Police and her responses suddenly made it very real and really upsetting.

Notes:

30.10.17
Absolutely shattered today. I had an e-mail from Fern. The Police are progressing the incident and she asked me to have a think about Stewart Kilbourne and making a statement. I'm just so tired.

Reflection: Fern told me that she hadn't fully understood the relationship with Stewart Kilbourne and she asked me to consider whether I would want to pursue this as a case.

Notes:

31.10.17
Charlie has been referred to CAMHS and I am so angry that Alan has done that to him. Charlie is full of anxiety, he's hearing voices. Alan shouting he said and having hallucinations. My baby boy and I couldn't stop him from being damaged and that devastates me. I'm sick to my stomach. The one thing I had to protect – my Son. I will do whatever I have to do to keep him safe and supported. I re-did my Will tonight.

Reflection: Again like my oldest Son, this was the hardest part. I could get my Son's voice heard, I could get all the support he needed, but I couldn't make my Son not be traumatised. I couldn't take that away. Only he could do that for himself and that is what sickened me. Had I been supported, would I still have been as traumatised? I don't believe so, but naively I think I believed at that time I could have taken all the pain away for my children for being there for them. Watching children in pain is almost unbearable.

Notes:

01.11.17

I met with my new Solicitor today. I really like her, she is a very strong woman. I trust her straight away, she has a very strong handshake and she is direct and when we disagreed with each other we both accepted each other's point. I really like her. Charlie asked me to talk to Sam and Elixabeth about what is going on. I told Sam about Charlie's anxieties, what was happening in relation to his hallucinations and voices and I explained why Charlie needs his television in his room to feel safe. Sam was so understanding and then he said that Charlie was 'doing it wrong'. He said by watching television in bed to cope he is just reminding himself about what has happened because he will know he is doing it to cope. He said what he needs to do is learn to relax in bed. Oh my, suddenly these little synapses are sparking in my brain. I know he was said something very profound and my brain is parking trying to make a connection.

It didn't take me long. For several months now I have been wearing a bracelet that says *"My story isn't over yet"*. It's a mental health, anti-suicide quote. You squeeze it because it is soft metal to fit around your wrist. I have been wearing this to remind me how hurt I have been and when I get stressed I squeeze it and I can feel it around my wrist. I have been wearing it to show how hurt I have been and how hurt I might still be. But wearing it is keeping me in that same hurt place. But all I really want to do is accept that I am hurting when I do, but when I'm not it's okay to let go. I don't need to keep hold of it. Nothing is hurting me now, so I can enjoy not being hurt. It doesn't mean it has to go away.

Reflection: Sometimes the wisest words come out of young minds. I was bowled over by what Sam had said to me. How incredibly profound for a 15 year old boy.

Notes:

02.11.17

I woke up this morning and looked at the bracelet and I took it off and put it away safe. When I hurt I hurt, I don't need to keep reminding myself just in case. I felt free to laugh at work today, I made other people laugh. I could because I didn't have that hurt reminder on my wrist. And when I hurt I will look after myself, because I deserve it and need to do it. I can look after my hurt on my own. I'm not scared to look at it, I can manage it by being so good to myself. I cannot believe how free that makes me feel.

That bracelet was a visible thing saying look at me I'm hurting, but I'm not scared of it any more. It's like I can suddenly look at it like an external thing. Separate from me. Meditation and practising meditation has taught me so well. I am not my thoughts. I can look at them like I'm watching a film and respond to them. So, if I feel sad today I can accept that I feel sad and think about what I need to take care of myself. Instead of panicking when I feel sad and wondering how long it will last and not knowing what to do.

Meditation is fantastic and it really works. I'm not scared of my range of emotions. None of them are negative because I accept them all at last.

Thank you Sam. What you said has massively opened up so much insight and understanding. You have made an incredible difference to me. You are truly amazing and I hope one day you get to read this and understand just what you have done.

Reflection: I still have that bracelet and I know if I ever get to a really dark place again I can wear it. That bracelet was My scar. But it was a scar that I could have when I needed it for comfort. When I took it off there was no evidence that it had ever been there. I don't believe I will ever get to that dark place again, because of how I have repaired myself, but that bracelet is my safety net. For a long time I needed a scar to show people and myself how much pain I was in. Then as I healed a little, I wanted the scar so people could see how much pain I had been in. But then I developed a little more insight and thought about a future where I no longer felt that pain and a scar would constantly remind me and I became troubled. That bracelet was My scar. I could wear it when I was in pain, so everybody including myself could see it, but when the pain went, I could take it off and there was no constant reminder. How cool is that!

Notes:

03.11.17-09.11.17
I have had six amazing days of being free. Free from associations, free from flash-backs, sad feelings, thoughts and bad memories. I have laughed at nonsense, lived in the moment. I have aired my opinions, I have expressed my emotions. I feel so good.

Reflection: Taking that bracelet off really did set me free. I didn't have to feel guilty about feeling happy. I could be myself without the reminder of the pain I would feel from time to time. I only needed to feel the pain when I was feeling it, I didn't need to be reminded of it when I wasn't.

Notes:

10.11.17

I couldn't put it off any longer. I have to look at what happened with Stewart Kilbourne. I talked to Jayne and we looked at the time-line and we decided that the easiest way to go through it is to look at the list of words I associate with him and you are going to go through it with me!

The first word we looked at was "*Trapped*". How did I feel trapped? I felt physically trapped because he tormented and tormented me until he wore me down, then he would rape me. It was so painful and he would rip me. He would withdraw his penis then force it straight back in and I would rip and it would sting like a hundred papercuts inside. He would rape me from behind and I hate people being behind me, it makes my skin crawl every time. It doesn't matter who is behind me, or where. And if I can, I will turn sideways.

He would lower himself over my face and rub his penis on my face and I couldn't push him off. I felt like I was going to suffocate. I felt emotionally trapped because I believed I was wrong to hate what he was doing because he told me I was wrong. He accused me of faking a period to avoid sex and would want to see my tampon to prove I was on my period. He made me feel guilty for being on my period, so much so that I would run out of sanitary protection and stuff tissue in my knickers. I desperately tried to deny my period because he moaned so much that I was making an excuse to avoid sex.

He criticised the way I looked, the way I spoke. He humiliated me, he put me down and I believed every fault he gave me. I felt trapped in my own head and body. My body because it was seen as an object to be violated. I hated my body for doing that. My mind because he told me I was wrong for not liking, for not enjoying what he did to me, so I felt a failure. I felt a failure because I didn't feel how he said I was supposed to feel, so I hated myself for not being able to cope with being raped, humiliated and criticised. I hated myself for not being able to feel different and not being able to cope. I hated myself because I failed as a wife, a woman, a human being. I hated myself because I attracted being used, hurt, violated, ripped apart.

And I hated myself because I couldn't even kill myself. I failed at everything. Body, mind and soul an absolute failure. An angry, hated failure. I was no good to anybody and no good to me. I was absolutely destroyed.

Reflection: The timeline came about as part of a review. I wanted to see if there was anything lurking in my mind that I hadn't addressed and Jayne suggested that one way of doing this was to draw a timeline. I didn't know exactly what she meant, but I understood it to be the events/experiences in my life in a chronological order. I left the appointment and went to work. Between appointments I looked at drawing up this timeline and it was as if my hand had become possessed. In hardly any time at all I had listed every emotional response my mind recalled on to that paper. It was incredibly powerful. (See Glossary).

Notes:

11.11.17
Didn't really think about what we talked about yesterday, but today was a busy day.

Reflection: Mind needing to do that healing thing again behind the scenes. Preparing itself for what was to come and I had no conscious idea it was coming.

Notes:

12.11.17
Felt a bit flat today. I don't like it when I don't have enough time to reflect on things.

Reflection: My mood was coming down.

Notes:

13.11.17
Another really busy day today, feeling a bit irritable.

Reflection: My mind was starting to process what Stewart had done and I didn't know it.

Notes:

14.11.17
I was in Court today. Alan continues to refuse to accept the harm he has done to the kids. He is so creepy, so sinister. He makes up disgusting lies to discredit me, abuses the children and then asked my Barrister if he can deliver the kids Christmas presents and asked if I could give him a Christmas list. He is utterly screwed up.

Reflection: Thankfully I was only in Court for about 10 minutes. The case was adjourned for the New Year. I was told I would need to make another report. Too much was now going on in my mind. Stewart was brewing.

Notes:

15.11.17
I didn't sleep last night worrying. I have to write another statement about Alan. Why? And what about? Why don't people just leave the kids alone? They have made their wishes explicitly clear. Why don't they just fuck off and leave them alone. I'm starting to feel trapped again. I am being forced to do something I don't want to do, which is to relive the horrendous time again. Relive the abuse, just so he can defend it.
Just like Stewart reminding me of Jack to defend his actions when he was raping me. The emotions, the flashbacks are exactly the same and I hate it. I fucking hate it!

Reflection: I didn't want to have to recount the abusive relationship I'd had with Alan, not on top of Stewart.

Notes:

16.11.17

Feeling very out of sorts today, it feels like I have too much to do. Statement for Stewart, Statement for Alan. A massive amount of being forced to relive abuse. Just like Stewart with Jack, just like Alan with all of it. Being forced to relive all the horrific abuse. I feel so sick and I can't lift it.

Reflection: It was becoming overwhelming. Although I wanted to pursue the case with Stewart, I hadn't come to terms which what he had done and it was frightening to have to go through it. Unlike with Jack, I had moved a lot further forward before I reported it to the Police. I hadn't really started with Stewart.

Notes:

17.11.17
I talked to Jayne about how I am feeling. She helped me to set myself mini goals, mini tasks and because they are so negative, to set myself some time for me. Some happy tasks. I hadn't thought of happy tasks just for me. Time-out just for me.
I feel so sick. My appetite hasn't come back since I was in Court in September, but I am looking after myself by putting a healthy salad for my lunch and several pieces of fruit, so I can eat little and often without feeling sick. And I am drinking plenty of water. I really am trying to look after myself, so much. I don't want to be dragged back to re-live the abuse, this horrifying abuse all over again. God! I could scream. I feel like it's happening all over again and I am being forced to go back and experience it. I feel so sick. So fucking sick.

Reflection: Jayne knew how big this experience with Stewart was and I didn't . I was trying to look after myself in terms of physical health, but I hadn't mastered looking after myself emotionally. I couldn't really see the point of mini goals, I didn't have any insight into how massive my experiences with Stewart had been. Thankfully Jayne did.

Notes:

18.11.17
This is so unbearable. I feel like I'm drowning in emotions, sensations, flashbacks. Every day now I am living with something that reminds me of being raped, or emotionally and physically battered. I have never addressed him because it affects everything I do.
Dealing with Stewart makes all the sensations I feel more intense, from people standing behind me, to being thanked for making coffee, to eating when I don't feel hungry and instead feel sick. I can't make the sensations go away. I feel sick and trapped and I want to scream and rip my hair out. I want to scream so hard to make it go away.

Reflection: The impact of Stewart was beginning to pick up pace. People standing behind me reminded me of being grabbed by Stewart and held and not being able to move. Being thanked for making coffee, reminded me of having to do something I didn't want to do and then that smile, that sickening smile he would make after he'd ejaculated either inside me, or all over me. When I told Stewart I was anorexic, he would humiliate me, force me to eat meals that I hadn't eaten for years and it made me feel so sick and panicked when I wasn't hungry. Other times, when my sugar levels dropped and I experienced hunger pains he would withhold food from me and tell me I was weird for needing to eat at a time he didn't agree with.

Notes:

19.11.17
I feel like I can't breathe. Consumed with sensations, I feel trapped. I have e-mailed a statement of events to Fern tonight. At least I don't have to do that again. All of my abusers have now been exposed. But when will I feel relief. When will I ever be at peace? Help me please, somebody please I just want it to be over. I can't breathe.

Reflection: Of all the abuse, I think Stewarts was the most damaging as it was repeated over and over again and I felt there was no end to it, only an end to me.

Notes:

20.11.17
Isolation is killing me. I believe it was 2 years ago today that I opened up about Jack. November always seems to be a significant month for me, but how do I open up about Stewart? With Jack and Stewart, Jason, Carl and the man in the park it all began with guilt, same and self-loathing. Now I have embarrassment. Reading about what I put up with embarrasses me. Because I can see now how depraved it all was. But as well as that it ripped me apart. It ripped my soul out and having to face it, having to come to terms with it feels like it is going to do it all over again. I feel so angry at the feelings, so frightened of their strength. I just hate being me.
I wish I wasn't here and then the pain would stop. All I want is for it to stop. I'm nearly 48 years old and I don't remember a life without torment, torture and horrific memories. It has to all end. I can't go on anymore.

Reflection: I was struggling to look at what Stewart had done to me. I wanted it to stop, because I knew I was about to go to a very dark place and I just didn't know if I could cope with that again, but I equally wanted it dealt with.

Notes:

21.11.17
I just want to get rid of this rubbish and live a life. Jason and Stewart are going to be investigated. Part of me feels incredibly strong and brave and part of me feels like I'm breaking. Reading back the response makes what they did so real. And even more devastating. I need to stop talking to people. I have to dig deep and find every ounce of strength to get through this. One way or another this is coming to an end. I'm so overwhelmed right now.

Reflection: The abuse from Jason and Stewart were being investigated at the same time. This was incredibly difficult. I wanted it done, I wanted to be free to move forward, but I was terrified of what was to come.

Notes:

22.11.17
Today was a very bad day. I e-mailed Jayne last night and explained how destroyed I feel. First Jack, then Jason, then the man in the park, Carl, then Stewart. Why did it have to get worse? Why did I have to be taught a lesson? Why did it keep getting worse until I was destroyed? Physically, mentally and emotionally destroyed. The monster inside me knows that if I destroyed me then I would have no more pain and nobody would be able to destroy me. I would win! But I have my children who mean everything to me. They are my reason to breathe. My reason to carry on. Without them, there is nothing here for me.
I heard from Fern today. I am going to get an appointment from the Police to be interviewed by them and videoed. I don't know how I am going to be able to do it. I feel so low. So helpless. So overwhelmed. I just want to be held and hugged so tight. I feel so scared. How am I ever going to be able to let it out? This was going to end my life and I coped by avoiding a relationship for 10 years. The problem with that was I kept myself safe only by avoiding men and not learning from what happened. Now it feels as raw as when it was happening.

Reflection: I was becoming overwhelmed and nobody outside of Jayne could see that. That 'monster' had returned. This was the part that wanted me to give up, destroy myself so I wouldn't have to live with any more pain. This was the 'monster' I believed was bigger than me. Not only was I being attacked with flashbacks of Jason and Stewart, the monster was attacking me to. I was holding on, but only just.

Notes:

23.11.17
I don't feel part of life. Every step is an effort, I need to get this out. I need to talk to Jayne, to tell her everything.

Reflection: I was starting to become disconnected again, that limbo between life and death. This was not a good place to be.

Notes:

24.11.17

I was so ready to talk to Jayne, but our appointment time got changed. I am focused at 9am, I know what I am going to talk about and I have no other distractions. 9am is the best time for me.

Anyway we talked about my thoughts this week. Suicide came up again. Not because I want to do it, but because so far it has been my door. My way to stop my pain. My children are my world and I would keep breathing every day to protect them. My fear now is the monster inside will convince me that they would be better off without me.

After our appointment I reflected hard on what we had talked about. And I decided the monster inside me is not my monster, it's his monster. The repaired part of my brain wants to be happy, live, love, be loved and grow. But it's sat next to a monster. His monster and he wants me to stay a victim, vulnerable and abused. When I try to expose the monster, it injects fear and anxiety into my veins and threatens me that if I tell, he will kill me, or hurt me badly. I felt this so powerfully this week, then when I realised I wouldn't be talking about it today, the monster quietened down.

Now I understand what he is trying to do. Just like I thought the world would come crashing down when I talked about Jack. But it didn't and I felt massive relief. But for now the monster is sitting on my chest, so I feel tight, tense and anxious. His monster is making sure I keep my mouth shut. When I text somebody he can't hear it, but to speak it out loud, he's going to try hard to stop me. This isn't my monster. I don't want to hurt me, or kill me. I want to live a happy life with my children. But he wants to get me drunk so he can convince me to hurt myself. Convince me that it will make me feel better. The worse I feel about myself, the harder I have to look after myself.

The monster is a bully, a threat and it has lived inside me for far too long. He knows it and he is going to try to do anything it can to stop me. I am going to have to be so strong to overcome this monster, because it doesn't deserve to posses me. It never did. This monster wants me dead, it wants to win and I have to want to live more. I have to trust that when I expose this monster, somebody will be there to pick me up off the floor because he is going to kill me. To convince me I would be better off dead, to convince me I am weak and he can kill me. Just like when I was about to expose Alan to Melvyn and Rachel and he suddenly blurted out I was suicidal and out of control. He tried to destroy me to stop me speaking out. He won't be able to do that in Court. He will be exposed too! This monster is making me shake and feel sick now.

I really need help to keep me strong. I have to stay strong or he will kill me! I'm so very frightened. Frightened of getting tired, frightened of getting so tired that I just give up. Frightened that he will wear me down just one time too many. I want to beat him, but I really need help. I really do!

Reflection: This is a really powerful entry. At the beginning of the journal I just wanted to end my life, I wanted to give up, there was no battle. But here, there was a battle, I believed, between two beings. Now the bigger being was the monster, the smaller being was healed me. When you have nothing to fight against, you give yourself over to others to hang on for you. Thankfully I had that and as you have read, those people, notably Jayne, did. This time though, I wasn't looking for others to hang on for me, I was battling myself. That was so much more dangerous and frightening, because the battle was within me and I wasn't looking outside for people to hang on to me, I was battling with myself for survival and at that time the monster was bigger.

Notes:

25.11.17

Absolutely petrified to go to sleep. Woke up at 2.30am this morning, heart thumping out of my chest, horrific nightmares. Then I had a panic attack. I tried to meditate, but I felt like I was suffocating. My heart was thumping so hard, I needed to breathe faster. The lid has come off Stewart Watts and I can't contain him. Friday feels like weeks away. Weeks away!

Reflection: How fascinating that I could see this coming reading through the previous entries. My mood was dropping and with each entry I couldn't see why, but reflecting on it, it is so plain to see. If only people could see that.
Friday was the day I saw Jayne.

Notes:

26.11.17
Slept soundly last night, kept really busy today to stop any thoughts, but it's bed-time again and I am panicking.

Reflection: I was doing everything I could to get through to that Friday.

Notes:

27.11.17
Bed time again. Terrified. Police came out to talk to the kids tonight. They will be video interviewed about Alan. I almost cried hearing them talk about how they felt. Now I must also be video interviewed about Jason and Stewart Watts on Wednesday next week. Both of them in one day. Shit…….. When the lid came off with Jack, it really came off. How am I going to get through this? This has probably got to be the worst time of my life. I just want to be free from this pain.

Reflection: It wasn't the worst time of my life, but it was the worst time since I had begun my journal, because so much abuse was being addressed at the same time. Even worse, it was not only me, but my kids too. It was one big melting pot of fire.

Notes:

28.11.17
Little sleep - nightmares.

Reflection: There was nothing else to dream about. It was all happening at once.

Notes:

29.11.17
Surprisingly good day. Bought Christmas presents. I was dreading it, but I did feel better.

Reflection: I've come to recognise those healing days now. I still find it incredible. I hope somebody who is reading this knows why this happens, either on a physiological, or psychological level.

Notes:

30.11.17
Very very anxious. I'm going to be talking about Stewart Watts tomorrow and I get stomach cramps, feel sick and dizzy just thinking about it.

Reflection: I remember this day and in my mind everything that had happened with Stewart was playing out over and over again.

Notes:

01.12.17

So today came at last and I did speak to Jayne about Stewart Watts, but it took me 20 minutes of talking about everything else before I could start. I had to say Stewart little before I could say his name, it was saying the name out loud. It made him a real person and I couldn't cope with his reality. I talked about when we began to have sex and I started to feel sick and my mouth went dry, but I carried on. I continued to talk about being raped and my heart was pounding and my mouth was dry, but I carried on. I talked about the physical pain, the mental torture and I feel really dizzy and sick. I didn't want to talk about it because I didn't know what was going to happen.

I was shaking inside, my legs were trembling. I talked about becoming anorexic to have some control, I talked about abusing alcohol to try to drink myself to death. I exercised to become so thin, so weak that my heart would give out! But it didn't. It never did and I tortured myself for it. I felt so dizzy when I stopped talking, I was shaking so much inside, but I needed to keep my shit together, the session was almost over.

The monster is out! He has been exposed and we talked briefly about me now being in control, me exposing my abusers. I began to feel angry. Angry and determined to destroy that monster, but mixed with that was a very angry monster. The monster trying to remind me that what he did was disgusting, soul destroying and absolutely breaking. Reminding me of my promise.

I've exposed the disgusting, life breaking episode and I need to block it out. Get rid of that disgusting feeling by getting drunk, slashing my arms to scrub out that evil filth. But to do that means damaging myself, reminding myself that the evil, disgusting feeling is still inside me. Still raping me whenever he wants. Reminding me that I'm re living it over and over again. This monster is now angry, so angry that I have exposed him. He wants to teach me a lesson. Teach me that he can make me feel pain, disgusting, smelly and injured, making me feel that I cannot cope with those feelings, those same feelings that made me try to kill myself before. This monster is so angry with me now, he's making me feel that nightmare over and over again. He's trying to destroy me. He's trying to win. I feel so sick, so very very sick.

Reflection: My promise was to commit suicide. I believed that that monster was him, Stewart, but it wasn't and I couldn't see it yet. I know now who that monster is and it was never trying to kill me, but I hadn't made the connection.

Notes:

02.12.17
Tension has been building all day. First having to get dressed before my shower. Feeling sticky and dirty, just like when I was raped. Flashbacks, nausea, irritation building all day. Finally I could go for a shower. I screamed, I cried, I relieved it all in the shower until I was so hot and exhausted. It's not right that I was told I was not special by my mum. It's not right that she told me she wanted a boy, it's not right I tried to find love elsewhere. It's not right Jack sexually assaulted me, it's not right my Cousin took advantage of my sexualised behaviour. It's not fucking right that I was raped twice by two unknown men because I believed that that's what happened and that their behaviour was normal. It's not fucking right that Stewart Watts took advantage of all of that and fucked me so hard I wanted to end my life. And finally it's not fucking right that Alan used my vulnerability to try to destroy me when I was trying to be strong. It's so not fucking right and I can't get my head around it and they all have to pay.
By the end of all this they will all fucking know, but just now I need to scream and cry and wail. And I am so exhausted, so fucking exhausted. Tired of fighting all the time. Tired of repeatedly having to recover from some bastards attempt to destroy me. Tired and so fucking angry. My healed brain will not let the monster silence me anymore. Do you fucking worst with the flashbacks - NO MORE!

Reflection: I had to get dressed before my shower because my kids had nagged and nagged me to put the Christmas lights up outside. I felt angry with them for forcing me to do something I didn't want to do (just like my abusers) and I felt angry for being made to feel like I did after I had been raped. I'd had to dress and have his disgusting ejaculate on my body, pain, bleeding, feeling so dirty, so unclean and my clothes would get sticky and I was reminded all of the time that I had just been raped. I always shower before I get dressed because I can't bare to put clothes on an unclean body. That's my perception and doesn't harm anybody. If I choose not to shower first, then that's my decision, but being forced to get dressed before showering makes me feel physically sick.

Notes:

03.12.17
Didn't really feel anything today. I suppose there is only so much my brain can take.

Reflection: I'm so lucky that my mind did that healing thing when it needed to. Not everybody has that I don't think, otherwise why would there be so many suicides?

Notes:

04.12.17
I've been told by a few people that I come across as cold, distant, or aloof. That makes me feel really sad because that's not me at all. But some days I have to dig deep to get through the day and that's everything I have. I can't remember a time when I wasn't filled with fear, dread and anticipation because of a life filled with flashbacks, sensations and association. I just want people to see me, because I am here amongst the nightmares.

Reflection: I felt so sad and isolated that nobody would approach me and ask me if I was okay. Instead they judged me and that made me feel even more sad and isolated. You're not going to open up to somebody who tells you that you are cold, distant and aloof. I wasn't anyway.

Notes:

05.12.17
Today was a real struggle. Such an effort to do anything. My hands are really dry and tingling. I think I am in denial still as I am not thinking about Stewart, or Jason, but my legs, arms and chest have felt like lead all day and putting one step in front of the other has been so heavy. Work has felt like a marathon. Tonight I was watching television, but biting the inside of my mouth all evening. The extent my emotions are being suppressed is incredible, but they're not surfacing. Tomorrow I fear is going to be a big day.

Reflection: This was the day before I gave my statements to the Police.

Notes:

06.12.17

I am writing this this morning before I go to make my statements. I felt like I couldn't breathe again in the shower, buy my healed part of my brain told me I can and I won't stop breathing. I am so pleased I have a healed part of my brain. Don't know what's going to happen today or what the consequences of that might be, but I do know that I want it out. I want it out so I can give life another go. Another go from a healed mind. Everything that has happened has been from a traumatised mind. Just one last push. I need to get it out irrespective of consequence or outcome.

Following The Statement: I made it out in one piece - just. Still shaking like an old car though. I kept my shit together until I got home and resisted the temptation to call somebody to be rescued from my emotions. I thought I was going to erupt, fall apart, scream hysterically, vomit all over the house. But I had a good cry, whacked the heating up so cosy and warm and had something warm to eat and drink.

It's so, so difficult talking about seven years of disgusting abuse and receiving no emotional response. I could have been talking about anything ordinary. I think that's what's messing with my brain most this afternoon. I half expected the Detective who interviewed me to say what happened to me wasn't rape, because he just responded so normally. Really bizarre.

I need to talk about Stewart a lot now. To pick apart that time in my life, just like I did with Jack. To lay it all out so no little bit is left hiding inside. This might sound bizarre, but to be perfectly honest, I feel like I'm letting the injured me down. I have hung on to Stewart for 21 years now feeling like I've been clinging on to avoid releasing the overpowering emotion.

It was a shit weekend and I cried and screamed in the shower. At times I felt like I couldn't breathe because my chest felt so tight. I could barely talk to the kids, but I didn't vomit, I didn't fain or wet myself. I held my shit together today and although shaking, I didn't cry for long.

I don't understand. He absolutely destroyed me and I had to shut that door down hard to survive, but now I've let it out, I feel like my response is not the same as the destroying impact it had. Why?

Part of me doesn't want to be okay because it wasn't okay and it wasn't okay for so long and it hasn't been okay for 37 years and it almost killed me. I don't understand at the moment.

(Light bulb moment - reading this again). I think what I expected when I let it out was to feel the emotions I felt then. Release the emotions I didn't release then. I did it once back when I was drunk by clearing a table of glasses onto the floor with a huge swipe of my hand. Oh and that felt amazing at the time.

Reflection: Letting my injured self-down. That sounds a bit like survivor guilt. Injured me, as I saw it was so traumatised and suicidal and couldn't cope, but healed me had just delivered a statement that didn't live up to what injured me was feeling, so I felt guilty. Flashbacks and memories are always so much more powerful and violent than the real thing because they come with images and emotions and feelings. It's like 2D and 3D.

If I told somebody I had been punched in the face and it really hurt. That would take the time if took you to read the sentence. That's 2D. If I had a flashback about it. I would see the person who punched me, maybe smell them, have an emotional response towards them. I would feel my fear before I was hit, I would feel the pain as I was hit and the emotions I was feeling and I would feel the pain after I was hit and the emotions I was left with. I would see what I was wearing, what the environment was like, how I was left feeling afterwards. I would see what I looked like and I could play that tape over and over again. That's 3D
One sentence to talk about it, Four sentences to have a flashback about it. Both the same experience. Yes I did feel guilty, but I didn't need to, I just didn't understand it yet.

Notes:

07.12.17
So here's the rub after 3 hours sleep last night. My injured self-wanted to commit suicide. But I don't now. My injured self-wanted to be rescued, held and cuddled after being raped, but I'm not being raped now. My injured self-wanted to tell people I have been destroyed, but I don't want to destroy myself now. My injured self wants to do all those things again to let people know I am destroyed because I didn't back then. I want all those things to happen now and make injured me back then better.
Injured me wanted to die. Injured me broke. Injured me did die and all that was left was a shell. And I survived and I feel so guilty for surviving because injured me needed to die and I'm not giving injured me any justice. I was terrified for all those years that if I faced what Jack did, Jason did, the man in the part, Stewart, Carl. If I faced all of that I would become suicidal. I would want to end my life, because injured me so desperately needed it all to end. I'm fighting an emotional battle in my mind. I'm desperate for this pain to stop.

Reflection: And the pain would have gotten a lot easier a lot quicker had I understood who 'injured me was'.

Notes:

08.12.17
I slept so badly last night, I woke having a panic attack. But I didn't panic because I knew what was happening. I just felt very tearful and shattered. I saw Jayne today and I tried to explain how I feel and what's going on in my mind and she drew me this diagram.

Here is how I understand it.

Healed me Injured me

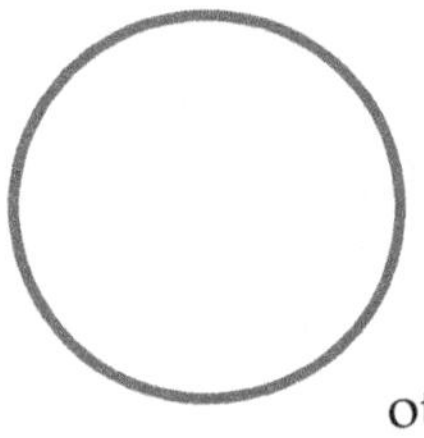

1.  Battling for power, but not connecting with each other. Suppressed emotions.

HM **IM**

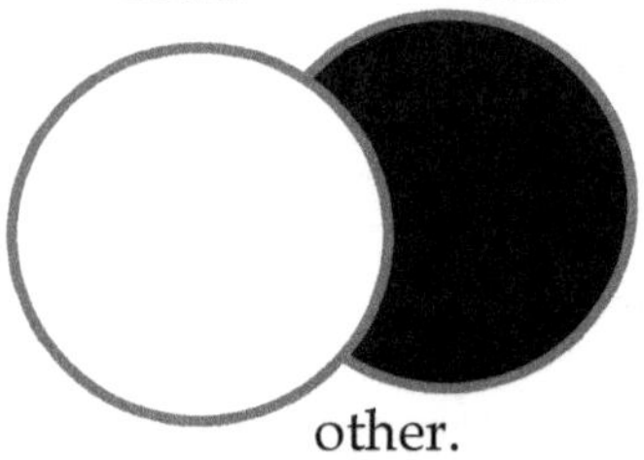

2. Trying hard to understand each other or even overpower each other.

Exposed. Emotions.

Whole Me

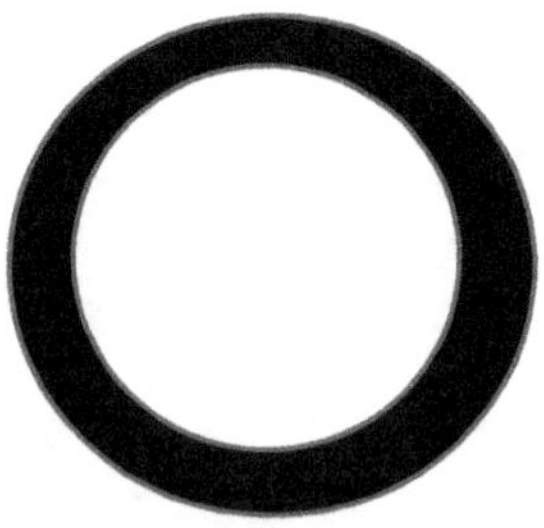

3. Accepting/Coming to terms with each other. Becoming whole, becoming one.

Before I exposed Stewart I was at diagram number 1. Now I have exposed Stewart, I am sitting here in number 2. Injured me is throwing a tantrum, screaming and shouting and demanding to be heard. Healed me is terrified of this tantrum. It's so strong, so powerful it wants me to self harm, it wants me to show it how injured it is, to injure myself to show it I understand how injured it its. My healed mind is trying hard to remain resolute. I know it would be the wrong thing to do to cut myself, to give in to the powerful tantrum, but it's so hard.

The healed me is so small and new and the injured me is so strong and loud and shouting and wants to be heard. It's screaming at me to listen, it's screaming at me to hurt myself so I can show injured me I understand how painful it is, so I can show injured me I understand how much it hurts. Injured me wants me to get drunk so I don't care, so my resistance is low, then I will self harm. I will cut myself so much, shred my arm to pieces just to satisfy injured me. To show injured me I know, I feel how painful it is. I told Jayne I needed her to know that this ferocious battle is going on in my brain and I'm trying so hard to stay strong, but injured me has been around for so long, that she is so very, very powerful and it is taking everything I have to stay strong. I just needed her to know it is taking everything I have got. Every ounce of strength. And she listened to me. She really listened to injured me telling her what I want to do and healed me telling her I am desperately trying not to give in. Trying to stay strong. She listened to all of me, accepted both of me. I left my appointment when we'd ended the session and went back to work. Injured me had to be quiet now.

A short while later I had to go out in my car, but I sat in my car and started thinking again, dreaming. Injured me is shrunk down and I am standing bigger, hands on hips, not shouting, but firm and saying to injured me *"What to you want? What do you want?"* Injured me is staring back, shocked, letting out little sobs. I continue to talk to injured me. *"I am not going to hurt myself, I am not going to self harm, I am not going to kill myself, I just won't! So what do you want? I've looked after you, protected you and kept you safe for 21 years, so what do you want?"* And there are little sobs and arms reach up for a hug. Such a sad, sad face reaching up for a hug, with sad tears and sad eyes and I reach out and I hug little me and I become whole. And that image played out in front of me over and over again and I cried and I cried every time the arms came up. Oh how I have cried today.

Then reality dawns on me. Oh my God! If I'd have tried to open this up without any healed brain I would have been absolutely demolished. I would have been utterly destroyed. I wouldn't have survived. Not with the power that injured me has. All injured me wants is to be heard, to be allowed to express every feeling and emotion and then be hugged. To cry and cry and cry whilst being hugged. Now that's what being truly accepted really means. That's having all those sad, devastating memories fully acknowledged, understood and accepted. That's what being listened to means. That's what being able to be me means. Such an overwhelming day today and so much hard work to do to keep injured me loved and safe, not ignored and pushed away. What a day!

Reflection: Every time I read that entry I cry. All the time I had sui, I had injured me, I had the monster. And all the time it was just me. All the time I was saying sorry and I was saying it into the darkness, I was saying sorry to me. I was recognising little me, the child that was me that had never been hugged, listened to, or cared for. All that time it was me. All that time I felt empty inside, it was because I hadn't seen me. All those tears crying to be heard and to be listened to and I was there all along, just waiting to be acknowledged. This has to be the most powerful entry of the whole journal.

Notes:

09.12.17
Very emotional today. I didn't suppress any emotions, some of it felt scary, but they all passed. I got angry at one point with the kids, but it passed. I got tearful at one point watching television and it passed. The tearful emotion was very loaded. Tearful about being rejected by my Mum. Tearful for never having that unconditional love, but the surge of emotion passed. I imagine this is going to be an emotional time. I need my friends.

Reflection: I had become whole and all that was happening was the whole of me was now grieving. There was no longer two minds, there was one complete mind that had joined at last. A bit like a group hug of tears.

Notes:

10.12.17
Still not sleeping great. Having nightmares, but not remembering what they were about. Just waking up trembling, I don't know why. Then during the day I feel like I don't know myself. Uncertain, like the stabilisers have been taken off my bike. I still dread going to bed. This is such hard work.

Reflection: Not remembering nightmares, this had happened before. Stewart was not going to go quietly.

Notes:

11.12.17

Woke up at 4m again today. Tried to hang on to my dream. I asked myself "*Why am I shaking?*" Then the answer came back "*Because you told.*" Emotional day, so spoke to a colleague about how I am feeling and it helped for a while. Until bed time again. I dread this time.

Reflection: This was about fear, about consequence. I didn't know what the consequence of exposing Stewart and Jason would be. Jason after all was my Cousin. Stewart, I didn't know anything about and that scared me, just like it did when I first reported Jack and I was anxious about the consequences.

Notes:

12.12.17
So it was 5am this morning. I'm so exhausted, I just need some time to sit with my thoughts.

Reflection: This was a time thing, it happened with Jack, it was happening again.

Notes:

13.12.17
I'm exhausted. And I think I'm doing okay, then somebody asks me how I am and I feel like I am going to cry. I just want to talk.

Reflection: I wanted to get it out, I felt like although I was talking about Stewart, it was too big to be aired only once. It felt like pressure inside of me.

Notes:

14.12.17
I feel like I'm drowning. I'm having panic attacks, I can deal with that. Nightmares won't stop and I just need to talk and talk and talk and cry until I can't cry anymore, but I have to keep a lid on it because I have to carry on, but it's just so big. This was always going to be just too big. Help somebody please, I just want somebody to be with me, I can't do this on my own. I just want to get drunk and fall apart with somebody.

Reflection: I couldn't come to terms with what Stewart had done to me, I never had. I couldn't comprehend that I had been so violated and destroyed and stayed alive.

Notes:

15.12.17
I had no sleep last night. The urge to self-harm is unbearably strong. So strong I'm terrified I won't be able to resist. I googled shit on my 'phone last night just to distract myself. I talked to Jayne today. I tried to explain that my injured self wants me to do it. I hugged her last week (my injured self), loved her, cared for her, but she wants more. She wants me to let her know how destroyed she is. If I self-harm I'm showing her I truly understand how damaged she is because of what Stewart put her through. He crushed her soul, she needs me to show her I understand that. Oh God, it is so powerful! We talked about directing the pain, the focus at Stewart, not me. I don't want to hurt me, I don't deserve to hurt me, but she just wants me to show her I really, really get it. Lack of sleep and a powerful force is almost unbearable to resist. I talked to a friend by messaging last night and the flashbacks came flooding in.
Being pinned down, having my legs forced apart and having a penis rammed inside me so hard I can't breathe. Being held so I can't move, or try to move to somehow make it less painful. It is the worst experience ever to have to live thought, not only once, but over and over again. And now to relive it through flashbacks over and over again makes me terrified to close my eyes. I have lived this real time and it almost killed me and now I am reliving it again, over and over and it's killing me all over again. I don't know how to make it stop and I'm broken all over again.

Reflection: Sleep deprivation really damaged my resolve. Everything I understood about not self-harming, becoming whole. I couldn't hold on to it when I was so down. Loneliness and isolation were making everything so difficult. I had never been able to talk whenever I needed to. I had either been silenced, or gagged, or only given permission to talk about certain things. When I was in Court I was told I wasn't allowed to talk about Sarah-Jayne and they wouldn't discuss my mental health. Nobody asked me about that. I was fully prepared to have my mental health discussed in Court and yes I did want to talk about Sarah-Jayne. I felt gagged. Even though I had given my evidence, I still hadn't been allowed to talk about it all. It was a game, the whole Court experience had been a sick game and I was a pawn.

Notes:

16.12.17
I managed to have 6 hours sleep last night, with shaking inside. It's been a busy day and we went to a Christmas Party at my Dads Care home and I just wanted to cry. I just wanted to talk to somebody. I don't want to do this on my own. Why do I have to do this alone? I wish I had somebody, I'm so lonely, so very lonely.

Reflection: I remember this day. Christmas music, decorations, Santa. I just wanted to sit with somebody quietly and tell them how sad I was and the music and jollity made me feel even more sad and alone. I wanted to tell somebody what I was going through and just weep whilst somebody held my hand.

Notes:

17.12.17
This is the content of an email that I sent to Jayne tonight:

Developing some clarity: I really wish I was sat next to you now having this chat. I'm calm and I'm back in the room. Thursday night before I saw you was one of the most difficult nights I have had. The urge to self-harm was unbelievably strong and I was in such a state of panic. I can't articulate how all-consuming that night was, but I am really going to try to from now on and I am going to try to explain.

On Saturday night (last night) the police came out to talk to my Son Sam. The Police Officer asked Sam how he was feeling and what he was thinking. Sam was just nervously laughing and I became so frustrated. I told him that it is absolutely fine to say exactly how he is feeling and what he is thinking, even if it is not okay to carry those thoughts and feelings out. The Police Officer told Sam he agreed with me and re-iterated the point and Sam then opened right up. Suddenly I had another light-bulb moment.

I have been plagued by flashbacks, thoughts, feelings and sensations and have been battling so hard not to act upon, at times incredibly overpowering urges to self-harm. What I have been doing is desperately trying to deny the thoughts. Thoughts of self-harm come, I try to distract myself from them, but the emotions take over. Thoughts of suicide, again I try to distract myself , but the emotions take over. Flashbacks the same. Last night I realised how if I deny the thoughts, can I expect the emotions to go away? That doesn't make any sense. I have been reading about flashbacks and I only found one piece that actually stated firstly that resorting to drugs and alcohol to cope actually prolongs the trauma. Well for me that put things right into perspective.

Also trying to ignore, or push away flashbacks is likely to make them stronger and more powerful as they fight for recognition. This actually made a lot of sense to me. We have spoken a lot about being congruent and I have felt really good about achieving this, but then as soon as I am faced with an emotionally charged challenge, I resort right back to trying to deny the thoughts, thinking that just because I anticipate them I can control them and then I want to know how long it will be before the feelings go away. When am I ever going to learn?

I was also messaging a friend and talking about how I felt and I sent her this (which probably didn't help her at all), but this is what I said. *"Being pinned down, having my legs forced apart and having a penis rammed inside me so hard I cannot breathe. Being held so I can't move or try to move to somehow make it less painful. Fucking hell, this is the worst experience ever to have to live through over and over again, both at the time and now. So much so that I am terrified to close my eyes. No wonder my heart is thumping out of my chest and I feel so sick, I'm constantly trying to get away"*.

That said everything that just saying I'm having flashbacks, didn't say, but instead it got it right out. After I sent that message I felt incredibly tired and I slept for 6 solid hours. I talk about flashbacks and try to deny them, but it's the detail I have to talk about. Really expose exactly what I am feeling, exactly what is going on in my mind. When I can do that it's no longer this massive pressure in my mind going over and over again. I do want to talk about it over and over again, to get it out to expose it. It's disgusting, it's dirty and it's sick, but I can't live with it in my head and I understand now that there is nothing wrong with exposing it. After all why shouldn't I? I have to. I have to talk about everything, not just the feelings.

I really hope you are going to be able to cope with this, not because I doubt you at all, or ever have, but because it is horrific, disgusting and depraved – at least for me and I am just trying to be considerate. I am trying so hard to be able to learn, to come to terms with this, but I think I understand now what I need to do.

A couple of years ago I called the Samaritans because I was really struggling and the person on the 'phone said that if I had been sexually abused just three weeks ago I would 't be expected to come to terms with it. So only talking about it a few weeks ago is exactly the same and should be given the same consideration. I remembered this also today and realised I have already done this with Jack, now I need to do it with Stewart.

Another couple of changes I need to make: Not writing in my journal just before I go to sleep. How can I expose all that emotion and then expect to have a peaceful sleep? Also trying not to leave it until bedtime to e-mail you, for the same reason, although this has more to do with having time to myself.

In relation to my Cousin, there is no denial here, but I just want to concentrate on one thing at a time and I have very difficult emotions about both. With my Cousin there is massive feelings of guilt, betrayal and abandonment, but I will be ready to talk about him afterwards.

Jayne, this is the hardest thing I am ever going to have to do. Nothing has ever threatened my life like this, but I know I have to clear it out, or it will never stop haunting me. If ever I needed your support, it's right now because I am going to expose everything and as long as I can do it slowly and thoroughly then I am ready to let it go, but at the same time I am feeling really, really vulnerable. I hope this is okay because I am really opening myself up to this and I just wanted you to know that I feel like I have some clarity. I am really trying so hard and I know I can't do it on my own and I know it's going to be really difficult. I feel even this new insight is a step forward, but I'm not celebrating like last week, I've certainly learned that lesson.
Thank you so much for your support.

Reflection: It kind of goes back to the 2D, 3D analogy I made earlier. Yes, saying I am having flashbacks about being raped, does not describe what I am feeling. I didn't have the same insight then, but I did recognise that I needed to pick the bones apart in order to come to terms with it and in order for the flashbacks to stop owning me, which at that time I really felt they did. I was at their mercy every single night.

Notes:

18.12.17
I feel slightly removed today, flat, lost desperately lonely. Sara came over for an hour and I talked about the message I sent her and said I was worried that I had exposed too much. She was amazing, she totally understands and encouraged me to keep going. I love Sara, to me she is a soul mate. She really is very, very special.

Reflection: And yet she wasn't. But that wasn't my fault. Sara let me down in the biggest way a friend could. I trusted her implicitly and that wasn't my fault. She actually wasn't particularly special at all. She was interested in me whilst my trauma served a purpose to help her feel better. Once that was no longer the case, she dropped me like a stone. Now I can't blame her for that, because before I had been able to face my trauma, I would associate with people who had been through trauma. Just so I could glean anything that would help me to understand why I felt the way I did. Or simply to not feel so alone with what I was feeling. I think I had started to recover in a way that she could no longer relate to. I'm sad that I lost her friendship, but I was honest with her, unfortunately she did not afford me the same respect.

Notes:

19.12.17
Oh dear God please help me. I can't do this, I'm so broken.

Reflection: Where was my mind healing day when I needed it?

Notes:

20.12.17

This morning, I have absolutely vivid images in my head of cutting and I am getting a rush just thinking about it, so much so my arms are aching. I have period pains because the images of being fucked so hard are so real that I can actually feel it. This afternoon I get Official confirmation that Alan, the perpetrator who abused my kids, is not proceeding with Court Action. It took a while, but the relief inside is huge and I feel like I can breathe. I want to celebrate with a drink, but of course I can't because if I do I will rip my arms to shreds. But for the first time since July 2016, when Jack was charged with two counts of sexual assault on a child under 13, I am not facing a looming dread. Seventeen months of dreaded anticipation. Now that deserves to be celebrated.

I am climbing to the top of the mountain and I am getting whiffs of pure air and then the images remind me and my stomach clenches again.

Reflection: The relief that my children were not going to be forced to be abused, was immeasurable. Being forced to do anything only ever brought flashbacks of being raped. The urge to self-harm was being waged against that pure air, that light, clean feeling that was creeping in and taking control.

Notes:

21.12.17
Today I spoke to my UAVA worker about Alan and she doesn't feel he will come back to the house. I will take that.

Reflection: I took any crumb of comfort at that time. I would have done anything that anybody would have suggested to make me feel better, or safer. I was very vulnerable and very fortunate to now only have supportive people around me.

Notes:

22.12.17
I spoke to Jayne today, I have no choice but to ride out the flashbacks. So the whole time I'm talking to her I have images of Stewart forcing me to perform oral sex, lowering himself over my face. If I didn't put his penis in my mouth I wouldn't have been able to breathe. Oh the smell, the awful smell. As soon as his penis swelled I would remove it and he would ejaculate all over me. God, the smell, it makes me feel so sick.

We talked about my son's and how they are both angry and having nowhere to vent their anger, so it manifests in other ways. One Son experiencing physical pain, another constantly re traumatising himself by going past the place he experienced the trauma and getting angry all over again. All three of us are stuck, but Jayne noticed I showed empathy for my Sons struggle and asked me where do I show myself any empathy. It really made me think. She told me the flashbacks will begin to lose their power and she told me I am much stronger than they are. I felt like she'd given me a death sentence. Especially as the afternoon was spent in the same place I have been video interviewed.

I took us all out for dinner tonight and we did have a good time. I loved seeing my kids happy and that made me happy.

Reflection: I felt like she'd given me a death sentence because I was still experiencing emotional pain and I believed her when she told me I was much stronger than the flashbacks. But, I hadn't made my mind up yet that I was never going to self-harm, or even commit suicide. I'd walked away from it and I'd begun to develop coping strategies, but I wasn't ready to dismiss them.
I spent the afternoon in the same building as I'd been in earlier that month making my statements about Stewart and Jason. My Son's were making their statements about Alan. It all came back to me and I felt like a victim all over again. If somebody had come and asked me if I wanted to talk, I would have done it all again. I wanted to be cared for, I wanted to be looked after. I wanted somebody to feel sorry for me.

Notes:

23.12.17
I fell asleep so quickly last night, but then the dog woke me up barking and I couldn't get back to sleep and the flashbacks started. I'm not brave, I'm not strong, I would do anything to take them away, but I have to keep keeping myself safe. I hate this, I hate it so much it's torture.

Reflection: The flashbacks were there because I was afraid. I was very afraid of confronting them. It felt like they were tormenting me.

Notes:

24.12.17
I woke up at 6am screaming because I was being raped. That burning sensation, like scraping off sand when it's stuck to wet feet. I woke myself up shouting *"no"*. Shouting *"I am going to tell Jayne"*. He stopped and stared at me.

Old friends came over this afternoon and were sharing 60 years of memories, of good times. I enjoyed listening, loved their company and it also made me want to cry. I am 48 years old and I have no span of happy memories. Yes good things have happened, but every event in my life has been tainted or had an association. Even waking up this morning. I went to bed thinking I would e-mail Jayne, but I didn't, I fell asleep. I just didn't want to experience that bad feeling on my own.

Reflection: Whenever I hear people reminisce about the past it provokes mixed feelings. I love hearing people tell stories and share experiences, but once I've heard them, I feel incredibly sad because I know I will never have those stories, or experiences to share. My stories have to stay locked away from people, I have nothing to say. I miss being able to talk to my children about my childhood, because the childhood I had is not one to be shared in that way. I dream of a childhood I wanted. I feel such loss.

Notes:

25.12.17
Five solid hours sleep. Absolutely shattered. But I did it again and the kids had a great Christmas.

Reflection: I did it again, meaning I made it so special and they were so excited. I have always wanted to love Christmas, but it's always held an association. Stewart raped me on Christmas Eve and then he videoed my behaviour on Christmas Day. I was devastated and he knew it and he caught it all on video. It was like the first time somebody is aware that they have done something wrong. That Christmas Eve was the first time that I had I told him to stop and he had completely ignored me. I cried and I told him he was hurting me and he ignored me. He ignored me and he raped me. It was every time after that.
Christmas time was when Jack sexually abused me and I had to pretend to be happy because everybody else was and I was dying inside. December always held that underlying sense of dread.
Christmas time was when Alan complained about my Birthday being so close to Christmas and always told me how difficult it was for him.
I stopped enjoying Christmas and my Birthday when I was 10 years old and I have been reminded of it every year since.

Notes:

26.12.17
I woke this morning after over 10 hours solid sleep. I had an amazing dream, every worry and anxiety I had somebody was saying to me *"You don't have to worry about that anymore."* It was bizarre, I couldn't work out if it was a male or female voice, but everything I said, work, Jack, Alan, Stewart, Jason, Flashbacks, friends. Every time I said *"What about this?"* the voice told me I don't need to worry about it anymore. I felt so peaceful when I woke Up. I felt guilty for being on edge with the kids, but I accepted that that's how I feel and I loved them all the more. I had no flashbacks to-day, no pangs of sadness. It was a good day, I think.

Reflection: The healing thing again.

Notes:

27.12.17
Absolutely shattered because my Son was up all night vomiting. I so loved that fresh feeling yesterday. I want it again.

Reflection: Inspite of what might have been going on in my mind, life carried on and had to be dealt with.

Notes:

28.12.17
Back at work today, tired, but I slept well. I fell asleep on the settee after work watching television with the kids. I felt so relaxed.

Reflection: I always felt safe around the kids. There was something about their implicit trust in me that made me feel safe.

Notes:

29.12.17
I spoke to Jayne today. I told her about my nightmare on Christmas Eve. I told her when I screamed at him to stop it, it wasn't me he had been raping it was the actors Kim and Vincent from EastEnders. They just stared at me, then told me they were just re-enacting what had happened. I told them no more and they just looked at me shocked by my outburst. I haven't had a flashback since. Sometimes I get the image of Kim and Vincent looking at me with that shocked look. I have reflected on this a lot. At first the memories were horrifying flashbacks, but then I think the flashbacks became more of a torment. A nasty deliberate reminder.

Jayne had reminded me last week that memories are not as strong as the actual event. They may be awful and really upsetting and frightening, but they are memories of a time gone by and not me now. That really made me stop and think. A memory can't hurt me. A memory isn't raping me. I have the physical response and feel as if I am experiencing the real physical pain, but I'm not. It is impossible for it to have more power than me, because as much as it feels real now, it isn't real now. I think me screaming at it to stop, is me putting it in it's place. Yes I have to come to terms with what happened, not to relive the trauma over and over again. I have done that this last few weeks. Now it's time to come to terms with it to move on from it, learn to let it become part of the past and not the continued part of the present, or even future.

Another insight I have developed is in relation to friendships. I have had little else to talk about since July 2015, other than the abuse I have suffered. A part of my relationship with friends has been because I needed to vent, to offload, because it was all too overwhelming for me to contain myself. Another part of my relationship with friends was to disclose as explicitly as possible to seek validation for just how destructive the abuse was and to articulate how broken I had become. The problem with that I now recognise is, not all friends will validate, some will only validate my feelings once or twice, some will avoid me because there is nothing else and by seeking validation from friends, I am not actually accepting, or considering exactly how I feel. I am relying on others to do it for me. So now it's time I did!

I have been hurt, I have been violated, I have had my heart ripped out and my mind, body and soul destroyed. Poor fucking me!! Poor, poor, hurt, scared, anxious, frightened and injured me. I deserve to love me unconditionally. I have been seeking unconditional love all my life. I had it with my Sister, she died. I believed I had it with Jack and Emily and he sexually abused me. I wanted it with Stewart and he sexually, physically and emotionally abused me and I wanted it with Alan and he abused me. And all the time unconditional love has been right here inside me. Because all these people rejected me and abused me, (with the exception of my Sister). When I was hurt I rejected and abused me. I have spent years wanting to be accepted unconditionally, yet I have never done it to myself. Well, no more. I have an inner voice and it's me who wants to take care of and love me unconditionally.
That poor voice has been gagged, abused, had vengeful anger directed at it. What have I done to myself? The only person who has ever wanted to love me, is me and I

have so violently abused me through self-destructive behaviour. The answer has been right in front of my eyes the whole time and it has taken until now. Of course I want unconditional love from somebody, who doesn't? but if I love myself unconditionally, then nobody can destroy me ever again. I don't need anybody else to validate my feelings anymore. I am me! And I am loved! And I am damn good enough just exactly how I am.

I need help, I need guidance to figure all this past behaviour out, but I need it to help me move forward. I listened to my friends talking about their life and ventures and I looked at my Mum, the same age, so full of self-pity and misery and I am resolute that I am not going to become her. I believe I have about as many years left as I have lived and I am going to make those years my life to live, my way, with all my love.

Reflection: The friends I am referring to were the friends who came over on Christmas Eve and reminisced about the past. They are the same age as my Mum and Dad. When they were there they talked about difficult times in their past as well as good, but they had their own self-respect and they had their love towards each other. My Mum has had all of that and rejected it, opting for a life of anger, misery and self-pity. I choose not to be that person. I choose to grab life by the balls and live it every single day. Inspiration comes from many different people and they don't even know they are doing it.

Notes:

30.12.17
I really don't recognise myself at the moment. Today my plan was food shopping, clean the house, so it's all fresh for new year. But Elizabeth had other ideas and decided to vomit all day. But instead of worrying and stressing about what I wanted to do, I accepted how the day was going to be. I cuddled up with her after I'd ironed and we spent the day together watching films. And I loved it. Really loved it. I accepted in the moment and allowed everything else to disappear. No worry, no stress, no nothing.

About 9pm my Mum turned up and moaned and moaned about just about everything and it didn't touch me. I wanted to have a bath and I couldn't in the end it was too late. But again I didn't stress, I didn't worry. I think I really do love myself. Before this, I thought loving myself meant external displays. Shaving my legs, or putting nail polish on, physically making myself feel nice and clean. And of course those things are lovely to do. But when self-love and peace are within, then when those things can't happen, it doesn't taint how I am feeling about myself. I feel like I can breathe properly for the first time.

Reflection: A reflective account that really shows how far I have come.

Notes:

31.12.17
Today was a lovely filled day. I took the kids, my Mum and Penny our dog to Liverpool. We went to the Albert Dock, took a ferry across the Mersey, saw my Auntie and Uncle and his boys. We came back later to the Albert Dock to celebrate New Year. It was a day filled with loveliness.

I still see Jack when I see a bald man, but it troubles me much less and I don't panic anymore. I accept it and the images and he's forgotten. Elizabeth and I also nipped into the Everton Store and I am keen to go back tomorrow.

Reflection: I am from the North West and have never lived in Liverpool, but when I go back there, I feel like I really belong. It's the only place I have ever felt that I belong. It feels like home, even though it never has been. I have a strong pull towards Liverpool.

Notes:

01.01.18
Am I glad to see the end of that year. I haven't looked at New year as New starts of years, I always thought it was a cliché, but I feel so differently. New Year, New week. Even a new me. We did go back to the Everton Store and I bought a few bits. I don't know why I really needed to be there. When we got home I laid it all out on my bed and then it hit me. Everton is a connection I have with my Dad and I felt a wave of grief flood over me, because although he is still here, he has gone. And those few little pieces I bought mean so much to me, because I feel near him. We were never really close, but we talked about Everton. I feel like parts of my brain are really opening up.

Reflection: My emotional connections were getting stronger. I had never had a very close relationship with my Dad. When I was growing up I hated him because my Mother used to tell me all sorts of horror stories about him. He never supported me emotionally, but he was there for every practical problem I had. He apologised for my unhappy upbringing too, where my Mother made it all about her and my rejection of her. I made peace with my Dad in my early 20's and we had a kind of understanding. When he developed Alzheimer's I cried, because I knew I was losing him. When he went into care I cried, because I knew he was deteriorating. Perhaps going to Liverpool made me feel close to him because he loved it. He loved Everton and he loved Liverpool people. My Dad only ever wanted to be happy. He never initiated a fight, but he never walked away from one. I was glad I was finally connecting with my Dad within myself.

Notes:

02.01.18
Another 12 hour sleep. Probably because of little sleep the night before. It was so noisy in a City Centre Hotel. Only to be expected on New Year's Eve. I had no anxiety about sleeping late. We went food shopping, went to the park with Charlie and Elizabeth and played football, then came home and had a lovely roast dinner and watched television together. I heard from Sara today' No anxiety or negative thoughts, just purely relaxed and enjoying my time off work.

Reflection: I really felt like I was bonding with my children. I had always loved them, but this was much deeper. We were all really getting to know each other, when I saw things in my kids that I hadn't seen before. Experiencing my own emotions, helped me to see the emotions in my children. How they really felt about things, how they all responded differently to things. I was really beginning to read them and it made me realise how much I had missed.

Notes:

03.01.18
Another good day, feeling relaxed and taking good care of myself.

Reflection: The good days were becoming more frequent.

Notes:

04.01.18
Felt really unwell today. I didn't sleep. Another crushing headache, but I took care of myself. I had a call tonight from a friend. She asked me about Court and Jack and I listened whilst she told me how I should feel. And I felt nothing, no pressure to agree and no desire to talk about it at any length. I accept that I feel how I feel and that is perfectly okay. I felt sad and reflective after the 'phone call, but I am sitting with that. Sad that since I have made a statement about Stewart and the rape and Jason and attempted rape. All the abuse makes me feel really, really sad. But I am not fighting it. I didn't want to talk about it because I am allowed to feel sad, so desperately sad.

Reflection: I didn't want to talk about it because I owned it. I owned how I felt and I no longer needed that validation. I felt appropriately sad, not panicked, or anxious because I had been told how I should feel. Perhaps that's where a lot of panic and anxiety came from. Not feeling how other people expected me to feel. So I felt wrong, abnormal, or different. Nobody wants to feel like an outcast and it causes anxiety when I do. I did not feel like that that night and it was good.

Notes:

05.01.2018

I slept really well last night, my headache gone. I saw Jayne today, we talked about the week, the positives, then towards the end we began to talk about relationships. I talked about how I feel betrayed by Jason. That lead on to talking about the mistakes I have made. I thought I was loved unconditionally when I was small, a young child. My Sister loved me unconditionally, then she died. I believed my Mum loved me unconditionally, but she made it clear after my Sister died that I was nothing special. Nothing could be clearer than actually telling me.

I loved Jack and Emily and Sarah-Jayne, but Jack betrayed my trust and sexually abused me. I loved Jason, I was prepared to have sex with him and because of that he later sexually abused me and Stewart who showed caring and kindness, just so I would disclose the sexual abuse, then he used that to betray me. And then Alan, who just saw my vulnerability to betray my trust. I have made such massive mistakes and I see a sexual act as a way of getting people to love me unconditionally. I have sold my soul to be loved unconditionally and now I think that's my worth.

Today, talking to Jayne I realised that it's not. I have been used for sex and without realising it, I have come to believe that sex equals being liked, being accepted. And now I know that it was all wrong. I believed sex made me wanted. Because sex is all anybody has wanted and now I feel so stupid and I have no internal voice telling me it's okay, because having it pointed out to me today makes me feel so, so stupid and utterly disgusting.

Reflection: Self-blame was still not that far away. Coming to terms with what has happened to me didn't just come in one wave. There were a series of waves, each one layering the other to help me to understand on every level why being sexually abused was not my fault. Some of those layers were there, but not all. Sometimes insight gave me another layer of understanding, but sometimes like this day it gave me grief and heartache.

Notes:

06.01.18
According to my Son I was shouting in my sleep last night. Today my heart felt light and it was yet another good day, but in between and having thoughts to myself I have been trying to understand. Trying to make sense of the fact that receiving comfort and love, listening and understanding is not paid for with sex. Is Jayne trying to tell me that that is not normal? I don't have to return the favour with sexual favours. Is that really the price I am paying. I've been so vulnerable, so low, so lost. Such low self-esteem, self-worth. My head is spinning, trying to make sense of this. I don't have to repay kindness with sex? I don't have to have sex to be listened to? But it does and it always has and it's all I know and now I'm being told that's not how it has to be.

I knew it, I knew it was starting to feel wrong. Only agreeing to talk to me if there was sex in return. Jayne has no idea what she has said. I have been so worthless. I feel so stupid. I feel so disgusting and so, so stupid. To use and exploit a vulnerable person for sex is disgusting, to allow it to happen is disgusting. How could I not know? How could I let it happen. How can somebody do that? Sexual favours in return for being made to feel loved. For fucks sake, what the fuck have I done to myself. I have always been used for somebody else's satisfaction and I have allowed it.

Reflection: What had happened was the day before we had been talking about relationships. Jayne had said that not everything has to end in sex. The conversation continued, but in that second my head stopped and I don't remember anything we talked about after that. I was too busy trying to comprehend that not everything has to end in sex. I was thinking she must be wrong, she must have this wrong. Everybody who has come into my life has used me for sex. Surely this is what sex is all about. Melvyn had been a friend and he had been a listening ear in return for sex and I thought it was my duty to provide that. I had been nothing more than a prostitute to him. I believed that because he was kind to me, I had to return the favour with sex. He kissed me, he fondled me, he had sex with me. I had to return the favour. If I wanted to speak to him and I didn't want sex, then it didn't happen. How could I have been so blind? When Jayne had pointed it out to me I felt sick. I had been 26years old and he was 42years old. That was a big blow to me and I felt absolute revulsion for myself and disgust at him and my head was spinning all over the place. It was so obvious, it had to be wrong.

Notes:

07.01.18
Still sleeping really well. But thinking about this during moments alone. I remember a time when he wanted to share me with his friend. He wanted me to come on to his friend for his entertainment and I was purely terrified. He thought it was funny and I was about to cry. All I could think of was I was going to be raped. I kept saying I don't want to, I don't want to, but he persisted and I was terrified, I was shaking. And all I felt when he backed down was relief and gratitude that he wasn't going to make me have sex with his friend. And I was so grateful that he didn't make me do it.

Today I am angry, so angry. Angry that he treated me like a piece of rubbish. Angry that all I felt was gratitude for him not making me do it. Absolute shock that I even entertained the notion that this behaviour was normal. Absolute disbelief that I had no concept at all that any of this was wrong before I spoke to Jayne on Friday. And now I can see it, it's so obvious, so fucking obvious that I feel only horror, disgust and so mind blowingly stupid. I have never been loved unconditionally. I have been used for sex. I have been so vulnerable, so damaged and he is such a clever person and I had absolutely no concept at all that it was wrong, because I was so grateful to be receiving love. Now I look back and all the time I was being used. He was playing on my vulnerability, my damaged, destroyed self and all the time I was just grateful for the attention.

I hate sex, I have always hated sex. It has always been used as a weapon, a bargaining tool, a payment. Please love me and I will suck your dick please love me and you can fuck me because I am grateful that you love me. I can't believe I didn't see it. I feel in shock! Everything I believed to be real is not real at all. This has hit me so hard, like a punch in the stomach. None of it was normal, none of it was right. My mind is spinning that wheel again, trying to land on an answer. No self-worth = no self-esteem = exploitation and no fucking insight! Absolutely unforgivable. I keep shaking, I feel dizzy, not like a panic attack, just shear disbelief. I feel like I can't breathe. Fucking hell I am so fucking damaged. I knew it felt wrong, but I didn't know why. I knew I wanted to stay away, but I didn't know why. Now I know why, it's so fucking obvious, but that sudden realisation did not come gently. It's smacked me so hard, I can't take it in. I'm trying to, but I just start panicking, my heart is thumping so hard. I can't take it in.

Reflection: I think that was the biggest betrayal. Somebody who knew I was so vulnerable, knew I could be manipulated. I was destroyed all over again. I didn't know who I could trust.

Notes:

08.01.18
Slept well again last night. I e-mailed Jayne my diary entry last night and kept reading it over and over again. Trying to figure out that somehow I must be wrong, but the more I am reading it, the more I can see it for what it was and the more humiliated I feel, totally degraded. My God I had no self-respect. I've been used all my life, I've been used. This is so powerful.

Reflection: Interestingly it wasn't affecting my sleep. This was a different enlightenment. It was a clarity, a real moment of truth. So shockingly eye opening and a massive relief. I didn't feel it right then, but as disgusted and used as I felt I knew I would never have to give myself for anybody ever again.

Notes:

09.01.18
The majority of my life I have made some catastrophic mistakes, or have I? I started off today full of self-loathing, full of self-hatred. Questions going round and round in my head. How could I let myself do those things? How could I not know it was wrong? How stupid and humiliated do I feel now I know it was wrong. Wrangling round and round in my head all day. My head has felt so tight, like it was being gripped in a vice. That wheel constantly spinning, trying to help me to understand, but always coming up with the same answer. I read a lot to try to understand what is going on in my head, to help me to understand what I am experiencing.

Tonight I read about vulnerability. The vulnerability that describes when you are open about yourself. There were various examples, but the one that stuck with me was when you expose your vulnerability (your real self) people will often warm to you because of your openness. However, what people respond to even more is when you are vulnerable and somebody judges you, or tries to manipulate you, but you are solid in your own boundaries and confidence in yourself, that you are able to dismiss them along with their judgements and values because you uphold you own and have the confidence to do so. I read this several times as I felt the tension begin to drain out of my head. I don't need to be angry at myself for any of this. I had no insight. I really had no insight. I have nothing to apologise for. I don't ever need to apologise for any of my behaviour in relation to the horrifying sexual abuse I had to endure. I have been so badly abused, so badly damaged and I have been so brave and strong. I have been used, rejected, humiliated, discarded and left to die. So I have absolutely nothing to apologise for. I read a lot about forgiveness and having to forgive in order to move on. Well, I think it's wrong. I will never EVER forgive those who abused me EVER. But what I will do is forgive myself. I forgive myself for all the mistakes I have made, because all those mistakes were made as a consequence of being neglected, physically, sexually and emotionally abused.

I forgive myself for it all and I am so, so sorry that I hurt myself so badly when it was never my fault. I am so, so sorry.

Reflection: I hope anybody reading this can find a way to forgive themselves for the trauma they have been subjected to. I read a lot about forgiveness and I still don't get it. It still doesn't sit right in my head. Apparently you have to forgive others in order to be able to move on. Well I have moved on now, I was moving on then, but the most important person I needed to forgive was myself. Once I was able to forgive myself I stopped taking responsibility for all of their actions.
I have also undertaken a lot of work understanding and analysing my abusers behaviour and once I could do that I was better able to move forward, but I still couldn't and can't forgive them for what they did to me, because as damaged and depraved as those people are, they still knew what where were doing was wrong.

Notes:

10.01.18
Feeling more at peace, but tearful and very, very down. I wish I had a close friend to talk to.

Reflection: Even though I had rediscovered myself, I was still incredibly lonely.

Notes:

11.01.18
I slept very badly last night. I had nightmares that I didn't remember today. I have been anxious about a course I am booked to go on in relation to mental health. It has made me want to cry when I thought about cancelling it, but equally it has also made me want to cry at the thought of going. I spoke with one of the midwives teaching on the day. It appears that it's about pathways and medication, not specifically about triggers to mental ill health.

In July 2015 I was going to commit suicide because of the explosion of emotion that I could no longer suppress about Jack. I felt like I had let everybody down, because I could no longer push the emotions away and because it completely overwhelmed me. I truly believed my children would be better off without me. Nobody was listening to me. I went to see my GP who prescribed Sertraline, but after 4 weeks I couldn't tolerate the side effects any longer and I have taken no medication since. I have completely exposed myself, stripped myself bare to expose everything. Everything that lead to that day in July 2015. Everything in this journal. I am anxious about attending the day because I don't want to hear people talk about the causes of mental ill health and what women do to cope. Because I am unique, I am learning my way and I don't want to be judged or generalised and I know I will get angry if I hear it. I also don't want to hear about mental ill health when I feel so down. I told somebody at work that I was apprehensive about going and they just said I will be alright. She didn't listen. I feel really down.

Reflection: It was and still is very difficult to hear people generalise about mental health. It's difficult to hear people put a label on it and Profess to know how people behave and what does and does not work. I feel very unique in my recovery. If it is the same as a million other people, then that's fine, but I don't want to be labelled, nobody does. Every person's recovery is unique to them and that should always be respected.

Notes:

12.01.18

I saw Jayne today, talked about how I have felt all week, trying to come to terms with what I have allowed myself to do. How I sold my soul for love. Everything was beginning to bubble out, but our appointment had to finish. I spent the rest of the day feeling stunned, shocked, very, very distracted and all I wanted to do was talk and cry and as always I couldn't. Tonight I had nothing left to keep me strong and I drank because I really did want to fall apart. I am sick and tired of always holding it together. But then after the kids went to bed I began to panic. I messaged two friends, but it was so late and I got no reply. I was scared, so scared so I e-mailed Jayne.

I'm two and a half glasses down a bottle of wine and this isn't going to end well. I have messaged two friends to see if they are awake, but had no reply. Tonight I have been a loving, compassionate Mum to tired tears, a cool Mum, a friend, a play mate, a counsellor, a negotiator and a responsible Mum. Every day I am at least 1 or more of those things, like any Mum. But tonight my heart is breaking. Tonight, whilst I am being all these things my heart is breaking. I have been so reasonable. I have been so reasonable about my Mum, Jack, Jason, not to mention the random rapes. Stewart and Alan. The Court verdict! Constantly working so hard to come to terms with it all. And now on top of that I have to accept all the humiliation of being fucked, albeit consensual fucking. A good oral, anal and vaginal fucking. Being fucked with a 5 day old baby. Bleeding, stitches, torn from arsehole to apex. Excruciating pain, but I took it because he came over and he comforted me because my mum ignored my pleas for help. He comforted me so I ignored the physical pain.

Being grateful for not being forced to be raped by his friend. Having to accept that I sold my soul for love. Actually sold my body for love. Having to accept that last week when you said not everything has to end in sex and all the time I'm thinking it was you that must be wrong. You must be wrong because all I have ever had is sex as a means of payment. You must be wrong, not me!! Because that's all I know and if I'm wrong then that means he used me too and all that time he was using me and I let him because that's all I know. And I know it's not my fault, but I still have feelings and I'm broken, I'm so broken. And all the time I'm trying so hard to work it out, be reasonable, be strong, be sensible. But nothing that has happened to me has been remotely near any of those things. Nothing – and I have feelings and I am broken and I have tried so hard, but I am broken and I am hurting so badly.

Reflection: And I was all of those things and I'm not going to take any of that away reflecting on it. It was a cold hard reality and I had to get through it, just like everything else.

Notes:

13.01.18
I woke up crying. I read and re-read that e-mail over and over again and it kept me safe. I read it until I couldn't keep my eyes open any longer and I cried myself to sleep. Jayne responded to my e-mail this morning. I felt so tearful all day. We went to a friend's 50th party and there were so many people, it was so loud and I knew nobody. I began a couple of conversations, but it was so difficult and I spent the whole time holding back tears.

Reflection: Now, I would never have gone to that party feeling so low, needing to resolve things in my head. But then, then I felt like I had to keep going, I had to keep moving forward, or I was afraid I would fall back and never stop falling. I was working hard, but I was also putting myself under so much pressure.

Notes:

14.01.18
I have slept little, but reflected over and over again, particularly on Friday and Saturday. I think I've realised that falling apart is actually not such a bad thing. I have been so frightened of falling apart because I have been too scared of how far I might fall. Given that just over two and a half years ago I was suicidal and self-harm has been a frequent thought. But self-harm and suicide came with hopelessness, no self-esteem, no self-respect. Not all of those apply all of the time any more. So falling apart on Friday night, as well as being terrifying, was also a huge relief of pressure. Pressure that had built up, being so damn reasonable, sensible and so fucking strong. Well I am glad I lost it on Friday night because I needed to. I was just too scared to realise it at the time.

Reflection: Another insightful entry. I didn't know it at the time, but I was reinforcing those layers of recovery.

Notes:

15.01.18
Numb and absolutely exhausted today. I went swimming after work. Good thinking time about me and what I need to do.

Reflection: Good old mind healing day. About time too.

Notes:

16.01.18
No real time to myself today. Very frustrating.

Reflection: I have found since that time, that I need time to myself every so often and I always find it. Even if it just means having a bath, where I can escape physically and mentally. I didn't quite have that confidence to do it then.

Notes:

17.01.18
E-mail from Fern today from the Police, asking for more witnesses to provide statements. I obliged, but I am totally focused on me now. My mind is scattered all over the place. Part of me wants to make my life unrecognisable. Part of me thinks if I do that it minimises what I have been through and I need time to work stuff through. I think both are right. I have decided to withdraw from the mental health training day. Two colleagues came and hugged me and I wanted to cry. Deep down I am not okay, but being busy pushes it away. That's okay as long as I am able to re connect with my emotions so I can untangle them.

I think I feel relieved that falling apart on Friday night, just meant a good cry. I have lost everything in terms of self-esteem, self-worth and the words I could find are self-respect. Whilst my self-esteem and self-worth are fragile, I have regained my self-respect. Because all of my life I have been disrespected and I refuse to accept that any more. If I have self-respect I can cling on to anything. I won't let anybody disrespect me again.

Reflection: I took care of myself by withdrawing from the course. I was beginning to understand what self-care really means.

Notes:

18.01.18
My head is doing that spinning thing again. Am I devastated by Melvyn and everything that's happened to me? Do I want to move on? I feel guilty about moving on and I should still want to self-harm, because if I don't, then that means it's not as devastating as it has been, or should be. My spinning thing said I can have all of them. I can be devastated by what's happened to me, I can accept that the things that happened to me are so bad they could cause me to feel suicidal and want to self-harm. I don't therefore need to be paralyzed by that fear or my experiences. I can move forward because I can accept all of those things. And I don't need to feel guilty about moving forward because I accept how all those things made me feel, even if I don't feel them now.

Where the hell did that insight come from? It's incredible.

Reflection: The entries are starting to become reflections in themselves.

Notes:

19.01.18
I talked to Jayne about this today. She helped me to understand that what I am feeling is because I am becoming me! I am beginning to accept myself on all levels and accept that I can hold and accept different thoughts and feelings all at once should they choose to arise. But not only accept them, but not judge them. So I don't become irritated with myself should a thought or emotion arise. I talked about the spinning wheel in my head. When I don't know what to do, or don't understand how I feel. I go to the spinning wheel and it gives me a rational, logical response. I asked Jayne how come when I don't know the answer and I spin the wheel, it does. She said because the wheel is me. And I do know the answer and what I am doing is turning in to myself. Looking within myself. How clever is that? How the hell did I learn that?

The first time the wheel appeared was Jacks acquittal verdict. It just appeared that night. It hasn't left me since. Jayne directed me to Carl Rogers Theory and it absolutely mirrored what I am doing. How absolutely amazing. I also talked about my going swimming and using weights to look after my body. I said it's not a fad, it's a way of life that I want. She helped me to understand that this is me, valuing me and recognising my worth and needs. My mind is changing and I don't know how it is doing it, or how it is doing it exactly like Carl Rogers explain it does in "*On Becoming a Person*". Wow! I'm becoming a real person. Oh My!! We talked about boundaries and how Sara was setting that boundary of friendship. I feel so relieved, so happy. I am beginning to understand boundaries and setting my own. I am so relieved that I will never have to have sex in exchange for compassion, during vulnerability ever again. I am setting my own boundaries - Get Me!

Reflection: Another reflective entry.

Notes:

20.01.18

I cannot remember a single day gone by without replaying what has happened to me over and over again. Mostly Jack. Today my mind felt so clear, I felt excited inside. What should I do? Read a book, watch television, Write? My lungs feel so clear, I feel like I can breathe again. I watched a film tonight, really watched it, engrossed. Anyway there was one scene where a young boy was lost in thought on a bus. Immediately the thought I thought of would be me thinking about Jack. Not chatting excitedly like everybody else on the bus. Not daydreaming excited thoughts. I was lost in reflection for a few minutes and my Son asked me if I was okay. It's funny how my face must reflect what I am thinking.

The moment passed, I was back in the film and I was reflecting on how amazingly free I feel, how present, alive I feel. I really don't remember the last time I felt excited and alive. 38 years I have carried Jack. Every single day he has taken me with him, to be part of what he did to me, or the living consequences of what he did to me. To understand that it's completely okay to accept thoughts and memories and not be crippled by them is astonishing. Liberating, absolutely tremendous beyond words I can articulate. I just feel so free, so excited. Flashbacks, I now understand they are just memories trying to torment me to keep me a victim. So if I accept them, not fight them and be completely open and honest and talk about them, they will have no power. They no longer have that threatening hold over me. Let the flashbacks play over and over if they need to. They are both as strong as me, too many years have gone, they've been talked to death. Like a great movie or programme. You can only watch them so many times and eventually they lose all that emotional influence they had over you.

I was trapped in time and it was all continually going round and round in my head. It had nowhere to go. But talking and talking, reliving, analysing, reflecting, exposing shame, guilt and grief. Doing it over and over again until each devastating memory, each sickening experience, each unrested emotion has been able to find a place to settle in my mind. And as all those terrifying, hauntings have left my soul to rest in the past, my soul has found me again. Or I have found my soul and I can begin to be me and I can't describe how that feels.

My final words to my inner demons. Rest in peace now all of you. You will always have a place in my heart, but my soul belongs to me now. If you ever feel angry or unsettled then you know I am always listening. I am always here, but you can't hurt me anymore. It's time to rest in peace.

Reflection: I felt like I had reached my level at this stage and to a degree I had. I had found myself. I had learned that coming to terms with what had happened to me was ongoing, because it was all a part of me and I was still growing. I wanted to push on just a little bit longer just to see how I developed before leaving my life to me.

Notes:

PART 3

BECOMING ME

18.03.18

It has been a little while now since I decided it was the right time to put my past to rest. To rest it because I have declared it, explored it and have found a place to be at peace with my past. This next chapter is purely about becoming me. I haven't known me since I was 10 years old. I feel like I have been beamed down from space and given a blank page to create a future however I want that to be. So first I will catch up on what I have experienced since I discovered my new found peace.

For about 3 weeks after I stopped writing I had only pure elation. My mind felt like it was totally clear and all I had was pure white space. I had so much energy, I felt I could breathe as deeply as I wanted and felt I could still inhale more air than my lungs could cope with. Everything suddenly felt clear and fresh and new, I felt like I could do anything, be anything. I no longer had that tight feeling in my chest, or my body that made me feel like I was being squeezed and needing to break out. I had so much energy, I felt elated, almost high. I was experiencing the best feeling in the world and then I became ill.

Horrible flu like pains, a cough, a sore throat, aching fatigue. I even had a couple of days off work. I slept an awful lot and during that sleep I began having nightmares about Jack. Jack and Court and I began to feel angry. During the day I didn't think about it, but I felt angry with everybody and everything, very angry, but I didn't know why. Then at night I would dream about Jack again and remembered being told in court about things I wasn't allowed to talk about. This dream became recurrent and I was getting angrier and angrier. Then the thoughts began to distract me during the day. But the thoughts didn't just stay with Jack and Court. The thoughts began to extend to all the people who have "gagged" me and then from all the people who have "gagged" me, stopped me from talking, to all the people who have let me down. My need to talk about this, to expose them is growing stronger and stronger.

I am so, so angry. With clarity has come absolute insight. Crystal clear insight and an incredible amount of anger. I had been completely satisfied when I made my statement to the Police on the 14th February 2016. That was because for the first time in my life I was able to talk. I could talk about absolutely everything. At no point was I told I couldn't talk about anything. Absolutely everything I said was written down and I was totally satisfied that I had given it back. Since being ill though I have gained even more insight and clarity and the degree of anger has arisen inside of me is phenomenal. More and more recognition that I have been let down, gagged, ignored and held down. Constrained from getting it out, getting to talk about, tell somebody who could have helped me, what has happened to me. All those people have been responsible for the devastating consequences of me being sexually abused over and over again and the devastating impact it has had on my physical and mental health.

I am so incredibly angry and I am going to expose each and every one of them so they are left under no illusion that they all played a part in either exploiting me, or being complicit with the sexual abuse that has devastated my life. Disgusting individuals every single one of them. As well as my personal determination to do this, I am also hoping to exhaust this anger when I take part in the National Inquiry into Child Sexual Abuse.

On the 11th April I will be going to Liverpool to be interviewed about my experience. I have already spoken with a support worker who has established where I am in terms of coming to terms with what's happened. I'm happy with the plan which is to discuss what happened to me, the impact it has had on my life and the people who let me down. This will be followed by me being able to discuss any recommendations I might wish to make. This fits perfectly where I am right now. I can vent all that anger, expose everybody and I am not going to be gagged. I really hope this is going to be enough to calm the beast.
Before I became angry I had so much energy. This was before I became unwell. I had started swimming several times a week after work and I was lifting weights at home. I felt so good and energised. Being unwell and becoming angry has sapped all that energy. I don't have restful sleeps any more, my anger is always re-energised in the evening. I meditate day and night, but my anger is fear and beneath fear is hurt and I do understand it. I understand that I am hurting so badly, because of everybody that let me down. Every single person that I told let me down. And if it's not about self-worth, or being worthless, then what is it about? Why did everybody from my mum and Dad to people in authority either ignore me, dismiss me or use me. Why? That's where I'm at right now. That's what I need to know. I need an explanation that satisfies my mind. But until it does I have to live with this fire raging inside me. I want my energy back, my white space!

Reflection: This anger crept up on me totally unexpected. I was enjoying the ride of becoming a fully functioning person, then this happened and I couldn't work it out.

Notes:

01.04.18
Anger is still inside me. I hate being angry because I hate the tension that is inside me. But I accept that I am angry. My Auntie called me recently because my Uncle is dying. She spent a long time talking about the past. The relationship my Mum had with her family. She talked about the arguments that my Mum started when she was drunk. Another validation for me. No I didn't make it up, I didn't exaggerate, I was spot on with my childhood memory. It's funny that we only have one word to describe it. "Memory". Memory suggest something we remember, but there is no word for something we have never forgotten. The two things are very different. Maybe momentous is the closest word? My Auntie was talking about a particular time and this time was my Cousins 18th Birthday and my Auntie said there was an argument about something. Well that something was about me! It was about my Auntie blabbing that she knew I was anorexic, because I wanted to die.
I wanted to die because I couldn't handle what Stewart was doing to me because Jack had sexually abused me. My Uncles were shouting at me to tell them who did it and I told them it was Stewart Watts and he lived in Liverpool. I was screaming back at them. At the same time the other night, my Auntie had no recollection of what that argument was about and my Uncle also said he didn't know I had been abused when I told him about the Court case. My Uncle who I have re-connected with and my Uncle who has now died. They were the Uncles who were screaming at me. Those bastards, every one of them complicit with what Jack did to me. As a consequence of that telephone conversation I began googling things about the New Town where I grew up. I was looking for places and areas from my past. When I found places from my past it gave me validation of what happened to me. That made me angry. When I couldn't find those places, that also made me angry. The flat Jack sexually abused me in no longer exists, it confirms my non-existence as a person, a body, a mind, a tormented child. It fuels my anger along with all those lying bastards who claim to not remember. Well to all you bastards, you all helped to destroy my life. You are all responsible in your own way. Well, I DO EXIST. And I did then too. And very, very shortly I'm going to remind you all explicitly what happened to me and you will never forget that I existed EVER again! My book will be called "I DO EXIST AND I ALWAYS HAVE". You will be named. You will all be named.

Reflection: As you can see, that isn't the title of my book, but my anger was coming from my absolute clarity into what had happened to me. I didn't understand it then, but I will try to explain using a different example.
People who smoke for example. They may smoke for years until one day they have a sudden realisation of truth and they decide to quit. They may have tried several times and not succeeded, but some wake up call, perhaps a health scare, or the birth of a child. Something really significant wakes this person up to quit and then they do after all those half-baked unsuccessful attempts. Then these newly enlightened people feel they have to share all their knowledge about these cancer causing sticks and point out to everybody within ear shot what a disgusting life limiting habit they are undertaking. They go on about the disgusting smell, the chemicals, the cost and they go on and on and on. Well in a way that's what was happening to me. I had

finally realised that all the abuse I had been subjected to was wrong, it was everybody else's fault and I wanted to shout it from the tree tops and the fact that I couldn't fuelled my rage.

Notes:

12.05.18

Anger is so tiring. I can't do anything about it, but it's wearing me out. I went to the Truth Project on the 11th April. I went to Liverpool to talk about my experiences and my anger. As if I couldn't get any more angry, I did.

I'm glad I took my friend Angela with me, I'm glad I didn't have to go through this on my own. On 16th April, Alan wrote a letter to my Mum telling her I was trying to ruin the lives of Jason and Sarah and Stewart, by alleging sexual abuse. He reminded her that she saw Jason as the Son she never had and told her to talk some sense into me before it's too late. Initially I panicked about what my Mum would think, but my sense of self very quickly kicked in. I love it so much that I have my own sense of self back after 38 years. I got to my Mums house and told her what he was saying about the sexual assault is true. She just stared at me shaking her head and said "*Are you starting all this up again*"? I couldn't hide my disgust, my revulsion at this statement. But all I could say was I wasn't starting anything up again, it had never ended.

She stared at me shaking her head and I left, taking my kids home. On 23rd April I took the letters Alan had written and spent over 3 hours at my local Police Station making a statement about his behaviour towards me and my children. When I got back to my Mums to collect the children Fern from the Police, was on the 'phone to my Mum taking a statement about Jason. My Mum told me she told me she didn't want to go to Court again. I took the kids home. I couldn't process what she had said. I was angry, sickened, devastated. She never EVER shows me any concern or compassion EVER. She will put my Cousin, that sick bastard before me.

I am devastated because she is supposed to keep me safe, love me, cuddle me, want me to be okay. I am angry because she is a bitch and cares more about my Cousin than she does about me. I am absolutely destroyed. Utterly, utterly devastated. I cannot express the raw emotion I feel inside. She held on to that statement for two weeks. She told me she didn't know if she wanted to sign it and send it back. Another knife in my chest. I would have nothing to do with her if I didn't need the practical support for the kids. She reminds me constantly that she has absolutely no consideration towards me, or my feelings AT ALL. I have gotten rid of all the toxic people in my life except her and I hate it.

Reflection: My Mother never fails to surprise me with the depths she can stoop to and she did it again that day. As if I didn't need anything else to fuel my anger.

Notes:

20.05.18

I have been sleeping really badly for the past couple of weeks. Keep waking up and my heart is pounding and I am panicking. I have tried to explore where this is coming from, I have tried to accept this feeling of anxiety, of dread, but nothing will come. Nothing that I can put my finger on. I talked to Jayne about all the different things that are happening. I am angry that I didn't consent to one of my children being weighed and they went ahead and did it anyway. I am angry that the hospital are ignoring my concerns about my Dad and drugging him up even though it's not addressing his aggression with personal care. I am angry that I was gagged in Court and couldn't say what I wanted to say.

Everybody has their own agenda and none of it is putting me, my children or my Dad first. My Mum won't agree to a care home that's too far away for her convenience. Irrespective of whether it's suitable for my Dad. It's like being abused all over again. Jack did what he wanted and ignored my pleas to stop. Jason did what he wanted to do, the same as the man in the park who raped me. Carl who raped me. Stewart Watts who raped me, used me for everything he wanted then left. Even Alan whose self-esteem was so low, he needed to keep me down to feel better about himself.

Every single person used me, then dumped me and wanted me to not make a fuss, or berated me for making a fuss. Now my Son and my Dad. I stick up for them and the same thing happens again. Bastards, all of them.

Soon the police investigations will be done and it will either go to Court, or the case will be dropped. I am so scared that when it all ends I won't know what to do. People who I have spoken to have just said I will get on with my life. In other words, shut up about it now the investigation is over, because there is nothing left to talk about. But I have spent 38 years of incredible energy suppressing it, then trying to come to terms with it, then trying to get justice for it. Court or no court. I was still hurt, I was still neglected, sexually abused, raped, and that still devastates me. That is still massive to me and people want me to shut up. Well, I can't anymore. I won't and I'm scared because I don't know what to do. What if people stop listening?

Reflection: Earlier I had stated that behind anger there is fear, and behind fear there is hurt and this was starting to emerge. I felt so desperately hurt by all those people who let me down. If I knew it then I believed they should know it too and tell me they are sorry for all the hurt and betrayal I have been through because of them.

Notes:

05.07.18
So on Monday, Fern called me to say the CPS are not pursuing the case because it's only my word against Jason. Jane, the person who disclosed to Fern about what happened with Jason has refused to make a statement. I try to be okay about it, but I'm not.
The Truth Project who said they would like to contact me to promote their service through my experiences have not contacted me. They have published 50 peoples accounts, but not mine. I feel so rubbish. For 35 years nobody would listen, I was sexually abused anyway. Now people do know, there is still no consequence for my life that's been destroyed. I don't want to waste my life, but I'm really struggling to move forward. I'm struggling so much. I don't know why it won't get easier. I just don't know what to do. I'm trying so hard, but I'm not getting anywhere. Please help me, somebody please help!

Reflection: It appears I was looking for something different now. I wanted a consequence from somewhere. Justice was not being done, so I wanted all those people who had let me down to pay some kind of price. I was struggling to accept that all this abuse had happened and nobody's life had changed. Nobody was feeling the pain that I was feeling. I had reported it, I had come to terms with it, but absolutely nobody else had been affected by what I had gone through. Even Jane who had given evidence for me in Court against Jack had let me down. I was no longer important enough to fight for what had happened at that time.

Notes:

06.07.18
I had a black episode when I got home from work today. I only came in to get Sam, have a quick wash and then take the kids to the hairdressers. I haven't had a black episode for a long time. I had no recollection where I left my keys. I looked in the car, the door, the kitchen, my work bag, everywhere upstairs. I sent the boys to the hairdressers and Elizabeth found my keys.
I was getting so angry because I had been in the house 5 minutes and it took 20 minutes to find my keys. I know why it happened, but I don't know why this is happening now. Last night I woke up having nightmares about being raped by Stewart. Now I haven't had one of those for a long time. I feel like somethings gone wrong and I'm falling backwards. I don't want to go to sleep. I wish it was morning. I wish I could enjoy my life. I wish I could say goodbye to this, buy my mind is tormented. Why now?

Reflection: I had the black episode because I was consumed with anger and absolutely distracted. I had the nightmare because I didn't feel like I was getting justice from anywhere for what Stewart had done to me and Jason had been let off the hook.

Notes:

16.09.18
I have been angry for a long time now. Angry with anybody and everybody who tries to dismiss me, or disrespect me or my family. Anybody who ignore their pain, or whose action will cause them pain. I have become that angry person who people have stopped listening to. And that isn't me, but I'm really struggling to manage my emotions.
All I have known in the past is either self-harm for feeling worthless, for being ignored. Hating myself for being a bad person that makes people want to hurt me, or more recently being angry and aggressive towards people because I'm learning that my feeling do count and I want everybody to listen to me. Both extremes are harmful to me. Both are negative and unproductive. I'm trying to access emotions that are positive and beneficial to me. This isn't about having people agree with me, just acknowledge my feelings and accept them.
Jayne asked me to try and look at the grey area in the middle and what that looks like. This really physically gave me a headache, but then the flashbacks came.

"Please don't go out and leave me, I'm scared" = ignored.
"I don't want to play anymore" = I'm sexually abused.
"Please stop, you're hurting me" = I'm raped.
"I'm really hurting inside" = Emotional abuse, degradation, rejection.

Those flashbacks crush me, make me feel like I can't breathe. They make me want to scream. They reinforce the negative behaviour, because that energy has to go somewhere. Self-harm, or attack. Am I ignored because I'm worthless, or am I ignored because they're not worthy of me? Am I ignored because I don't shout loud enough, or am I ignored because I'm shouting too loud? Am I trying too hard and like anybody who tries too hard, it pushes people away?
I have so much energy inside when I want to be heard. That energy is overwhelming and I just want to scream *"Listen to Me, please listen to Me, because when you don't, I feel 7 years old and frightened. I feel 10 years old and abused, discarded, worthless"*. I'm reading this over and over again, trying to see the other side, but all I can see is the side I know and that's pain. And I don't know what to do and it's eating away at me. All I ever wanted was to feel solid, safe and secure. Unconditionally loved and accepted as a valued person. But I'm not, I'm empty, I don't feel safe or secure. I have no foundations, no roots. I'm constantly searching for that absolute belonging, but the flashbacks are winning. I just want to feel like I've arrived and I'm okay. But instead I'm lost and completely empty. I just want to feel relief, peace.
Okay, I'm reading. Be kind to myself, love and accept myself fully. Stop trying, notice what makes me different. Embrace the truth of who I am. I don't feel understood - I'm isolated. Communicate feelings better, listen, accept change, put myself out there.

I feel so lost.

Reflection: The issue I have here is being ignored. If I am too loud people ignore me, if I am not loud enough, people ignore me. I was struggling to find a balance and all I was doing was repeating the same behaviour. I hadn't developed the skills I needed to be listened to.

Notes:

21.09.18

I thought to have self-confidence/self-esteem I had to be sorted. I had to never get angry, to be perfect, to always be helpful. Now I realise it's about self-belief. With self-belief I don't need to judge others, I don't need to be angry. I can be more confident, I can have a high self-esteem. No self-belief came from always being put down, mocked, laughed at, even lied about. So I was and have been always trying to improve myself. I felt I needed to be absolutely perfect to be accepted, to be loved, to be just good enough. Because I couldn't achieve this I hated myself, because I truly believed I was not as good as everyone else. I believed it was true what all those people were saying about me. Now I understand none of that is true.

I am good enough because I am a good person and nobody can ever break that now I have finally discovered self-belief. Those that try to destroy me, put me down. They are far more damaged than me, than I will ever be. Because I believe in myself, I will never need to destroy anybody to make me feel better about myself. I finally believe I am absolutely fine just how I am, flaws and all. And I think I might finally be finding some peace. I recently started believing in myself and my opinions. I didn't see it as self-belief at first. I saw it as me shouting *"I am important, my feelings do matter"*. But I was shouting it at everybody else, but I soon realised nobody is really bothered, or listening. Either because they didn't care, or they already know it. I have suddenly realised I don't need it validating. I have started to become self-reliant I have started to develop a real sense of myself. Self-reliance and reflection make me feel a whole lot better than the need, or often in the past the desperation for somebody else to say it.

I believe in me and I love that more than anything. And that makes me feel happy because everything I do is coming from a good place and that makes me feel great. What that does mean also is that I am no longer a victim. Wow! That's a massive thing to write. That's a huge, freeing statement to make. That claustrophobic tight feeling lifts just writing that sentence.

My lungs feel like they can't expand far enough, there feels like so much space my head feels light and spacious, not tight and cramped with anxiety. This is what it must feel like to be high. I can't imagine anything better. I feel like I can accept any emotion. If I am sad I can reflect on it, angry, the same. If I feel angry I can reflect on it and if I feel justified in my anger it won't necessarily take it away, or it might, but as long as I understand the emotion and why I feel it, then I can accept it. And if I can accept it I don't feel stressed or tense about it. Accepting it eases it because It's part of me and my feelings, so I can console myself.

What I have found in reality though, is I am less angry, really not angry at all about anything. I no longer need anybody to validate my feelings. Of course it's lovely to get a compliment, or receive support, even an opinion. The realisation for me now though is I no longer need it. I no longer search for it. This for me means I no longer feel the urge to tell my story. Equally, I feel relaxed when I do tell my story, or talk about my experiences because I accept them now and all the emotions that come with them. I have finally accepted me and I have a huge clear space in my mind. I feel free, clear, light. I have me and I will always validate me. I really couldn't feel more love.

Reflection: Finally the penny dropped. Once I was fully able to accept myself I no longer needed people to validate me. I no longer needed to feel sad, or angry if they didn't. What a massive relief.

Notes:

14.10.18
Since writing this journal I have had a few challenges. I have felt intimidated by my ex-husband, I have felt angry at things that have gone wrong and initially I felt I'd failed. Failed in all the beliefs I have come to recognise, but what I forget to remember was with each of these challenges I have reflected. I have reflected on the way they made me feel the way I do, accepted they make me feel the way I do as frustrating as they are, but ultimately because I am able to reflect and I am self-reliant. I have not felt the need to be rescued or validated and that in itself is helping me to become even more confident. It's helping my self-esteem to develop further. I am beginning to feel whole, whereas I have always felt hollow and fragile.
I am finally becoming me.

Reflection: I am finally becoming me.

Notes:

22.10.18

Everybody has something, don't they? Something they need or rely on to make them feel better about themselves. For some people it's material things, like a car, a house, flash clothes, power dressing. Or perhaps it's something more related to the self. For instance wearing jewellery, or not being able to go out without make up on, or that 'special' lipstick that gives you confidence.

With me, it had always been my hair. When I was young I have very long blonde hair. That attracted a lot of unwanted attention. I always used to say I wanted my hair dyed black and cut really short. Of course that produced nothing but amusement to my parents, but I hated the unwanted attention. The touching, like I was a piece of meat. When I was deemed old enough to be allowed to choose, I had my hair cut very short. I looked like a boy and the attention changed to being mocked for looking like a boy.

I hated my hair and my looks as much as I hated myself. Then the perm came in and I loved it. I idolised Kylie Minogue who had big curly hair, although I think hers is natural and she did what was perceived to be a 'mans' job in her TV character. Kylie Minogue's character was everything I wanted to be. She was beautiful, confident and knew what she wanted and did it without concern for anybody else's opinion. She also had a boyfriend in the show who was kind, gentle and considerate and he adored his girlfriend.

I had the perm. The perm showed the world I was confident. It showed the world I was strong, even though I was dying inside. The perm was my mask. The worse I felt, the bigger I would dry my perm. In the early 90's a hairdresser straightened my hair, he told me perms were no longer fashionable. I felt like my strength had been sapped, just like Samson. My hair was beginning to go darker and started to resemble a dirty blonde colour, so I lightened it myself. A tutor at the University where I was studying commented on my hair. Annie Cropston her name was. I didn't want to admit I had lightened it myself, I don't know why, so I said I had washed it. Her retort was to say I should wash it more often.

Not only did I feel exposed in terms of my vulnerability without my perm, I also felt the dirt and filth that I had inside had also been exposed. I felt physically revolting as well as emotionally revolting. I continued to colour my hair to hide the filthy disgusting person I believed I was.

Then I met my second husband Alan. He complained bitterly about my long hair. Remarking frequently that it was too big, too thick, too long. He bought me hair straighteners and I tried relentlessly to get my hair to be as smooth and flat as I possibly could. But when I looked for validation, he continued to remark that it was still too big.

He left in September 2016 and since then I have gone from strength to strength. Early this year, as part of becoming me, I had my hair permed again. It was a kind of two fingers approach to those who had told me the hair I believed I loved was outdated. I wanted it back and I got it back. It was also two fingers to Alan, as I tipped my hair upside down and fluffed that perm right out. Then recently something changed, when I developed the sense of myself.

I wanted me back. I didn't know what me even looked like. I've spent most of my life trying not to be me. I have issues with going to the hairdressers. I associate it with pain that was inflicted by my mother when she did my hair. Pain and being burnt by tongs. I'd rather go to the Dentist than the hairdressers. It's less painful and over quicker. So I decided to speak to my hairdresser about my fears. Catherine, she was brilliant. I explained that I didn't want to carry on trying not to be me any longer. So on 18th October 2018 13 years after my unborn baby died, I became me. I had my hair cut to shoulder length, my perm straightened out and my colour dyed back to my natural colour. I finally look like me. Yes my hair has still to grow to get rid of the colour and residual perm. But I am also still to grow. I am physically becoming me as well as emotionally becoming me.

Reflection: I was experimenting with how I wanted to look. How I believed I should look and not how everybody else thought I should look. It was a very exciting time.

Notes:

19.11.18
So I finally get to hear the outcome from the Police and I am to blame. They are not taking further action against Stewart Watts for six years of rape, because I came off the pill and was allowing myself to get pregnant.

Reflection: This was a crushing blow to me and I was told I had the right to appeal and I did. I couldn't be left with the blame. I had exposed all my abusers and now Stewart was trying to give it back to me. I really couldn't be left with the blame.

Notes:

20.11.18

Detective Inspector Mason called me today. I told her the only difference was me stopping the pill. I told her I was raped 3-4 times a week. It was never consensual, it didn't make any difference whether I wanted him to leave me alone. If he wanted it, he had me. She told me my Mum said I had anorexia when I was 14 years old. Again I pointed out that there was no medical evidence to support this, no photographs to support this. But there is medical evidence to prove I was anorexic when I was with Stewart. I weighed 6 stone and the aggressive GP who weighed me, told me that if I dropped below 40KG I would be hospitalised. She told me to tell my family and I did and they humiliated me and Stewart called me a freak, ugly. He said I was a freak because my body didn't work properly. There are also photographs of me when I was anorexic. DI Mason advised me to appeal her decision. I told her nobody had clarified any points with me when she asked me why I hadn't mentioned this before. I have appealed, but I've also found out that nobody will talk to me until after the appeal. What then, is the point of the appeal?

Reflection: Good old Mummy to the rescue again. That woman didn't have a clue I was anorexic until she had to have it pointed out to her when I was in my early 20's. Then she could abuse me even more. I was incandescent with rage.

Notes:

23.11.18
I am broken.
Half of my brain is angry at the Police because of their total lack of insight into Domestic Violence. Why did I marry him? Why did I move to another part of the country with him? Why did I come off the pill to allow myself to get pregnant through rape? That would have given the rape a purpose hey!
The other half of my brain is angry at myself. 36 years of believing I'm no good, I'm worthless, I'm only good for being used and abused. Repeatedly having this message reinforced. My Mum telling me I wasn't special, being emotionally neglected. Looking for love and Jack sexually abusing me, looking for love and Jason sexually abusing me. Looking for love and being raped. Looking for love, looking to be wanted, desperate to be wanted and receive comfort and safety and marrying a man who used all that knowledge to rape me abuse me and humiliate me because I didn't know normal and he told me it was normal. He told me I was abnormal because I didn't like what he was doing. I felt abnormal.
Brenda Smith said "*These things happen*". I had to let it happen to be 'normal'. I didn't want to be rejected again. Nobody has ever wanted me, I'm only here to be used. Melvyn and his listening ear. Finally I'm loved, I'm accepted. But no, here comes a cock in the mouth, oral and anal sex. All payment for being listened to, but I allowed that too. I allowed it because he told me I was special. Just like Jack did. Then the narcissist Alan. He loved me because I was a victim. This made him feel good about himself, but as soon as I stopped being a victim and didn't want to be controlled, he turned on me and tried to destroy me. All of this reinforces all the reasons I believe my worthlessness. How can my kids be proud of me, because everybody else believes I'm worthless?
I only fight for them. But they are going to notice, nobody really wants me. Nobody ever has. I've tried so hard to recover, to understand, to discover my worth and now the Police are reinforcing that I am completely worthless. I came of the pill, therefore I must have wanted to be raped. Nobody understands. Nobody understands that when all you know is rejection and abuse, eventually you believe you are worth nothing at all. The only fight left is self-destruction, anything can be going on around me, but I am no longer in there. I no longer feel anything because my soul is broken. Everything becomes disconnected and I exist only in that space somewhere between life and death, hoping the end will be quick.

Reflection: Now there was a whole lot of damage done by the Police in how they delivered their decision. In one sentence they had reduced me to that suicidal, broken individual I had been three years previously. It was delivered in a savage fashion and there was no support. Everything I had worked so hard to understand was beginning to unravel.

Notes:

29.11.18
I've been very low. Nobody to talk to when I have asked and in addition to that I find out that somebody who I considered a friend actually only saw me as a problem. Now she is focusing on somebody else and channelling her angst into them. She has dropped me. I thought we were friends. I thought she wanted to be with me because she like me, not because I was a charity, or someone to pity, or someone she could invest her time in.
It takes me straight back to being rejected. I am here at the convenience of others only. I am going out for a meal tonight, but only because I suggested it. If I don't suggest it she doesn't ask me. I really wish I knew what it is about whatever I do that people only see my presence as an inconvenience, or to use me, then ignore me when it suits them.
I wish I knew what I do wrong. How can I not dislike myself when it's clear that nobody else values me? I've learnt to like myself, I've learnt to be self-reliant, I'm not needy. So why when I ask for help do people turn their back on me, or ignore me or see me as an inconvenience, unless they want to use me? I'm so confused. I've only ever wanted to give, but nobody wants me.
Why do I have to be here? My kids are my everything. They are lovely, lovely kids and I would give anything to keep them safe and happy and they love me. So why does nobody else? Please somebody tell me.

Reflection: The answer was I just hadn't found the right place. I needed to connect with likeminded people and making connections with other people wasn't a bad thing, it was what I probably would have done if I'd had the opportunity to explore my identity as a young person. I was reaching out to people and at that time, it just wasn't the people who necessarily had the same interests as me. But I couldn't see it at the time. I'd spoken to Jayne about it and she told me to hold on and she had faith that it would come.

Notes:

11.04.19 – Everything finally comes together.

This is going to be my last entry, but for me the most significant one.

On 5th March 2019, I received an e-mail from the Criminal Justice Change Management Team. In it was an attachment to a letter detailing the outcome of the investigation into Stewart Watts and the rape, physical and emotional abuse I was subjected to.

The letter was savage. It put the responsibility for what happened to me firmly back in my court. I read this e-mail when I was at home with my children and I was broken and devastated.

I needed a scar, a scar for every bastard that tore me apart and got away with it. A scar that shows how devastating and destroying what they did, did to me. A scar that shows how badly I have been hurt. I started waking up shaking inside, or numb and for a split second feeling everything was okay, but then realising it wasn't.

I felt I had been gagged all over again. I had very strong thoughts for those people who kill themselves over this, who self-harm. I felt anger at the lack of understanding, no worse, the cruelty of those who deliver these outcomes in such a callous way. They have no idea at all what it feels like to experience abuse, to live with the impact it has on every sinew of your being. To be destroyed when I had the strength to speak out rally messed with my head.

On 07th March 2019, the overpowering thoughts of self-harm got the better of me. I sat on my bed with a pair of scissors whilst messaging Jayne, urging her to reply. I wanted to use them. I wanted to cut myself so deep, so deep that I would feel the excruciating pain, to match the emotional pain I was feeling inside. My thoughts weren't clear, everything was racing in my head. All I knew was I was in so much pain that I needed to see it, physically see it. Let everybody physically see it.

But I was bargaining with myself. A tiny part of me was saying, *"give it a week and if you still feel bad then do it"*. But a week felt like a year away, a mountain to climb and I was tired of bargaining with myself. But then a nagging thought kept reminding me that if I did self-harm to get that scar, then when I didn't feel bad it would serve as a constant reminder that I wouldn't then want. I was so overwhelmed, my mind was spinning. Then Jayne messaged me. She said *"I've got you"* and my mind stopped spinning. I put down the scissors. I didn't self-harm.

On 11th March 2019 I responded to Fern in relation to the Report. I had to go through everything that had been written. I needed to go through everything. I was fighting to be heard, fighting to let her know that what Stewart did to me was wrong. I needed her to understand the devastating impact the Report had had on me and how the savage way it had been delivered had caused me to consider self-harming. Self-harming to physically show everybody what he did was evil, depraved, inhuman. I told her I didn't need to hear from her. She had let me down so significantly. I needed to scream and shout to everybody what he had done. It felt like the DCI who wrote the Report had normalised what had happened by comparing rape and depravity to normal behaviour. I couldn't cope with that.

Then Jayne went off sick and I had to bury it, but the nightmares got worse. I couldn't always remember them, but I was waking up in the early hours absolutely terrified and shaking. I would try so hard to calm myself down, meditate and go back to sleep, but the nightmares were getting worse and I was beginning to feel really, really tired.

On 19th March 2019 Somebody visited my home when I was at work and put a note through the door. An Adult Mental Health Intervention Worker. Fern had contacted them, NOT ME! Concerned for my welfare. I told him I was fine. He asked me what had prompted me to talk about self-harming and I told him briefly about the investigation and how the outcome had been delivered. He said he understood how I must have felt and enquired as to whether a Liaison Officer at the Police had been round to talk to me, at which point I laughed and stated nobody had been round. He told me I didn't need to self-harm. I was so angry. Some faceless individual who knew nothing about me turns up unannounced at my door and then tells me over the 'phone that I don't need to self-harm. My immediate thought was "*What does he know? What does anybody know about how I am absolutely broken and falling apart inside*". I really, really needed to self-harm right then to show them all. To show them all that they know nothing.

I e-mailed Jayne and she was with me again. I didn't self-harm. I told her I needed to explore everything about Stewart because there was still something inside and I didn't know what it was. She told me I could explore anything with her and she would support me.

On 28th March 2019 I was watching a television programme where a victim wanted her abuser to be physically scarred for life as she was emotionally. My client group self-harm as a result of being victims of abuse. Everything around me at that time was pointing to scars. Everything suggesting that this is the expected behaviour and I was fighting hard to avoid it, but with no other outlet. My mind continued to be destroyed. I was becoming absolutely tormented by nightmares. I was waking up every night shaking, but unable to remember. I was beginning to feel really low. I was determined not to self-harm, but every thought in my head was telling me I would feel better.

After all, why not? It appeared to be an acceptable expectation. I felt like the happier I wanted to be, the worse the scar had to be. I felt like I had a little demon inside me that didn't want to let go.

I knew there was some really bad stuff inside me, but I didn't know what it was. I felt like I needed to keep telling people what has happened to me. My mind was desperately trying to find the bit that has really broken me, so I could fix it. But right then it felt like I was experiencing the abuse over and over again and I needed to talk about it, to get it out because I was reliving it every night and really, really struggling.

In addition to all this I had stopped eating properly. When I had a particularly bad day, the pain of hunger and the rubbish feeling that goes with hunger matched exactly how I was feeling emotionally. I really felt like this was all getting the better of me, so I e-mailed Jayne again and I told her about not eating.

I had another nightmare. What I had been doing was meditating to get back to sleep, but because I knew I was going to be able to talk to Jayne, I didn't meditate this time. I lay awake to allow the thoughts back in. To allow the memory of the nightmare to come back.

It was horrifying. The nightmare was about suffocation, it was about Stewart lowering himself down onto my face so I couldn't breathe. I couldn't breathe until I opened my mouth and he forced his penis inside it. I was gagging and desperate for breath and I could only breathe once he had his penis in my mouth and he would lift himself up. I was gagging, horrified, terrified. I had rushes of anger, I just wanted to bite it off. He would ejaculate in my mouth, or all over my body. It was the most horrific, claustrophobic, powerless, silencing experience of my life. And now I knew what the nightmares were about. And then there was anal rape. Flashbacks, but no clear memory of on particular experience. Trapped, unable to move. Overwhelmingly savage, incomprehensible.

After I allowed the nightmare to materialise, I was spiralling. I was unable to focus or concentrate. I was functioning on automatic pilot, but I only had a day or so until I could talk to Jayne. I just needed to hang on, but I was losing myself. I believed this was going to take forever to work though.

I saw Jayne that Friday and I told her about my nightmares in detail. I told her the outcome of the investigation being no further action was beginning to make be believe what Stewart had done was normal. I explained how I am in an amazingly beautiful relationship for the first time ever and my mind can't understand how what's happening now can be the same as what happened with Stewart.

Jayne explained it brilliantly and I will try to make it as clear as she did with me. She said my very positive experiences and very negative experiences are like 2 balls of wool and my mind has been tangling the thread of both balls together. So we talked about my very positive experiences that are healthy, safe, fun, consensual and extremely enjoyable. Then we talked about Stewart and how that was rape, abuse, threatening and violent. The two things are completely disconnected.

One is love making, the other is rape. There is absolutely no connection. What my mind had done in my head because the Police had normalised it by not processing it as a crime. It had made connections between the two. How could I love love making, but hate what Stewart did if the two are the same? Well the answer is because they are not the same. Ice-cream and chilli are not the same. Cars and trains are not the same. Rape and love making are not the same.

The penny dropped! By Jayne talking to me about Stewart. Talking about rape, violation, abuse, humiliation. I severed the thread in my mind between those two balls of wool. There is no connection between love and rape. Finally I got it. I had allowed Fern to influence my mind. To make me feel that what Stewart had done was okay. To question my understanding of what happened Somebody who doesn't know me, who hasn't lived it with me like Jayne.

Jayne reinforced my self-belief and that's what it came down to. I believe what Stewart did to me was wrong. I know it was wrong. Fern derailed me and I allowed her because my self-belief is so new.

I now know why I had the sudden urge to tell everybody what Stewart had done. Because I needed external sources to validate my self-belief, because my self-belief is still quite fragile. All I needed in the end was Jayne. Jayne to reflect back to me what I already knew to be true. That I knew all along what he did to me was wrong.

All of a sudden the last few pieces fell into place. I don't ever need to self-harm. There will never be self-harm because I know now, really know that what he did was wrong. I finally have enough self-belief to know that it doesn't matter anymore. There will be no starving or anorexia, because I no longer need to prove to myself physically that what he did was wrong. I no longer need that scar, I no longer need to feel that pain. Everything is going to be okay. I am going to be okay.
All this time holding on to guilt, shame, low self-esteem. I have at last completely severed the link between rape, sexual abuse and it ever being perceived as anything other than a sadistic, perverted act of horrific violation. Violation of a person's mind, body and soul. An act that I now know only ever requires the victim to love, honour and cherish their whole being to allow healing. In exactly the same way you would if you were to suffer any other insult, or injustice.
I am finally free. It has taken me 39 years to put my abusers exactly where they need to be. In the deepest, darkest basement of my mind. I have a bright future to look forward to now. I know those memories are in the basement, I know they can pop up whenever they feel they have an opportunity. But I have got me back. I own me now, they don't own me. So if and when they might need airing in the future, it will be on my terms, not theirs. I own them now as well as me and they can't hurt me anymore. I can finally let go.
I am finally free. 13/04/2019 owned by Paula Pearce.

Notes:

And Finally……………

When I began writing this journal, I didn't know what to expect. I didn't know what the outcome would be. It was possibly that final suicide note. I had no idea what I would do with it when I had come to the point that I no longer needed to narrate my recovery.

Once I had come to that point, I decided to type it up. That was a good review for me, to check that there were no underlying issues I still hadn't dealt with. There wasn't. As I was typing the journal up, I thought the entries I had made might help other people who have experienced similar traumas, or who have reacted to their trauma in a similar way I had. I thought it might help them to not feel alone. I thought this might have the right format to become a book. The more I typed and the more I could see how I was recovering, the more I thought that it would be a good idea to be able to reflect on those entries. To put what I was saying into context, or to demonstrate my understanding now. So after nine arduous months of typing up the journal, I went back to the beginning and started to reflect on those entries. This gave me a much deeper insight into my recovery and also tested out whether there were any issues still lurking in the dark corners of my mind. There wasn't.

Throughout the whole journal, there was only one entry I had no recollection of, not bad going considering the depth of trauma I was dealing with. Moving on to that. Whilst I didn't become affected by what I had written, I did become really exhausted going through those reflections. Every single entry apart from that one, I immersed myself back into the feelings I had then. So as I was typing up the reflections I was feeling angry, scared, abused, panicked, crushed, frightened, hopeless, to name just a few. At the beginning I was slightly anxious that I might get stuck back in one of those emotions, one of those traumas I was reliving. To add more confidence to my recovery, I didn't. Though interestingly on the occasions where I was describing my urge to self-harm, my arm would physically ache where I had self-harmed and I had to rub it. That was the only physical reaction I had, but it left just as quickly as the others as I moved through each entry.

There were a couple of other things that really stood out for me during the reflection process. I'd like to share with you now:

I recognised that mirroring, if that's what it is called, is really dangerous. By that I mean when somebody reflected the trauma back to me that I was experiencing, it felt like I was experiencing it for the first time and it shocked and horrified me each time that happened. It was a sickening blow, every time.

There are several entries where I felt totally numb. I could see that those times were the times my mind was doing some maintenance all on its own. I wasn't consciously working on anything, I wasn't distressed, I really didn't feel anything on those days, but usually I had a better day after that. It was like my mind was knitting together a little bit more and whilst it was concentrating on itself, it had no time to make me consciously try to work harder, or even be distressed. I found that really incredible and I have a big respect for my mind. (Even though it's mine).

And finally the title of my book "*Dying to be Heard.*"
In the beginning I was dying to be heard, just like we might say we are dying for a drink, or dying to go to the toilet. I was dying to be heard for thirty five years. I was shouting and screaming and doing everything I could to be listened to, to be heard. But after thirty five years I had hit the end of the road. I couldn't shout and scream anymore, I didn't have any more energy inside me to make people love me unconditionally. I didn't know how to love me unconditionally. I had nothing left and the saddest thing of all was I had to be dying, to be heard.
I hope you have enjoyed this book, I hope you will be able to take something positive away from reading it. I hope somebody reading this book will find the strength to carry on, to get help and support, because believe me it is out there. But you do have to scream and shout very loud to get it. Not because you are not worth it, not because nobody cares, because they do. I am living proof that they do. If you take anything from this book please let it be the belief that you don't have to be dying, to be heard.

Glossary

Witness Impact Statement.

Emotional

Being Sexually assaulted by Jack has destroyed my ability to live a full life. On the worst of days wishing I was no longer alive. Jack robbed me of my ability to sleep peacefully due to continuous nightmares of being trapped, held down and sexually assaulted, then waking up and wishing I was dead just to escape the constant torture. By day being tortured by flashbacks of what he had done to me, constant feelings of being trapped, then dreading going to bed again, terrified that Jack would climb into my bedroom and sexually assault me again, lying trembling in bed terrified to go to sleep, yet terrified to be awake.

I became obsessed with thoughts of suicide to escape the torture of flashbacks. I made attempts to end my life by deliberately abusing alcohol to such an extent I was hoping to drink myself to death. I became anorexic, first to gain some control, but later I could see it as a way out, if I could just get thin enough I knew, I wished, I hoped I would go to sleep and not wake up again. I longed for my heart to give up, my body to give up, just so I could have some peace, some rest from the constant feeling of being trapped and abused, from constant flashbacks and sensations.

I became 'spaced out' during the day, disconnected from everything – friends, school. Unable to concentrate, unable to learn, constantly distracted. I was so clever at primary school, but failed to achieve at secondary school and left with no discernible qualifications. I was a disappointment to my family, I was a disappointment to myself. I felt guilty for not being liked, I felt guilty for introducing myself to Jack and Emily, I felt so guilty for being with them when I realised they didn't want me to be. I believed that Jack sexually assaulted me because he didn't like me, he didn't want me there. He sniggered at me when I told him I didn't want to play anymore, when I asked him to stop, I felt like a piece of rubbish, worthless, not a person, just an object for him to play with or to punish me, to make me stop being with them. I hated myself for being a bad person, for getting in the way.

I developed a fear of being alone with men, believing that this was what men did, but not understanding why it didn't feel right. I grew to hate my body, hating a protruding stomach. Hated being 'touched', because of constant flashbacks of Jack touching me, making me touch him. I exercised obsessively to stay small, invisible, un-noticeable and continued to drink excessively to try and block out flashbacks and awful sensations. I grew to believe that my body was worth nothing, but for the use of other men, to do with what they wanted and hating myself for being just a body to be used. Constantly wishing I was dead. My self -esteem and self-worth was destroyed and I self-harmed to feel something, anything other than the sensations I was feeling of being sexually abused by Jack, something else to focus my mind other than flashbacks. I have lived with a constant dread, a constant fear that this might happen again, because I am aware of a danger that wasn't there before. Jack robbed me of my childhood and destroyed my innocence. He robbed me of any exciting unknown experiences and opportunities that I might have encountered and instead filled my life, my thoughts and feelings with terror and dread, despair, mental torture and absolute hopelessness. Leaving me to encounter my life ahead with fear, anxiety, stress and uncertainty.

Physical

I don't know what the long term effects of alcohol abuse and 8 years of anorexia will be as yet. Self-harming has left no physical scars, but I continue to have issues with food and body image. I also find it very difficult to be present and focused. After years of dissociation and hyper vigilance it is incredibly difficult to be in the moment, rest and be at peace. This is exhausting and debilitating and often distressing because I cannot enjoy the full experience of what is happening around me and cannot immerse myself in positive experiences and recall of recent events. My inability to learn and process information due to this, destroyed my potential at school and therefore this has had a massive impact throughout my life both socially and in relation to employment. I have been unable to engage in meaningful conversations, which has further affected my self -confidence and self-esteem.

Social

My relationship with my mum deteriorated after Jack sexually abused me. My education suffered and my mum would tell me frequently how disappointed in me she was. I felt enormous guilt, then anger at her for not keeping me safe, for not noticing I was suffering. I grew up feeling I was not good enough, feeling I had let everybody down, feeling a failure and a disappointment for being a bad person.

I went on to have two failed marriages, both abusive. Both knew about my past abuse and used that to manipulate me. I was told I was abnormal for not liking sex being forced upon me, or being touched, or abused in ways that humiliated or demeaned me. My thoughts and feelings didn't count and I was mocked, belittled and humiliated and told I was abnormal for protesting if I didn't like what was happening. I continued in both marriages for a number of years because I grew up believing that was what men did and I couldn't understand why it didn't feel right so my self-hatred deepened.

In relation to my own children, I was unable to connect emotionally when pregnant. I hated my growing stomach and felt exposed again to others touching me and every time somebody touched me I had flashbacks of Jack. I hated being pregnant and disconnected from any emotion in relation to it. I felt I was the property of others – to be done to and it ignited flashbacks of Jack. I couldn't accept pain relief during childbirth because I couldn't bear to be numb whilst being touched and not able to move, trapped again. I have become an overprotective parent, trying to shield my children from any potential threat, or danger and that has tarnished my enjoyment of them growing up.

Employment

I will never know what my true potential could have been. I will never know what direction my life could have taken. I work with vulnerable young people. I do this because I want to give them the voice I never had. I treat them with the upmost respect and uphold their dignity because I believe everybody deserves to be respected. I am trying to achieve for them what I didn't have, what was taken from me. Finally in July 2015 I broke down and I couldn't suppress the enormity of emotion I had always felt any longer. I was off work for 6 months and I don't know how this has affected my career prospects. I have carried Jack with me throughout my life and he has tarnished everything along the way. He has invaded my first experience of every significant life event, because there has always been an association.

Timeline

1969	1977	1980/81	1981	1983	1986	1990-1996	2005-2016
Born wrong sex	Sister died	Jack Kilbourne	Jason Jones	Man in the park. Held his hand.	Carl Collins	Married Stewart Watts	Relationship Alan Barton
Not good enough	Told nothing special anymore. Used. Not good enough. Worthless. Frightened. Sad. Lonely.	Sexually abused. Trapped. Used. Mocked. A good girl. Special. Loved. Worthless. Terrified. Suicidal thoughts. Dread. Self-hatred. Defenceless. Isolated. Lonely. Sad. Discarded. Nightmares. Disconnected. No sleep.	Sexually abused. Trapped. Mocked. Used. Discarded. Worthless. Forced. Angry. Suicidal thoughts. Self-hatred. Hopeless. Defenceless. Nightmares. Flashbacks. No sleep.	Raped. Trapped. Used. Special. Forced. Terrified. Alcohol Abuse. Suicidal thoughts. Self-hatred. Dread. Nightmares. Flashbacks. No sleep.	Raped. Trapped. Used. Discarded. Worthless. Forced. Terrified. Alcohol abuse. Suicidal thoughts. Self-hatred. Hopeless. Defenceless. Nightmares. Flashbacks. No sleep. Physical injury. Pain. Bleeding.	Raped. Physically abused. Emotionally abused. Anorexia. Trapped. Claustrophobic. Demeaned. Humiliated. Not good enough. Rubbish. Used. Discarded. Mocked. Controlled. Physical pain. Physical injury. Bleeding. Worthless. Forced. Terrified. Alcohol Abuse. Suicidal. Dread. Self-Hatred. Hopeless. Defenceless.	Emotional Abuse. Mocked. Belittled. Discarded. Trapped. Not good enough. Controlled. Worthless. Frightened. Suicidal. Dread. Self-Hatred. Blame. Hopeless. Defenceless. Isolated. Lonely. Sad. Nightmares. Flashbacks. Poor sleep. Trying to please. Trying to be good enough.

<table>
<tr><td></td><td></td><td></td><td></td><td></td><td></td><td>Isolated.
Lonely.
Sad.
Desparate.
Destroyed.
Nightmares.
Flashbacks.
Poor sleep.
Trying to please.
Trying to be good enough.</td><td></td></tr>
</table>

Parents. Mocked, laughed at, criticised, put down, not good enough, used, neglected emotions, controlled, a disappointment, worthless, alcohol abuse, ignored, isolated, sad, lonely, trying to please to be good enough.

Flashbacks now.

Raped, pain, trapped.
Used,
Discarded,
Not good enough.
A disappointment,
A failure,
Being forced to do something.
Anxiety, afraid of letting people down.
Sad, can't talk about childhood experiences to kids, questions = flashbacks.
Can't talk about school – disconnected – flashbacks – groped, touched.
Can't talk about past relationships – flashbacks
TV causes flashbacks
Work causes flashbacks
In Court – defenceless – flashbacks
Disconnected
Sad, can't remember chunks of life

Nightmares,
Poor sleep,
Lonely
Claustrophobic
Insecure.
Dread.

www.ingramcontent.com/pod-product-compliance
Lightning Source LLC
LaVergne TN
LVHW060214210926
848481LV00009B/2744
* 9 7 8 1 7 8 3 8 2 5 2 7 1 *